Biomedical Signal and Image Processing in Patient Care

Maheshkumar H. Kolekar
Indian Institute of Technology Patna, India

Vinod Kumar
Indian Institute of Technology Roorkee, India

A volume in the Advances in Medical Technologies and Clinical Practice (AMTCP) Book Series

IGI Global
DISSEMINATOR OF KNOWLEDGE

Published in the United States of America by
IGI Global
Medical Information Science Reference (an imprint of IGI Global)
701 E. Chocolate Avenue
Hershey PA, USA 17033
Tel: 717-533-8845
Fax: 717-533-8661
E-mail: cust@igi-global.com
Web site: http://www.igi-global.com

Library of Congress Cataloging-in-Publication Data

Names: Kolekar, Maheshkumar H., 1972- editor. | Kumar, Vinod, 1951- editor.
Title: Biomedical signal and image processing in patient care / Maheshkumar H. Kolekar and Vinod Kumar, editors.
Description: Hershey, PA : Medical Information Science Reference, [2018] | Includes bibliographical references.
Identifiers: LCCN 2017010730| ISBN 9781522528296 (hardcover) | ISBN 9781522528302 (ebook)
Subjects: | MESH: Telemedicine--methods | Signal Processing, Computer-Assisted | Image Processing, Computer-Assisted
Classification: LCC R855.3 | NLM W 83.1 | DDC 610.285--dc23 LC record available at https://lccn.loc.gov/2017010730

This book is published in the IGI Global book series Advances in Medical Technologies and Clinical Practice (AMTCP) (ISSN: 2327-9354; eISSN: 2327-9370)

British Cataloguing in Publication Data
A Cataloguing in Publication record for this book is available from the British Library.

For electronic access to this publication, please contact: eresources@igi-global.com.

Advances in Medical Technologies and Clinical Practice (AMTCP) Book Series

Srikanta Patnaik
SOA University, India
Priti Das
S.C.B. Medical College, India

ISSN:2327-9354
EISSN:2327-9370

Mission

Medical technological innovation continues to provide avenues of research for faster and safer diagnosis and treatments for patients. Practitioners must stay up to date with these latest advancements to provide the best care for nursing and clinical practices.

The **Advances in Medical Technologies and Clinical Practice (AMTCP) Book Series** brings together the most recent research on the latest technology used in areas of nursing informatics, clinical technology, biomedicine, diagnostic technologies, and more. Researchers, students, and practitioners in this field will benefit from this fundamental coverage on the use of technology in clinical practices.

Coverage

- Medical informatics
- Neural Engineering
- Medical Imaging
- Biometrics
- Telemedicine
- Biomedical Applications
- Clinical Studies
- Clinical Data Mining
- E-health
- Clinical Nutrition

IGI Global is currently accepting manuscripts for publication within this series. To submit a proposal for a volume in this series, please contact our Acquisition Editors at Acquisitions@igi-global.com or visit: http://www.igi-global.com/publish/.

The Advances in Medical Technologies and Clinical Practice (AMTCP) Book Series (ISSN 2327-9354) is published by IGI Global, 701 E. Chocolate Avenue, Hershey, PA 17033-1240, USA, www.igi-global.com. This series is composed of titles available for purchase individually; each title is edited to be contextually exclusive from any other title within the series. For pricing and ordering information please visit http://www.igi-global.com/book-series/advances-medical-technologies-clinical-practice/73682. Postmaster: Send all address changes to above address.

Titles in this Series

For a list of additional titles in this series, please visit: www.igi-global.com/book-series

Table of Contents

Section 2
Biomedical Image Processing

Detailed Table of Contents

Section 1
Biomedical Signal Processing

This section elaborates signal processing approaches on different biomedical signals such as Electroencephalogram, Electrocardiogram. Chapter 1 addresses the clinician's perspective of biomedical signals interpretation. Chapter 2 and Chapter 3 focus on Focal seizure detection based on EEG signal processing approach. Chapter 4 describes the classification and compression of ECG signal based on discrete wavelet transform which can be used for holter device.

The field of Biomedical engineering has brought two apparently diagonally placed poles of academia of excellence, i.e., field of medicine and the field of state of art engineering science to a closed proximity. Now a day most if not all of the state of art diagnostics in the field of medicine are almost totally dependent upon biomedical signal analysis. Whole of the biological systems are run by nothing but the bio-signals. The process of signal analysis depends upon the types of signals, recording methods, data types, need of compression and portability and possibility of artifacts. The important areas of the clinician's prime concern are the reliability of the data generated, the utility of the data produced in the real clinical settings in making a diagnosis and interference of the diverse type of equipment's signals with each other and its impact upon the final output. Physiologists act as a bridge between the biomedical engineering and the clinician's need assessment and product delivery process.

The chapter presents a new approach of computer aided diagnosis of focal electroencephalogram (EEG) signals by applying bivariate empirical mode decomposition (BEMD). Firstly, the focal and non-focal EEG signals are decomposed using the BEMD, which results in intrinsic mode functions (IMFs) corresponding to each signal. Secondly, bivariate bandwidths namely, amplitude bandwidth, precession bandwidth, and deformation bandwidth are computed for each obtained IMF. Interquartile range (IQR) values of bivariate bandwidths of IMFs are employed as the features for classification. In order to perform classification least squares support vector machine (LS-SVM) is used. The results of the experiment suggest that the computed bivariate bandwidths are significantly useful to discriminate focal EEG signals. The resultant classification accuracy obtained using proposed methodology, applied on the Bern-Barcelona EEG database, is 84.01%. The obtained results are encouraging and the proposed methodology can be helpful for identification of epileptogenic focus.

Epilepsy is the most common neurological disorder with 40-50 million people suffering with it worldwide. Epilepsy is not life threatening but it disables the person to a greater extent due to its uncertainty of occurrences. Epilepsy is detected by repeated occurrences of seizure. Seizure can be generated in brain due to abnormal activity of group of neurons caused by brain tumor, genetic problem, infection, hemorrhage etc. Seizure can be detected by observing the variation in Electroencephalogram (EEG) signal. Focal seizure is defined as seizure localized in one lobe of brain. In this chapter discrete wavelet transform and Hidden Markov Model based focal seizure detection method is proposed for epileptic focus localization. EEG signal was decomposed up to level 5 using dual tree complex wavelet transform and entropy features such as collision entropy, minimum and modified sample entropy were extracted. Hidden Markov model was used for classification purpose. Maximum 80% accuracy was achieved in detecting focal and non-focal EEG signal.

ECG signal processing for holter monitoring of heart patients is still exploratory. Many signal processing techniques have been evolved for classification and compression of ECG signal. Despite an increase in research in this area, many challenges remain in designing an efficient classification and compression algorithm for ECG signal. These challenges include classification accuracy, good compression ratio with acceptable diagnostic quality etc. This chapter addresses a classification and a compression algorithm based on discrete wavelet transform. Classification algorithm uses discrete wavelet transform based feature to classify abnormal heart beat from ECG signal. Support vector machine is used as a classifier to detect abnormal heartbeat. The compression algorithm utilizes discrete wavelet transform and run-length encoding as a compression tool. Proposed classification and compression algorithms can be employed in monitoring of cardiac patients using holter device.

Section 2
Biomedical Image Processing

This section includes different topics of medical image processing which are MRI denoising, medical image and text report retrieval system, image registration in ultrasound assisted brain surgery, retinal, blood cell, and smear tuberculosis image analysis.

Biomedical Image processing is an important research domain which contributes to the human health care. Magnetic resonance imaging (MRI) is the most popularly used medical imaging modality for its ability to scan any organ or tissue of a body without causing health risk to patient. Because of immense potential of MRI in health care it is very popular with the researchers. Along with improvisations in MR machines, the researchers are exploring different de noising filters, implementation techniques, and platforms so as to improve the MR image quality and enhance accuracy of diagnosis. The chapter discusses all the aspects of MRI - its physics, image attributes, rician noise pdf, different denoising filters and their implementation aspects. The performance analysis being significant in evaluating image quality, different quality measures used are discussed in details. The chapter also briefs about possible opportunities of research in the said domain.

Medical images are vital part of diagnostics and patient treatment. With the advent of technology, there is a rapid increase in the number of radiological images produced every day. Attempts have been made to use a Content Based Image Retrieval (CBIR) approach for assisting in radiological diagnosis. However, this approach suffers from the semantic gap problem. Few text retrieval systems are in place for assisting the radiologist to retrieve similar past cases. However, for the least experienced radiologist it is hard to describe the unknown case using text query. Therefore, the aim of this chapter is integrating the radiological CBIR and text based reports retrieval in order to support radiological diagnosis. The proposed technique is described in three stages: a) retrieval by image similarity, b) retrieval by text, and c) fusion of image and text retrieval for better diagnosis. Number of experiments are demonstrated along with their evaluation techniques on mammogram image database.

Image registration is an essential step in the image guided brain surgery. A preoperative magnetic resonance (MR) image guides the neurosurgeon about the size and the location of the tumor inside the brain of the diseased person. Due to several reasons, brain shift occurs during the surgery, results in the shift of the actual position of the tumor. Intra-operative MR imaging is expensive and may not be financially viable for many hospitals. An effective intraoperative US can be used in replacement of MR. For performing registration of US and MR images, the most of the state-of-the-art methods use a suitable similarity or dissimilarity measure, a spline based deformation model, a smoothing technique and an effective fast optimization method. This chapter starts with a discussion on various types of brain tumors and their clinical significance. It also covers on various similarity measures, optimizations and the available database of US and MR brain images.

Diabetic Retinopathy, a condition in the person affected by diabetes, is most common cause of blindness in the world. Recent research has given a better understanding of requirement in clinical eye care practice to identify better and cheaper ways of identification, management, diagnosis and treatment of retinal disease. The importance of diabetic retinopathy screening programs and difficulty in achieving reliable early diagnosis of diabetic retinopathy at a reasonable cost needs attention to develop computer-aided diagnosis tool. Computer aided disease diagnosis in retinal image analysis could ease mass screening of population with diabetes mellitus and help clinicians in utilizing their time more efficiently. The recent technological advances in computing power, communication systems, and machine learning techniques provide opportunities to the biomedical engineers and computer scientists to meet the requirements of clinical practice. With proper self-care, management, and medical professional support, individuals with diabetes can live a healthy and long life.

Acute Lymphoblastic Leukemia is a cancer of blood caused due to increase in number of immature lymphocyte cells. Detection is done manually by skilled pathologists which is time consuming and depends on the skills of the pathologist. The authors propose a methodology for discrimination of a normal lymphocyte cell from a malignant one by processing the blood sample image. Automatic detection

Foreword

Research, development, and innovation by biomedical engineers and scientists over the past five decades have led to the establishment of the computer as an indispensable tool in medicine and healthcare. Whereas the detection of heart beats via the application of digital signal processing (DSP) techniques to the electrocardiogram (ECG) was a research topic of great interest in the 1960s and 1970s, heart-rate monitoring tools are now incorporated into consumer devices such as mobile phones, watches, and fitness gadgets. Regardless of such advances, the variety and complexity of the biomedical signals and images that are being gathered and used in clinical diagnostic and monitoring applications, combined with the expanding array of diseases and exasperating conditions that afflict the human body, continue to pose more and more difficult challenges to researchers. In this context, the book *Biomedical Signal and Image Processing in Patient Care* edited by Maheshkumar H. Kolekar and Vinod Kumar makes a useful and timely contribution.

At the early stages of development, the aims of biomedical signal processing were limited to filtering for removal of noise and interference, Fourier spectral analysis to analyze the frequency characteristics of signals, and mathematical modeling for parametric representation of physiological systems. Current efforts are aimed at quantitative analysis of biomedical systems and processes via signal analysis. Biomedical signal analysis has advanced to practical application of signal processing and pattern analysis techniques for improved diagnosis, monitoring, and rehabilitation. Methods and systems developed by biomedical engineers and scientists are gaining wider acceptance by practicing clinicians and healthcare institutions, and their role in diagnosis and treatment is gaining much-deserved acceptance, recognition, and respect.

A major application of computers in biomedical signal and image analysis is the design and development of DSP and modeling techniques for quantitative analysis. Analysis of signals by human observers is subject to perceptual limitations, inter- and intrapersonal variations, errors due to fatigue, and environmental distractions. Computer analysis of biomedical signals can add objective strength to the interpretation of an expert in the mode of operation known as computer-aided diagnosis (CAD).

The chapters in the book deal with DSP techniques for analysis of not only various biomedical signals such as the ECG and the electroencephalogram (EEG), but also computational methods to process and analyze biomedical images. The book includes material related to multiple imaging modalities such as magnetic resonance imaging, ultrasonography, and sputum-smear imaging.

The chapters in the book describe various theoretical aspects and demonstrate practical applications of advanced techniques such as hidden Markov models, multifractal analysis, empirical mode decomposition, intrinsic mode functions, multimodal image registration, wireless computer-controlled drug delivery systems, and virtual reality for treatment planning and rehabilitation. Details of DSP techniques that can detect epileptic seizures via analysis of EEG signals are presented; such methods could assist in providing early warning of a potential seizure to the patient and prevent injury.

The chapters describe computational methods and models to address major healthcare problems that affect large populations across the world, such as diabetic retinopathy, tuberculosis, and leukemia. It is shown how research and development contribute to progress from signal processing to signal analysis, and onward to improved diagnostic decision making with CAD. It is also possible to advance further to computer-aided planning and design of patient-specific and personalized therapy, drug delivery systems, point-of-care healthcare systems, assessment of a patient's response to treatment, and rehabilitation.

The evolving techniques of CAD and computer-aided therapy are essential tools in healthcare. It is gratifying to witness practical applications of engineering in the amelioration of human health and wellbeing. I wish the authors who have contributed to the book, researchers working in related areas, and readers of the book further success in their endeavors in the service of humanity.

Rangaraj M. Rangayyan
University of Calgary, Canada

Preface

There is huge demand of the portable, wearable, implantable, wireless, miniature, medical devices because of modern and healthy living and in this scenario, biomedical signal and image processing raised up as vital need for clinicians and researcher to offer better care to the patients by providing concise information. Basically, Human body parameters provide constantly altering information about our health and this information is measured by physiological sensor or devices that measure heart rate, nerve conduction, brain activity and so forth. Conventionally, such parameters are measured at specific points in time recorded on the patient's chart and all the medical devices have main function that is the acquisition and analysis of physiological data either offline or real time. Development of every new biomedical sensor and diagnostic devices generates abundance of biomedical data in every second and it left caregiver with substantial number of data streams which can only be decoded by clinicians and researchers. In healthcare system, medical devices help physicians and specialist in diagnosis, prognosis, and therapeutics. For them, clinical decision making is a complex task due to tremendous amounts of complex patient data. Actually, it is very difficult to interpret patterns of physiological signal and images from the human eye specially in case of any neurological disorder. Thus, high quality of the signal processing algorithm is an important part of such processes. Biomedical signal and image processing includes the analysis of such physiological patterns to provide useful information upon which clinicians can make decisions. Researchers are developing innovative ways to process such information using a variety of mathematical formulae and algorithms and software computation of signals acquired from traditional bio-measurement tools also assist physicians with real-time data and greater understandings in clinical assessments. Quick diagnostic and therapeutic assessment aidfast clinical decision in case of urgency situation. It is clear that healthcare providers require innovative signal and image processing algorithms that can create recommendation and faster predictions to facilitate clinicians. In the research, validation of a medical device is only possible by accurate signal processing. The performance of such algorithms need to be enhances with diverse quantitative approaches. Thus, Biomedical Signal and Image Processing plays vital role in the modern days.

The field of biomedical signal and image processing has contributed immensely to human healthcare systems. In order to improve health and quality of human life, Signal and Image processing has played a significant role in a wide range of health care system by identifying the meaningful features from different image diagnostic sources like X-ray, Magnetic resonance imaging (MRI), Computer-assisted ECG, EEG, EMG, Audio and Video monitoring, Ultrasound, Tomography, Scans, Continuous physiological monitoring, tele-healthcare, tele-medicine. Signal and Image Processing has played vital role in the development of intelligent healthcare systems and devices such as Image reconstruction and modeling techniques allow instant processing of 2D signals to create 3D images in case of EEG or CT-Scan. In case of simple x-ray based eyeball test, image processing software assists to recognize and investigate problem with the human eye. Computerized algorithms can make available temporal and spatial analysis to detect patterns and characteristics revealing of tumours and other ailments. Different diagnosis can be considered depending upon the imaging technique. Image processing and analysis can be utilized to determine the diameter, volume, and vasculature of a tumour or an organ. The objective of this book is to bridge the gap between signal processing and healthcare system and present a collection of high-quality research work that report the latest advances in the area of Signal and Image processing techniques in healthcare. Learning this book can provide skills to the student that can be immediately applied in real-life technological inventions.This book mainly focus on advanced topics in biomedical signal and image processing and its recent applications in medical and research field.

TARGET AUDIENCE

The impact of the contribution through this edited book is going to be widespread considering the very fact that advanced biomedical signal and image processing techniques are being needed and are of utmost importance in the development of health-care systems.

Potential uses

1. The researchers will be able to know the latest application area of the biomedical signal and image processing in developing tools for health-care systems.
2. Various novel quantitative approaches will assist clinicians in improved and faster decision making.
3. The business users will get to know how of advanced biomedical signal and image processing techniques for health-care systems.
4. Learning this book can provide skills to the student that can be immediately applied in real-life technological inventions.

ORGANIZATION OF THE BOOK

The book is organized into 12 chapters. A brief description of each of the chapters follows:

Chapter 1 covers basis of biomedical signal processing. It addresses the clinician's perspective of biomedical signals interpretation. Biomedical signal basics such as action potential, previous verse present recording techniques, and common artefacts in biomedical signals, compressibility and ethics in biomedical signal recording are covered in this chapter.

Chapter 2 focuses on automatic focal seizure detection based on bivariate empirical mode decomposition and least square support vector machine classifier. Bivariate bandwidths namely, amplitude bandwidth, precession bandwidth, and deformation bandwidth are computed for each obtained IMF. Interquartile range (IQR) values of bivariate bandwidths of IMFs are employed as the features for classification. Higher accuracy is achieved for focal seizure detection.

Chapter 3 focuses on focal seizure localization. Dual tree complex wavelet transform and hidden Markov model (HMM) were used for focal and non focal seizure classification. Entropy features were used as biomarker for auto diagnosis. Classification accuracy achieved is encouraging.

Chapter 4 describes ECG signal compression and classification which can be used in monitoring of cardiac patients using holter device. This chapter addresses a classification and a compression algorithm based on discrete wavelet transform. Support vector machine classifier is used for classifying normal and diseased ECG signal. Run-length encoding is used as a compression tool.

Chapter 5 discusses all the aspects of MRI - its physics, image attributes, Rician noise pdf, different denoising filters and their implementation aspects. The performance analysis being significant in evaluating image quality, different quality measures used is discussed in details. The chapter also briefs about possible opportunities of research in the said domain.

Chapter 6 aims are integrating the radiological CBIR and text based reports retrieval in order to support radiological diagnosis. The proposed technique is executed in three different stages involving retrieval by text image similarity and finally fusion of both for better diagnosis. Different experiments are performed on mammogram image database to prove efficiency.

Chapter 7 describes the different types of brain tumors and their clinical significance, the image registration problem along with the issues related with registering brain images; a common setup for image guided neurosurgery and outlines the challenges in US and MR image registration.

Chapter 8 focuses on developing a system for reliable computer aided disease diagnosis in retinal image analysis for diabetic retinopathy thereby increasing efficiency of the doctor and decreasing workload for this retinal disease diagnosis. This chapter covers definition and classification of diabetic retinopathy, the epidemiology, automatic screening of retina by computer aided diagnosis and teleophthalmology tools. With proper self-care, management, and medical professional support, individuals with diabetes can live a healthy, long life.

Chapter 9 proposes methodology for automatic detection of malignant lymphocyte cells as compared to normal lymphocyte cells. To identify prominent 16 shape features, Correlation based Feature Selection is applied. Principal Component Analysis is applied on the texture features to reduce their dimensionality. Support Vector Machine is used for classification. Accuracy achieved was 92.23%.

Chapter 10 attempts have been made to automate the analysis of positive and negative Tuberculosis (TB) sputum smear images using multifractal approach. The images are subjected to multifractal analysis and the corresponding spectrum parameters are extracted. Most significant parameters are selected based on principal component analysis. Further, these parameters are subjected to classification using support vector machine classifier with different kernels.

Chapter 11 chapter explains VR as an innovative platform in the sector of medical & others such as military and sports for assessment as well as for training.

Chapter 12 describes the development of a wireless controlled iontophoretic drug delivery system which employs ZigBee communication protocol for control purpose. The developed drug delivery system was tested successfully. It offers minimal error with high efficiency.

Maheshkumar H. Kolekar
Indian Institute of Technology Patna, India

Vinod Kumar
Indian Institute of Technology Roorkee, India

Acknowledgment

We would like to acknowledge the help of all the people involved in this project and, more specifically, the authors, reviewers and editorial board members. Without their support, this book would not have become a reality.

We received total 40 book chapters and out of that we selected 12 book chapters based on reviewers and editorial board members' comments. We are thankful to reviewers for reviewing book chapters and giving their expert opinion. We wish to acknowledge the valuable contributions of the editorial board members regarding the improvement of quality, coherence, and content presentation of chapters.

We would like to mention our special thanks to IGI Global publisher for giving us an opportunity to edit this book. We also extend our special thanks to Maria Rohde, Assistant Development Editor, who helped us at every stage of the development process of the book.

We would like to mention special thanks to Prof Pushpak Bhattacharya, Director, IIT Patna for his support and fruitful discussion which has helped to enhance the quality of this book. We are also thankful to our friends, colleagues, PhD scholars at IIT Patna and IIT Roorkee for their encouragement, and support at various stages of the book.

We are thankful to our family members who cooperated with us during the whole book development process. Dr Maheshkumar Kolekar would like to thank his mother Sushila, wife Priti, daughters Samruddhi and Anwita for their encouragement and support which has helped him in completing this book. Dr Vinod Kumar would like to thank his wife Dr Reena who was always very supportive and helpful in completing this book.

Last but not least, we would like to thank almighty God and everybody who has directly or indirectly helped us in completing this important book.

Maheshkumar H. Kolekar
Indian Institute of Technology Patna, India

Vinod Kumar
Indian Institute of Technology Roorkee, India

Section 1
Biomedical Signal Processing

This section elaborates signal processing approaches on different biomedical signals such as Electroencephalogram, Electrocardiogram. Chapter 1 addresses the clinician's perspective of biomedical signals interpretation. Chapter 2 and Chapter 3 focus on Focal seizure detection based on EEG signal processing approach. Chapter 4 describes the classification and compression of ECG signal based on discrete wavelet transform which can be used for holter device.

Chapter 1
Biomedical Signal Analysis and Its Physio-Clinical Perspectives

Kamlesh Jha
All India Institute of Medical Sciences, India

ABSTRACT

The field of Biomedical engineering has brought two apparently diagonally placed poles of academia of excellence, i.e., field of medicine and the field of state of art engineering science to a closed proximity. Now a day most if not all of the state of art diagnostics in the field of medicine are almost totally dependent upon biomedical signal analysis. Whole of the biological systems are run by nothing but the bio-signals. The process of signal analysis depends upon the types of signals, recording methods, data types, need of compression and portability and possibility of artifacts. The important areas of the clinician's prime concern are the reliability of the data generated, the utility of the data produced in the real clinical settings in making a diagnosis and interference of the diverse type of equipment's signals with each other and its impact upon the final output. Physiologists act as a bridge between the biomedical engineering and the clinician's need assessment and product delivery process.

INTRODUCTION

A signal in biomedical jargon is any physical quantity that varies as a function of one or more independent variables. According to the number of variables it may be one dimensional, two dimensional or even multidimensional signals.

Our biological system is a dynamic state device that works upon a complex pattern of multidimensional signals called biomedical signals. The basic source of the biomedical signals lies in the membrane properties of the various living cells of the biological system.

Objective of the chapter is to have an introduction to the clinician's perspective of biomedical signals, address the issues related to patient care linked with the biomedical signal analysis and interpretation and the physiologists point of view regarding the alteration in the behavior of biological signal generators and its effect on the signal data output.

DOI: 10.4018/978-1-5225-2829-6.ch001

CELL AS A SOURCE OF BIOMEDICAL SIGNALS

Most of the electrophysiological studies involve bioelectrical potentials generated by sources inside the body such as nerve, brain, pacemakers, muscles etc. The body as a whole acts as volume conductor and it helps in the extracellular spread of current (i.e. volume conduction). The source of current lies in the cell membrane where millions of voltage gated and ligand gated ion channels are placed which is being operated under dynamic equilibrium with various neuro-hormonal regulatory systems of body. The intricately tuned regulatory control system changes the behavior of the membrane property by changing the permeability of the membrane to a particular ion which in turn is being controlled by the variable expression of the channels for those particular substance or ions over the cell surface. The change in the channel behavior alters the potential difference between the two surfaces of the cells, alters the Calcium or other ionic level inside the cell and may also create a train of propagating impulse without any decrement in the voltage called action potential.

One of the important determinants of the current strength and its initiation is the intracellular versus extracellular ionic distribution and its balance. For example a small change in potassium concentration extracellularly may cause cardiac emergency or flaccid paralysis because of the change in the cardiac or skeletal muscle ionotropic properties. As many of the ion channels are voltage gated channels, a slight change in the ionic concentration gradient across the cell membrane may cause a significant change in the resting membrane potential or the threshold local potential to generate action potential. In other words, it may cause a change in the membrane excitability. Tetany may be cited as a good example of similar change in the membrane property. Tetany is a condition in which the skeletal muscle becomes hyper excitable resulting in the spasmodic contraction of a group of skeletal muscles upon very trivial stimulation. The condition is caused by slight decrease in the extracellular ionic Calcium concentration. The ionic Calcium in its normal extracellular concentration is responsible for the stability of the skeletal muscle membrane Sodium channels. When it decreases due to any reason, the membrane Sodium channel becomes unstable and even a trivial stimuli is capable of opening sufficient number of Sodium channels to create a threshold voltage for generation of action potential resulting in the hyperexcitability of the skeletal muscles.

Action Potential

The basic activity that is responsible for the generation of biological signals in almost every biological cell or system is action potential. This is defined as the change in the membrane potential across any semi permeable biological membrane, which can travel along the membrane without any decrement in the intensity and which follows all or none law. Another term that is often in use along with action potential is the graded potential or local potential, which is the local change in the membrane polarity which doesn't follow all or none law and which can't travel along the muscle or nerve membrane. As discussed above, the generation of action potential depends upon the membrane property which is the function of various ion channels present in the cell membrane, their permeability and the concentration gradient of various ions across the membrane. Besides it is also dependent upon the excitability of the membrane which is under dynamic control of various neuro-hormonal factors present in the biological system. The duration of action potential also determines the reactivity of the membrane to second successive stimuli. If the duration is longer, the membrane will remain in the period of relative or absolute refractoriness and will render the second stimuli futile. This makes the basis for certain very important biological functions and phenomena like tetanus and clonus.

Generation of action potential:

To know about the action potential first one should get to know about what resting membrane potential is and how is it formed? The Resting membrane potential is the difference between electrical charges of inside and outside of a biological membrane because of the differential distribution of ions, selective permeability of the membrane and the presence of non-diffusible charged particles (Proteins) inside the cell. The distribution of ions across a typical reference human cell is as shown in Table 1.

These values may even vary to some extent from cell to cell. Here one can see that there is considerable variation in the distribution of various ions across the cell. Furthermore the cell consists of large amount of protein particles, significantly greater that the plasma or interstitial proteins (the extracellular proteins). This protein is a negatively charged non permeable particle which influences the movement of other charged particles across the cell membrane in a predictable way first time hypothesized by Gibbs and Donann. According to Gibbs and Donann, the movement of ions is predictable and can be quantified. Finally the electrical disequilibrium created due to this ionic movement across the cell membrane and chemical disequilibrium due to unequal distribution of the ions across the membrane, balance each other to reach a new equilibrium called Donnan equilibrium or Gibbs-Donnan equilibrium. This equilibrium potential, as said earlier, could be quantified, and is called resting membrane potential because the cell membrane is at resting state at this potential owing to the equilibrium status. The main contributors of this equilibrium are:

- The high permeability of K+ ions across the cell membrane.
- Presence of the electronegative non permeable protein particles inside the cell.
- The sodium –potassium pump present over the cell membrane which of electrogenic nature (pumps two K+ inside the cell in lieu of 3 Na+ ions outside the cell).

Na+ ions as such can't permeate across the cell membrane, hence don't contribute directly to the resting membrane potential. But when sodium channel are activated, they open up and permits large quantity of Na^+ ions to permeate inside the cell. This large sodium influx inside the cell results in generation of action potential. The amount of sodium influx is determined by the equilibrium potential of $Na^{+,}$ also called Nerst Potential which is calculated by computing various determinants including the molecular weight, valance, intra and extracellular concentration of the ion and some constants. The Equilibrium potential for Na^+ is + 61 mV (considering normal intracellular and extracellular concentration of Na^+).

Table 1. The distribution of ions across a typical reference human cell

Ion	Intracellular Concentration (mEq/L)	Extracellular Concentration (mEq/L)
Na+	10	142
K+	140	4
Cl-	4	104
HCO3	10	28
Ca++	0.0001	2.4
Mg++	58	1.2

This is followed by opening of voltage gated K^+ channels to restore intracellular negativity i.e. resting membrane potential (RMP). Furthermore Na+ K + ATPase pump get activated to restore the RMP and marks the end of the depolarization process.

Various tissues of our body behave differently in context to the generation of biological signals depending upon the interplay of various factors discussed above. Some of the important organs and their characteristic action potentials are discussed below in brief:

- **Cardiac Muscle Action Potential:** This is characterized by the explosive Na+ entry causing depolarization, followed by slow depolarization along with a plateau phase owing to the opening of slow Calcium channels (see Figure 1). The prolonged plateau phase is an important provision with cardiac muscle which imparts it with long refractory period and renders them resistant to tantalization (Cheitlin *et.al 2003*) (Bers, D. M, 2002) (Brutsaert, D. L, 2003).
- **Nerve Action Potential:** This is characterized by a depolarization from its Resting membrane potential (-70 mV) followed by the quick repolarization due to opening of voltage gated K+ channels and action of Na+ K+ ATPase pump (Figure 2). The sub threshold stimuli results in the generation of graded potential without action potential. Once the strength of stimuli crosses the threshold level, action potential sets in.
- **Muscle Action Potential and Muscle Contraction:** The action potential in muscle generates in a similar way to the nerve but the mechanical process of muscle contraction follows the electrical event and has the different curve (Figure 3). Thus by the time muscle contraction effectively starts, the repolarization process already get completed. This renders the muscle excitable to next stimuli. In other words, the muscle could be tetanized if stimulated with certain frequency of repeated stimuli.
- **Pacemaker Potential:** Many tissues of biological system are having the capability to generate spontaneous impulse without any external stimuli. They are called the pacemaker cells. Example of pacemaker cells includes conduction system of heart, interstitial cells of Cajal in stomach and nerve cells responsible for generation of ramp signals for respiration in brain. The mechanism of the setting in of action potential is almost similar to any other tissue except that the major role played in depolarization is by Ca++ ions rather than Na+ ions (Kaupp *et.al* 2001). Secondly during hyperpolarization phase, the leaky K+ channels get closed and slow Na+ - Ca++ channel opens up to attain the threshold voltage for next action potential (Figure 4). This process is spontaneous and continuous (James, T. N, 2002).
- **The Cortically Generated Potentials:** In human brain the potential generated by a population of neuron is equal to the sum of potentials generated in the individual neurons. In the cerebral cortex the generators of the spontaneous EEG activities, the pyramidal neurons are arranged in sheet with the axes of the dendrite trees are parallel to each other but perpendicular to the cortical surface.

A small group of axons, usually simultaneously excite those pyramidal cells to produce either inward or outward current depending on whether the activated synapse is excitatory of inhibitory in nature.

Figure 1. Cardiac muscle action potential

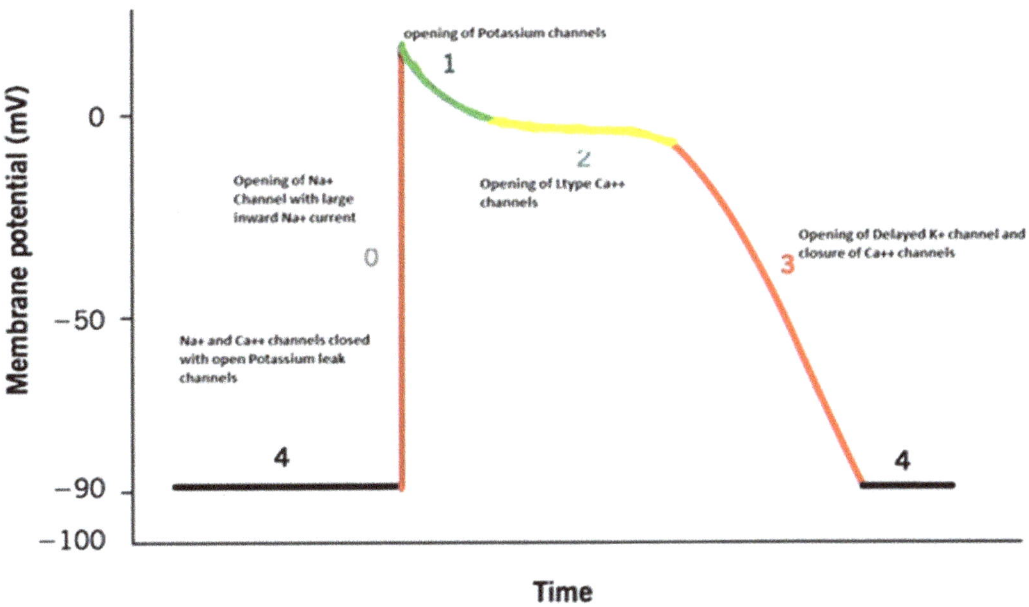

Figure 2. Nerve action potential

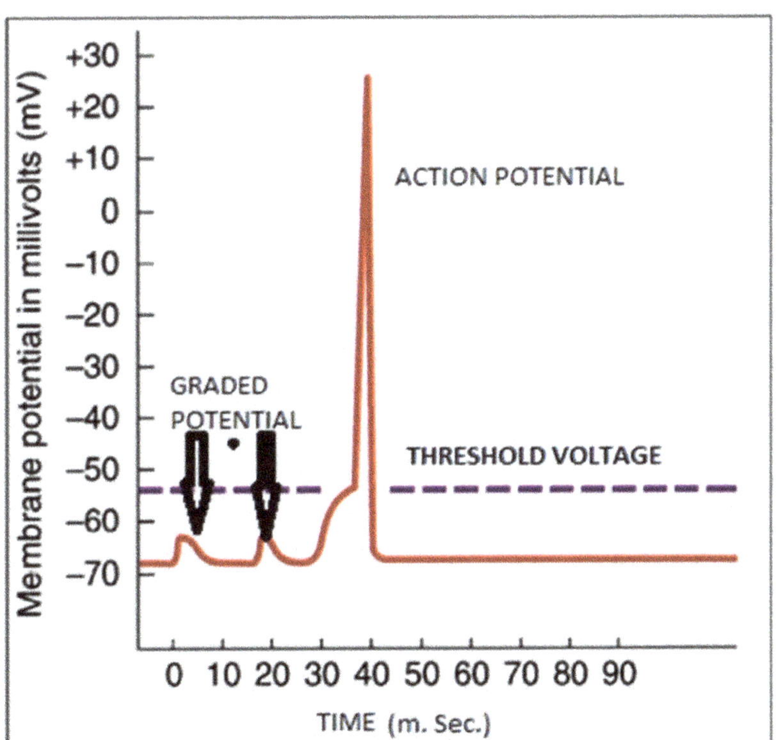

Figure 3. Skeletal muscle action potential and simple muscle curve

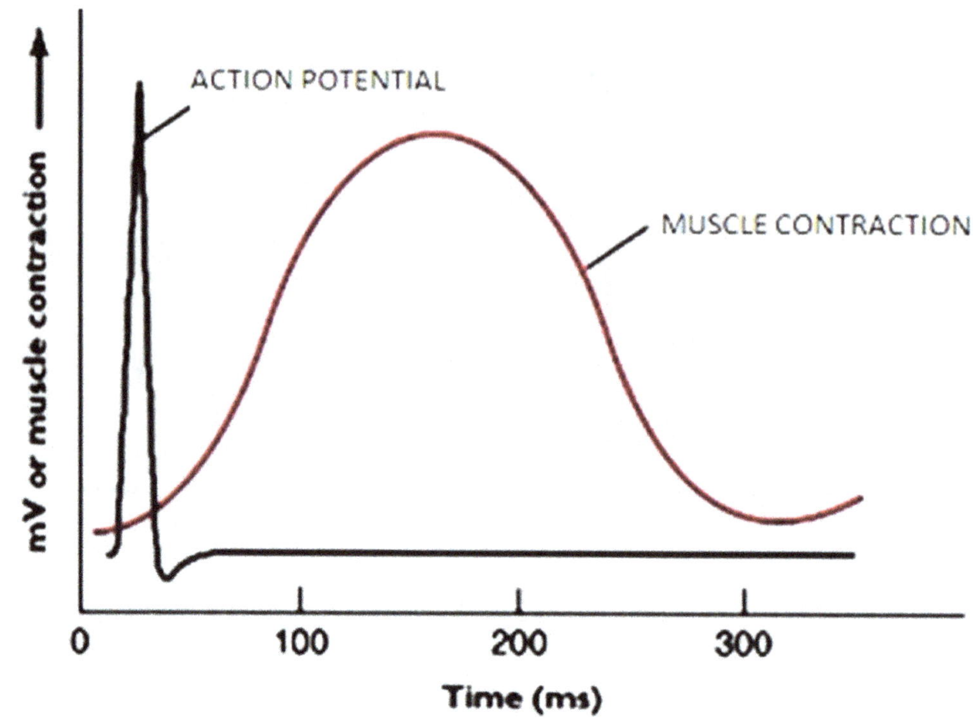

Figure 4. Pacemaker potential

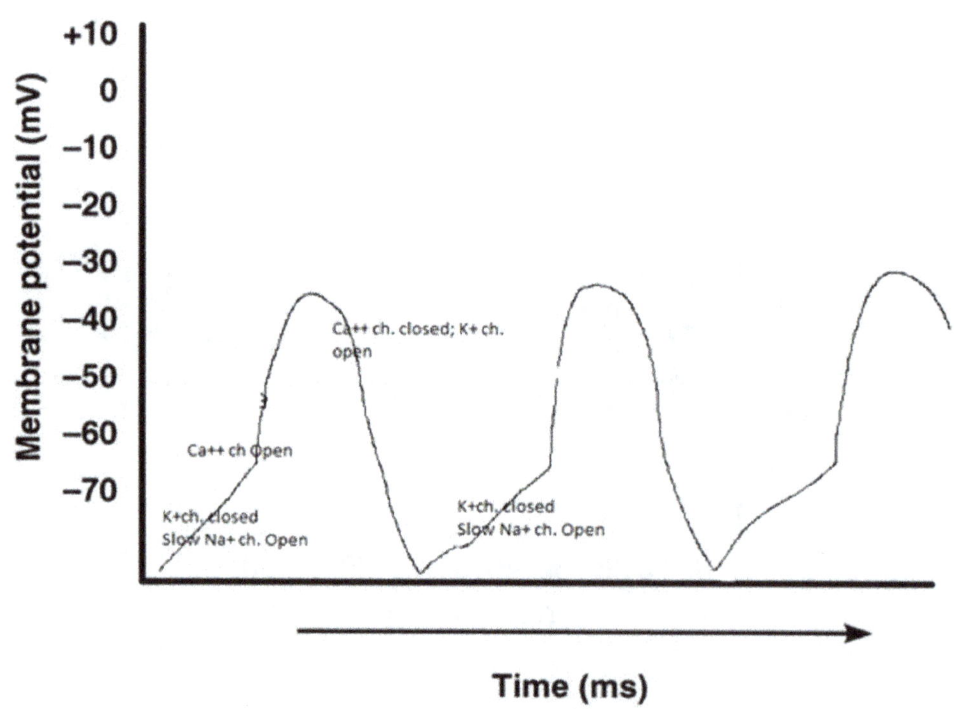

ANALOGUE VS DIGITAL SIGNALS

The Analogue signals represents the potential of an electrical activity in quantitative terms i.e. the potential is directly proportional to the physiologic quantity represented by the signal. It is generally continuous in nature i. e. the potential varies continuously as a function of time. These types of recordings are more suitable for manual interpretation.

In contrary to this, the digital signals are the discrete and discontinuous recordings with only one of the two possible states i.e. 'yes' / 'no' or 'zero' / 'one'. They store the physiological signals as binary numbers. This is the only format in which digital devices store information. It is most suited for performing most complex and accurate mathematical operations.

Digitization is a process by which analogue signals could be converted to digital signals. This is done by a complex circuit called analogue to digital convertor.

ARTIFACTS IN THE BIOLOGICAL SIGNALS

Artifacts are one of the most important sources of error in the biomedical signal based diagnostic endeavors.

The artifacts are best defined as the electrical activities of no clinical significance originating from non physiological sources. The artifacts could be of two types:

- **Physiologic Artifacts:** When the source of artifact is the signals originating from living tissues.
- **Non-Physiologic Artifacts:** When the source of artifact is the signal coming from some other sources.

Example of physiologic artifacts includes the ECG and EMG artifacts or movement of electrically charged structures like eye, tongue etc producing artifacts during EEG recording. The source of non physiologic artifacts may include the wire connecting the apparatus, interference between metal electrodes and skin surface etc. Besides the artifacts due to sweating, salt bridges on the skin surface, 50 or 60 HZ interference due to electrical interference etc may be the other common source of non Physiologic artifacts.

The continuously occurring artifacts are called noise. A high signal to noise ratio increases the likelihood of eliminating the artifacts by averaging the signals. The following table depicts the source of artifacts, generators and the appearance of artifacts especially seen in EEG records (Mariappan *et.al* 2016)

PORTABILITY OF BIOMEDICAL SIGNALS

The importance of biomedical signals lies in the data sharing and portability. In the era of globalization and telemedicine it is of paramount importance. The portability of the properly acquired biomedical data depends upon:

- Data volume
- Compressibility of the content
- Digitization
- Ethical issues: The data governance

Table 2. Source of artifacts and their appearance in the record

Source of Artifacts	Appearance
Eye movement	Slow positive lateralized
Eye blink	V shaped positive
Pacemaker in heart	1 Hz spikes at regular interval
ECG	Regular sharp spike like localized
Muscle movement	Rapid intermittent spikes
Perspiration	Slow undulation
Electrode movement	Irregular, rapid spikes
Wire movement	Slow waves
Electrical switch artifacts	Multiple rapid spikes

DATA VOLUME

This is an important aspect of the data portability. As is obvious, a high volume data is more difficult to port from one system or place to other in undistorted form. Reduction of data volume is also required as a cost cutting and performance tool as too much data being created and retained on the live database often causes rising IT costs, complex system management and decelerated system performance. For a large volume data several techniques of compression is utilized to reduce its volume without any significant impact upon the quality of the data.

COMPRESSIBILITY OF THE CONTENT

The data generated from biomedical signal recorder equipments are quite varied in nature. It may be a big pile of paper strips as in case of analogue data or could be in the form of images, videos, digital signals, audio records etc. Storing such a varied data base of diverse types for long term without distortion is a big challenge especially in a setup where such a huge and varied data are being generated on daily basis like big hospitals and educational Institutes.

There comes the idea of compressibility of data without actual distortion or loss of information. There are various ways in which medical data could be compressed. As an example a few of them could be described as follows:

- **DICOM:** This is digital imaging and communication in medicine, used largely for handling, storing, printing and transmitting information related to medical imaging. Initially it was developed by the American College of Radiology and National Electrical manufacturers Association (USA) for sharing radiological data but later on it became an essential tool for sharing variety of image generating bio-investigative equipments ranging from X-Ray and Ultrasonography to MRI and angiography.

- **Compressive Sensing:** This is another compression technique used for compressing EEG data. As the volume of data generated by multichannel EEG equipments are quite large, it essentially requires a robust compression mechanism to reduce data volume without compromising with its information.
- **Multimodal Compression:** This technique is used for compressing diverse types of data including images, and multichannel bio-signal data effectively (zeybek et.al 2012) . Long term monitoring of ECG is necessary for cardiac patients. Arrhythmia patient requires holter monitoring which produce large amount of data to be stored for future use. So ECG compression technique is required to store data in less memory without compromising with its information (Jha *et.al* 2015).

DIGITIZATION OF BIO-MEDICAL DATA

Earlier the clinicians and researchers used to record the biomedical signals in analogue forms and study. It was a big hindrance in data sharing, portability and analysis. The data required manual handling which was quite cumbersome, time consuming and also carried an inherent risk of mistakes. As stated earlier, storing the data safely for long time was another problem with the analogue records. The technique of digitization came as a big boon to this problems related to the analogue data. It is a technique by which images, sound clips, documents or other signals are represented in a digital manner by generating a series of numbers that describes a discrete set of its samples. It works by converting the continuous signals i.e. analogue signals) in to discrete signals. This not only helps in easy sharing and transportation of data but helps in preservation and storage of data for long term maintaining its quality. This also makes the data handy for statistical analysis using computers and representation in various formats by easy manipulation.

Digitization has made a large difference in disease monitoring and diagnosis by continues monitoring and analysis of bio-medical signals. EEG has a major role in Epileptic seizure detection. Digital analysis of EEG can help doctor to diagnose and predict seizure beforehand. Many processing techniques have been used for automatic seizure detection (Kolekar *et.al* 2015) (Absishek et.al 2014). Machine learning algorithm such as support vector machine classifier (Kolekar *et.al* 2017) and Bayesian classifier (Kolekar *et.al* 2015) can be used for auto diagnosis of the disease.

ETHICAL ISSUES: THE DATA GOVERNANCE

One important and pertinent issue in the context of biomedical data is the ethics involved in it. As all the data are related to human subjects, many things come to the way of data handling right from the basic human rights to the data sharing norms, copy right issues, portability issues, benefit sharing among the involved investigators, conflict of interest etc. If the data is stored at a bigger platform using cloud based technologies, the issues may involve the data safety too. Individual may ask for access to the data base for their personal health benefits or for the larger biomedical research projects. Many countries or unions like European Union (EU) practice a transparent and reliable data protection regulation system where an individual can legally ask for a copy of data which involved him personally, for further use (Mittelstadt *et.al* 2016).

BIOMEDICAL DATA: CLINICIANS PERSPECTIVES

The final destination of biomedical equipments is the clinician's office or the lab of researchers. Therefore it is imperative to consider the concerns of the end users.

The important areas of the clinician's or researcher's prime concern especially related to the data generation are:

- The reliability of the data generated.
- The utility of the data produced in the real clinical settings in making a diagnosis or formulating a hypothesis.
- Interference of the diverse type of equipment's signals with each other and its impact upon the final output.

Thus in a nut shell, they are concerned about the output generated in a real clinical/research setting, may be a jam packed Outpatient department and ICU of a tertiary care centre or a highly sophisticated state of art research lab packed with hundreds of signal generators.

In research settings it is relatively easy to maintain the standard set of conditions to acquire a 'pure' data with minimum of noises or artifacts.

But, in contrast, in real clinical settings, the devices are prone to numerous interferences from signals generated from varieties of biological and non biological signal generators. One of the most common culprit in this regard now a days is the cell phone devices, which emits strong electromagnetic energy affecting thereby the functionality of many medical equipments of vital importance including ventilators, ECG monitors, cardiac monitors and even the implantable devices.

Besides, many medical devices can interfere with the other devices in the nearby locations owing to its electromagnetic properties. Other interference may include those coming from electrical wiring, air conditioning apparatuses, and mechanical vibrations etc.

These problems can significantly alter the output of the electro-diagnostic and management devices which may sometimes prove detrimental to the patients especially in the ICU settings.

To take care of the issues, modern device manufacturers, especially those of the wireless devices, make sure to design it in such a way that the interference remains minimized. The devices normally come with guidelines regarding the minimum interinstrumental distances and other safety instructions. Provision of various filters is another way of handling such issues.

The clinician's way of handling the issues includes, maximizing the use of clinical cues for diagnosing or prognosticating a condition and minimizing the blind dependence upon the gadgets where ever possible or use it as an adjunct to the clinical findings instead of using it in exclusion.

SUMMARY

The field of Biomedical engineering has brought two apparently diagonally placed poles of academia of excellence i.e. Field of Medicine and the field of State of art engineering science to a closed proximity. Now a day most if not all of the state of art diagnostics in the field of medicine are almost totally dependent upon biomedical signals. Recording and interpreting the signals accurately, therefore, is an important aspect and requirement of the field. Whole of the biological systems are run by nothing but the bio-signals. Right from nerve signals to the membrane receptors everything is dependent upon the voltage changes at the membrane level and a process of signal transaction. These signals make the basis of hyper, hypo or normal functioning of every cell to system in the body of an individual living being. The signals are prone to artifacts and needs various states of art processing techniques to get rid of that. Besides, data get recorded or converted in the digital format for the ease of storage and portability. The digitization also makes it easy to compress the data without change in the data quality. Ethics is another important aspect which needs to be taken care of while data handling and data processing. India, being a developing country with a population of more than 1.25 Billion and an overburdened health care system provides an apparently golden opportunity to the field of biomedical engineering where a robust team work of physiologists, clinicians, and experts from engineering background can take the challenges of developing sophisticated man -machine interface modules with highly specific signal analysis system.

REFERENCES

Article 18: council of Europian Union. (2015). *Draft data protection regulation.* Retrieved from http. data.consiliun.europa.eu/doc/documents/ST-9565-2015-INIT/en/pdf

Bers, D. M. (2002). Cardiac excitation–contraction coupling. *Nature, 415*(6868), 198-205.

Brutsaert, D. L. (2003). Cardiac endothelial-myocardial signalling: its role in cardiac growth, contractile performance, and rhythmicity. *Physiological Reviews, 83*(1), 59-115.

Cheitlin, M. D., Armstrong, W. F., & Aurigemma, G. P. (2003). ACC/AHA/ASE 2003 Guideline update for the clinical application of echocardiography: Summary article. A report of the American College of Cardiology/American Heart Association Task Force on Practice Guidelines (ACC/AHA/ASE Committee to Update the 1997 Guidelines for the Clinical Application of Echocardiography). *Journal of the American Society of Echocardiography*, *16*, 1091. PMID:14566308

James, T. N. (2002). Structure and function of the sinus node, AV node and his bundle of the human heart: Part I—structure. *Progress in Cardiovascular Diseases, 45*(3), 235-267.

Jha, C. K., & Kolekar, M. H. (2016, January). Efficient ECG data compression and transmission algorithm for telemedicine. *International Conference on Communication Systems and Networks*, (pp. 1-6). IEEE. doi:10.1109/COMSNETS.2016.7439988

Kaupp, U. B., & Seifert, R. (2001). Molecular diversity of pacemaker ion channels. *Annual Review of Physiology, 63*(1), 235-257.

Kolekar, M. H., Dash, D. P., & Patil, P. N. (2017). Support Vector Machine Based Extraction of Crime Information in Human Brain Using ERP Image. *International Conference on Computer Vision and Image Processing* (pp. 163-174). Springer. doi:10.1007/978-981-10-2107-7_15

Kolekar, M. H., & Sengupta, S. (2015). Bayesian network-based customized highlight generation for broadcast soccer videos. *IEEE Transactions on Broadcasting, 61*(2), 195-209.

Kolekar, M. H., & Dash, D. P. (2015, November). A nonlinear feature based epileptic seizure detection using least square support vector machine classifier. *TENCON 2015- Region 10 Conference* (pp. 1-6). IEEE.

Mariappan, P. M., Raghavan, D. R., Aleem, S. H. A., & Zobaa, A. F. (2016). Effects of electromagnetic interference on the functional usage of medical equipment by 2G/3G/4G cellular phones: A review. *Journal of Advanced Research, 7*(5), 727-738.

Mittelstadt, B. D., & Floridi, L. (2016). *The ethics of biomedical big data*. Springer. doi:10.1007/978-3-319-33525-4

Zeybek, E. H., Fournier, R., & Na, A. (2012). Multimodal compression applied to biomedical data. *Journal of Biomedical Science and Engineering, 5*(12), 755–761. doi:10.4236/jbise.2012.512094

Chapter 2
Automated Classification of Focal and Non-Focal EEG Signals Based on Bivariate Empirical Mode Decomposition

Rajeev Sharma
Indian Institute of Technology Indore, India

Ram Bilas Pachori
Indian Institute of Technology Indore, India

ABSTRACT

The chapter presents a new approach of computer aided diagnosis of focal electroencephalogram (EEG) signals by applying bivariate empirical mode decomposition (BEMD). Firstly, the focal and non-focal EEG signals are decomposed using the BEMD, which results in intrinsic mode functions (IMFs) corresponding to each signal. Secondly, bivariate bandwidths namely, amplitude bandwidth, precession bandwidth, and deformation bandwidth are computed for each obtained IMF. Interquartile range (IQR) values of bivariate bandwidths of IMFs are employed as the features for classification. In order to perform classification least squares support vector machine (LS-SVM) is used. The results of the experiment suggest that the computed bivariate bandwidths are significantly useful to discriminate focal EEG signals. The resultant classification accuracy obtained using proposed methodology, applied on the Bern-Barcelona EEG database, is 84.01%. The obtained results are encouraging and the proposed methodology can be helpful for identification of epileptogenic focus.

INTRODUCTION

Electrical activities related to different pathological conditions of brain are commonly measured using electroencephalogram (EEG) signals. EEG signals are frequently used for assessment of the different mental states of a person for example (Ahmadlou and Adeli, 2014), autistic spectrum disorder (Ahmadlou

DOI: 10.4018/978-1-5225-2829-6.ch002

et al., 2010), Alzeimer disease (Adeli et al., 2008), epilepsy (Adeli et al., 2003) etc. The epilepsy is of two types generalized epilepsy and focal (partial) epilepsy (Badawy et al., 2007). In case of focal epilepsy, limited area of brain gets affected by onset of the epileptic seizures. With the time, approximately 20% patients of generalized epilepsy and 60% patients of partial epilepsy grow immunity for drugs during medication (Pati and Alexopoulos, 2010). For such patients, surgical resection of affected brain region is considered as the therapy option in order to reduce seizure occurrence frequency or get cured (Rosenow and Lüders, 2001). The identification of the epilepsy affected brain region from EEG signals can serve as vital step prior to surgery.

BACKGROUND

Many methods are developed for assessment of the characteristic changes in EEG signals related to epileptic seizure activities. These techniques can be helpful for localization of epileptogenic zone. In (Gutiérrez et al., 2001), the electrocorticography (ECoG) recordings of the 21 patients are studied and processed with wavelet packet functions to characterize the spikes in ECoG segments. The frequency-entropy templates are computed by wavelet packet decomposition and the best basis algorithm for each electrode (Ben-Jacob et al., 2007). It is suggested that epileptogenic focus can be associated with the locations of high template similarity of ictal template. In (Panet-Raymond and Gotman, 1990, Marciani et al., 1992), delta band activities based asymmetry measures are shown as significantly reliable indicator of epileptogenic focus. The EEG recordings acquired from 23 patients are analyzed and it is found that epileptiform oscillations in high-frequency range (60-100 Hz) may be clinically important to localize seizure onset zone in patients affected by neocortical epilepsy (Worrell et al., 2004). In another study (Sabesan et al., 2009), intracranial EEG signals from four epileptic patients are analyzed using surrogate analysis of the transfer entropy to localize the epileptogenic focus. Interelectrode synchrony is studied in (Schevon et al., 2007) and it is speculated that local synchrony can indicate the epileptogenic cortex. In (Warren et al., 2010), neural synchrony measures such as linear mean phase coherence and cross-correlation of local field potentials are investigated using the intracranial EEG recordings, and it is observed that brain region affected by epilepsy is functionally isolated from the remaining brain regions in patient with partial epilepsy.

Several nonlinear parameters are used to quantify the change in dynamics of the cortex like correlation dimension and measurement of complexity loss (Lehnertz and Elger, 1995, Widman et al., 2000). Functional connectivity patterns obtained by analyzing EEG signals are used to predict the seizure activity and localization of the seizure onset zone (van Mierlo et al., 2014). In (van Mierlo et al., 2013), effective connectivity patterns are computed for the first 20 seconds of ictal intracranial EEG signals from eight patients and ictal onset zone is localized considering the highest total out-degree. The focal and non-focal EEG signals refer to intracranial recordings acquired from the patients of pharmacoresistant focal epilepsy (Andrzejak et al., 2012). The focal EEG signals and non-focal EEG signals are denoted by X_F and X_{NF}, respectively. It should be noted that X_F signals refer to the recordings of electrodes where changes related to seizure onset are detected. The EEG recordings of the electrodes from other brain areas that are not associated with the seizure onset referred as X_{NF} signals (Andrzejak et al., 2012). By performing classification of X_F and X_{NF} signals one may identify focal and non-focal regions. Therefore, it can help in determination of epileptogenic focus.

Several techniques based on empirical mode decomposition (EMD) (Huang et al., 1998) have been presented with the goal of epileptic seizures detection in EEG signals. These techniques analyze and classify the EEG signals by computing features from the intrinsic mode functions (IMFs) obtained from EMD of EEG signals. Mean frequency of IMFs obtained using Fourier-Bessel series expansion (Pachori, 2008), spectral peaks, spectral entropy, and spectral energy of IMFs (Martis et al., 2012), weighted mean frequency of IMFs (Oweis and Abdulhay, 2011), ellipse area parameter of second order difference plots (SODP) of IMFs (Pachori and Patidar, 2014), fluctuation index and coefficient of variation computed from IMFs (Li et al., 2013), ellipse area parameter of 2D phase space representation (PSR) and interquartile range (IQR) of Euclidian distances parameter of 3D PSR of IMFs (Sharma and Pachori, 2015), multilevel local patterns (Kumar et al., 2014) are some of the features which have been studied for analysis of epileptic seizure EEG signals.

The X_F and X_{NF} signals are analyzed using EMD (Sharma et al., 2014, Sharma et al., 2015a), discrete wavelet transform (DWT) (Sharma et al., 2015b, Sharma et al., 2017), combined EMD and DWT approach (Das and Bhuiyan, 2016) and tunable-Q wavelet transform (TQWT) (Bhattacharyya et al., 2017). The EMD method operates on the univariate data. Multivariate recordings from adjacent channels enable to establish interrelation between simultaneously recorded EEG signals. However, the EMD method may not exploit the cross-channel relation, and number of resultant IMFs can be different for both signals of bivariate data (Ahrabian et al., 2013). Due to these reasons, we have used bivariate EMD (BEMD) method for decomposition of EEG signals.

Our main contribution is to use bivariate bandwidth features namely, amplitude bandwidth, precession bandwidth, and deformation bandwidth computed from bivariate IMFs for classification of X_F and X_{NF} signals. In this work, entire dataset containing 3750 pairs of X_F and X_{NF} signals is used. The schematic flow chart of proposed system for classification is depicted in Figure 1. Firstly, decomposition of EEG signals is performed using BEMD in order to get equal number of relevant IMFs for both time series of bivariate signals. Bivariate bandwidth parameters are computed from these pairs of IMFs. Finally, these obtained parameters are used as the input features to the least squares support vector machine (LS-SVM) classifier.

METHODOLOGY

Dataset

Bern-Barcelona EEG database (Andrzejak et al., 2012) is used for this study which can be obtained online at www.dtic.upf.edu/~ralph/sc/. Dataset includes the intracranial recordings from five patients. These patients had the pharmacoresistant temporal lobe epilepsy. Sampling frequency of EEG data is 512 Hz. In the dataset, there are 3750 EEG signal pairs corresponding to each X_F and X_{NF} signals. Each

Figure 1. Flow chart of the system proposed for classification

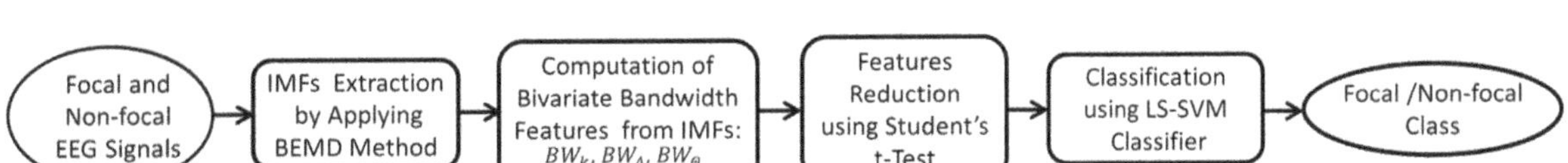

pair composed of two signals indicated as '*x*' and '*y*', each of length 10240 samples. These '*x*' and '*y*' signals are recordings of two adjacent EEG channels. Please refer (Andrzejak et al., 2012) for more information about the dataset. In this work, complete EEG dataset is used for study.

Bivariate Empirical Mode Decomposition

In order to analyze univariate data EMD can be a suitable choice, on the other hand bivariate empirical mode decomposition (BEMD) (Rilling et al., 2007) is specially proposed for analysis of bivariate data. The X_F and X_{NF} recordings are bivariate in nature, since these signals are simultaneously recorded from the neighboring channels (Andrzejak et al., 2012). Therefore, we suggest using the BEMD for decomposition of these EEG signals. On decomposing a signal using EMD the outcome is a set of band-limited, oscillatory components known as IMFs. The IMFs satisfy the two basic conditions mentioned in (Huang et al., 1998).

The BEMD method is applied on bivariate signals and it uses the rationale underlying the bivariate framework (Altaf et al., 2007, Rilling et al., 2007), and it extracts the zero mean rotating components from bivariate signals. The decomposition using BEMD is based on the principle that fast rotating components superimposed over slow rotating components (Rilling et al., 2007). If a bivariate signal represented as the complex signal z(t), then the algorithm of the BEMD can be explained in the following steps (Rilling et al., 2007, Amoud et al., 2008, Park et al., 2011):

Algorithm 1: BEMD

1. For $1 < \boldsymbol{k} < \boldsymbol{N}$
   a. Corresponding to direction Ψ_k find projection of signal $\boldsymbol{z}(\boldsymbol{t})$ as:

$$\rho_{\Psi_k}(t) = \Re(e^{-j\Psi_k} z(t)).$$

   b. Obtain the maxima of $\rho_{\Psi_k}(t)$ as $\left\{t_i^k, \rho_i^k\right\}$.

   c. Obtain the envelop in the direction Ψ_k by interpolating points $\left\{t_i^k, e^{j\Psi_k}\rho_i^k\right\}$ as $e'_{\Psi_k}(t)$.

2. Extract the mean value of all tangents as: $p(t) = \frac{2}{N}\sum_k e'_{\Psi_k}(t)$.
3. Compute detail component as $d(t) = z(t) - p(t)$.
4. Check if $d(t)$ satisfies the criteria for bivariate IMF or not.
5. Continue repeating steps 1-4 on $d(t)$ and examine if it meets the requirements of bivariate IMF.

Once bivariate IMFs are obtained, then the bivariate signal $z(t)$ can be expressed as (Amoud et al., 2008, Mandic et al., 2013):

$$z(t) = \sum_{k=1}^{M} I_k(t) + r_M(t). \tag{1}$$

where $I_k(t)$ and $r_M(t)$ represent the kth bivariate IMF and a residuals, respectively. In this work, the number of directions is taken as four to decompose bivariate EEG signals. Figure 2 and Figure 3 depict the X_F signals and their corresponding eight IMFs for 'x' and 'y' EEG signals, respectively. Similarly, the X_{NF} signals and their corresponding eight IMFs for 'x' and 'y' EEG signal are depicted in Figure 4 and Figure 5.

Features Extraction

A description of extracted features namely, IQR values of amplitude bandwidth, deformation bandwidth, and precession bandwidth is presented in this subsection.

A real valued bivariate signal can be defined in the form of time-varying modulated ellipse as follows (Lilly and Gascard, 2006, Lilly and Olhede, 2010):

$$s(t) = e^{j\Theta(t)}\left[C(t)\cos\varphi(t) + D(t)\sin\varphi(t)\right] \tag{2}$$

where, $C(t)$ and $D(t)$ are semi-major and semi-minor axis of the time-varying modulated ellipse, respectively. The parameter $\Theta(t)$ is instantaneous semi-major axis orientation in respect of the x-axis and parameter $\varphi(t)$ is called orbital phase which is a measure of instantaneous position of the particle around the ellipse perimeter in respect of semi major axis (Lilly and Gascard, 2006, Lilly and Olhede, 2010).

The expression of bivariate bandwidth for a bivariate signal in terms of ellipse parameters can be written as follows (Lilly and Olhede, 2010):

$$BW_s^2(t) = \left|\frac{d\ln[k(t)]}{dt}\right|^2 + \frac{1}{1-\wedge^2(t)}\left|\frac{1}{2}\frac{d\wedge(t)}{dt}\right|^2 + \wedge^2(t)\omega_\Theta^2(t) \tag{3}$$

Figure 2. 'x' Time-Series of X_F signal pair and corresponding first eight IMFs obtained using BEMD

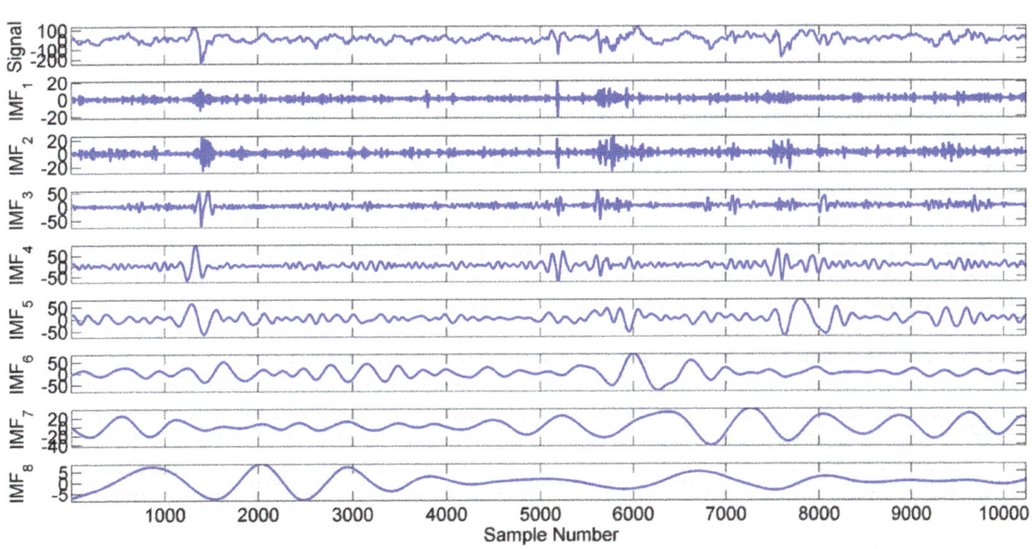

Figure 3. 'y' time-series of X_F signal pair and corresponding first eight IMFs obtained using BEMD

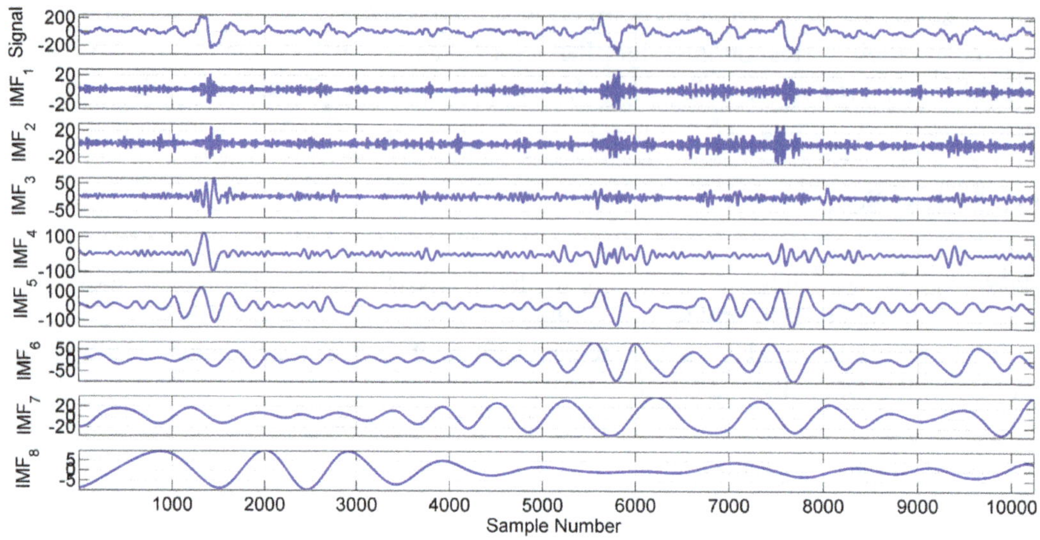

where, $\omega_\Theta(t)$ is called precession rate, and can be expressed as follows (Lilly and Olhede, 2010):

$$\omega_\Theta(t) \equiv \frac{d\Theta(t)}{dt} \tag{4}$$

The $k(t)$ is called root-mean-square amplitude and can be shown as (Lilly and Olhede, 2010):

$$k(t) \equiv \sqrt{\frac{C^2(t) + D^2(t)}{2}} \tag{5}$$

Figure 4. 'x' time-series of X_{NF} signal pair and corresponding first eight IMFs obtained using BEMD

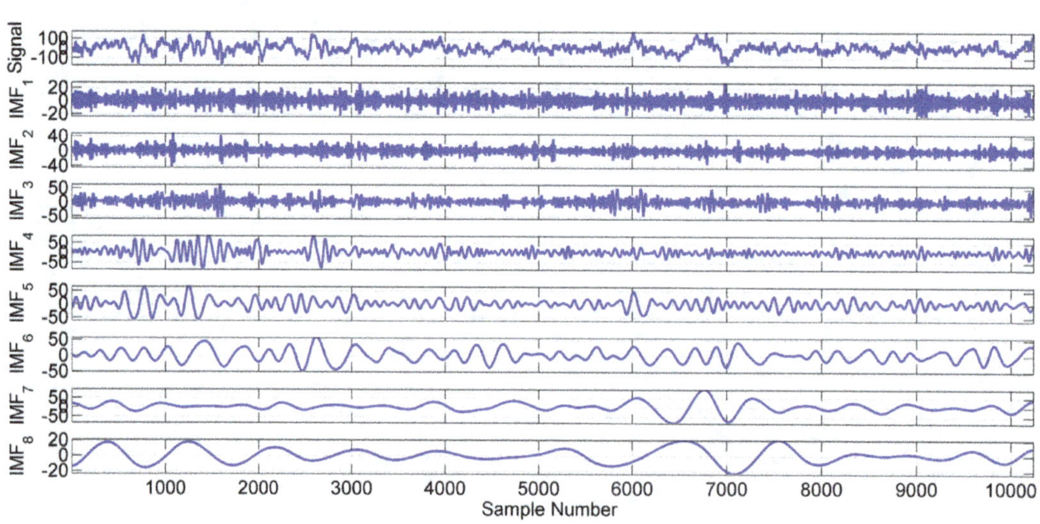

Figure 5. 'y' time-series of X_{NF} signal pair and corresponding first eight IMFs obtained using BEMD

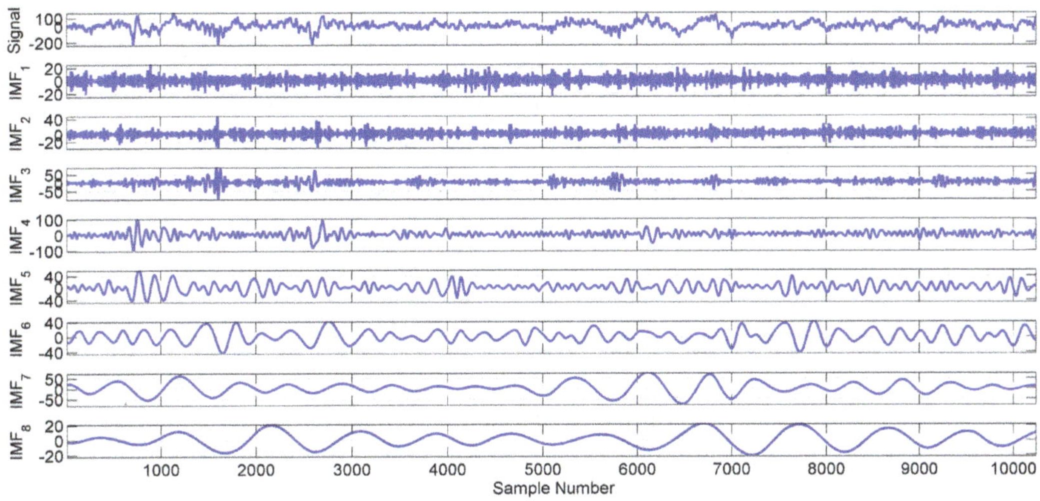

The $\wedge(t)$ in (3) is known as eccentricity, and it can be given as follows (Lilly and Olhede, 2010):

$$\wedge(t) \equiv r_s \frac{C^2(t) - D^2(t)}{C^2(t) - D^2(t)} \tag{6}$$

where, r_s is direction of rotation of the particle around the time-varying modulated ellipse and can be defined as follows (Lilly and Olhede, 2010):

$$r_s \equiv \operatorname{sgn}(D(t))$$

The expression in (3) can also be defined as follows (Lilly and Olhede, 2010):

$$BW_s^2(t) \equiv B_k^2(t) + B_\wedge^2(t) + B_\Theta^2(t) \tag{7}$$

where

$$\boldsymbol{B_k}\left(\boldsymbol{t}\right) = \left|\frac{\boldsymbol{d}\ln\left[\boldsymbol{k}\left(\boldsymbol{t}\right)\right]}{\boldsymbol{dt}}\right|$$

$$B_\wedge(t) = \frac{1}{2\sqrt{1 - \wedge^2(t)}}\left|\frac{d\wedge(t)}{dt}\right|$$

and

$$B_{\Theta}(t) = \wedge(t)\omega_{\Theta}(t)$$

The terms $B_k(t)$, $B_{\wedge}(t)$, and $B_{\Theta}(t)$ are called amplitude bandwidth, deformation bandwidth, and precession bandwidth, respectively. The IQR (Manikandan, 2011) values of $B_k(t)$, $B_{\wedge}(t)$, and $B_{\Theta}(t)$ are termed as BW_k, $BW_{\wedge}$, and BW_{Θ}, respectively, and used as the features. The parameters BW_k, $BW_{\wedge}$, and BW_{Θ} computed from bivariate IMFs are given as input features for classifier. These bandwidth parameters can be computed using the JLAB toolbox which is available at http://www.jmlilly.net/jmlsoft.html.

Student's *t*-Test Based Features Selection

In this work, Student's *t*-test is used for dimension reduction of feature set. The Student's *t*-test indicates weather the two sets are statistically different or not (Acharya et al., 2013, Boneau, 1960). This test results the *p*-value which indicates the similarity between two classes (Acharya et al., 2013). Lower *p*-value indicates more separability between two groups. In this work, features are ranked according to the Student's *t*-test. The classification is performed considering different number of ranked features. In this way, best combination of features is obtained for classification of X_F and X_{NF}.

Least Squares Support Vector Machine Classifier

The support vector machine (SVM) (Vapnik, 1995, Suykens and Vandewalle, 1999) is a technique for classification of signals of two different categories or groups. SVM classifier has been employed in different studies (Patidar and Pachori, 2014, Siuly et al., 2011, Patidar et al., 2015, Kolekar and Dash, 2015, Kumar and Kolekar, 2014) to classify EEG signals. The LS-SVM formulation considers equality type constraints in place of inequality constraints as used in SVM. In turn, instead of quadratic programming problem the LS-SVM deals with linear equations. The LS-SVM can be briefly described as follows:

Considering training data points $\left\{x_p, y_p\right\}_{p=1}^{k}$ where $\boldsymbol{x_p} \in \mathbb{R}^n$ denotes input and $y_p \in \left\{+1, -1\right\}$ indicates p^{th} label of output class. Decision function of LS-SVM can be shown as (Suykens and Vandewalle, 1999, Li et al., 2013, Siuly et al., 2011, Sharma and Pachori, 2015):

$$w(x) = \operatorname{sgn}\left[\sum_{p=1}^{K} \alpha_p y_p \Omega(x, x_p) + \beta\right] \tag{8}$$

where $\Omega(x, x_p)$ represents a kernel function and β is a bias. Used kernel functions can be defined as:

1. The radial basis function (RBF) kernel (Siuly et al., 2011, Khandoker et al., 2007):

$$\Omega(x, x_p) = e^{\frac{-\left\|x - x_p\right\|^2}{2\sigma^2}} \tag{9}$$

2. The Mexican hat wavelet kernel (Zavar et al., 2011):

$$\Omega(x, x_p) = \prod_{k=1}^{K}\left[1 - \frac{(x^k - x_p^k)^2}{a^2}\right] e^{\frac{-\left\|x^k - x_p^k\right\|}{2a^2}} \tag{10}$$

3. The Morlet wavelet kernel (Zavar et al., 2011):

$$\Omega(x, x_p) = \prod_{k=1}^{K}\left[\omega_0 \frac{(x^k - x_p^k)^2}{a}\right] e^{\frac{-\left\|x^k - x_p^k\right\|}{2a^2}} \tag{11}$$

In (9)-(11), x_p^k represents the pth element of kth training set. The kernel parameter σ is a scaling factor which determines width of the RBF kernel. Similarly a is a scaling factor for Morlet wavelet and Mexican hat wavelet kernels. The parameter ω_0 defines the oscillations present in Morlet wavelet kernel.

The performance of LS-SVM classifier is evaluated using different performance parameters namely, accuracy (*ACC*), sensitivity (*SEN*), specificity (*SPF*), negative predicted values (*NPV*), positive predicted values (*PPV*), and Matthews correlation coefficient (*MCC*) (Azar and El-Said, 2014, Yuan et al., 2007).

RESULTS

The BEMD is applied on these signal pairs which results in bivariate IMFs. The examples of BEMD of the X_F signals are depicted in the Figure 2 and Figure 3. The IMFs corresponding to '*x*' and '*y*' signals are equal in numbers. In this work, first eight pairs of IMFs are considered for feature extraction because each EEG signal pair of the dataset results in minimum eight pairs of bivariate IMFs. The parameters BW_k, $BW_\wedge$, and BW_Θ are computed for first eight pairs of bivariate IMFs of EEG signals. The box-plots for BW_k, $BW_\wedge$, and BW_Θ are shown in Figure 6, Figure 7 and Figure 8. These three parameters BW_k, $BW_\wedge$, and BW_Θ computed from eight IMFs form the feature set comprises of twenty four features. These twenty four features and their corresponding range (Mean $\pm$ standard deviation) are shown in the Table 1. In order to reduce the number of features for classification, the Student's *t*-test is employed on these features. The *p*-values are analyzed for each feature and listed in the Table 1. It is observed that twenty one out of twenty four features resulted the significant *p*-value ($p < 0.05$). The features are ranked according to the Student's *t*-test. The ranking order of these features are as follows: BW_k of IMF_3, BW_k of IMF_6, BW_k of IMF_5, BW_Θ of IMF_3, BW_k of IMF_2, BW_k of IMF_4, BW_k of IMF_1, BW_Θ of IMF_2, BW_Θ of IMF_6, $BW_\wedge$ of IMF_6, $BW_\wedge$ of IMF_3, BW_Θ of IMF_5, $BW_\wedge$ of IMF_5, $BW_\wedge$ of IMF_2, BW_k of IMF_7, $BW_\wedge$ of IMF_7, BW_Θ of IMF_7, $BW_\wedge$ of IMF_4, $BW_\wedge$ of IMF_1, BW_Θ of IMF_8, $BW_\wedge$ of IMF_8, BW_k of IMF_8, BW_Θ of IMF_1, and BW_Θ of IMF_4. Various experiments are performed using different features by combining them in their ranking order for classification of X_F and X_{NF} signals. We start our experiment by combining first two features and performed classification. Then, first three features are combined for classification of X_F and X_{NF} signals. Further, next feature is included in the features set. In this way, classification accuracy is obtained for each combination of features. The number of features used in the combination of features varies from 2 features to 24 features. The classification accuracies obtained using LS-SVM classifier are depicted in Figure 9. The 10-fold cross-validation (Kohavi, 1995) procedure is employed for evaluating classification performance. It can be observed from Figure 9 that the maximum classification accuracy is obtained when first 20 features are selected for classification with Morlet wavelet kernel is used as classifier kernel. The performance measures of LS-SVM classifier corresponding to different classifier kernels are mentioned in Table 2. The optimum kernel parameters also specified in the Table 2, which are determined by trial and error experiments. Figure 10 shows the receiver operating characteristic (ROC) (Khandoker et al., 2007) curves for different kernels of LS-SVM classifier. The area under ROC curve (AUC) (Khandoker et al., 2007) is found to be 0.9105, 0.9159, and 0.9057 for RBF kernel, Morlet wavelet kernel, and Mexican hat wavelet kernel, respectively.

Table 1. Range of bivariate features for first eight IMFs extracted from X_F and X_{NF} signals (given as: Mean ± standard deviation)

IMF	Bivariate Features	X_F Signal	X_{NF} Signal	*p*-value
IMF_1	BW_k	0.1737 ± 0.0199	0.1673 ± 0.0256	6.97×10^{-3}
	$BW_\wedge$	0.1383 ± 0.0255	0.1405 ± 0.0359	0.0027
	BW_Θ	0.1261 ± 0.0250	0.1255 ± 0.0322	0.3376
IMF_2	BW_k	0.0757 ± 0.0103	0.0717 ± 0.0114	3.85×10^{-56}
	$BW_\wedge$	0.0663 ± 0.0112	0.0636 ± 0.0166	1.1102×10^{-16}
	BW_Θ	0.0543 ± 0.0089	0.0513 ± 0.0122	8.2×10^{-34}
IMF_3	BW_k	0.0334 ± 0.0052	0.0288 ± 0.0053	8.5×10^{-291}
	$BW_\wedge$	0.0274 ± 0.0059	0.0256 ± 0.0082	3.61×10^{-26}
	BW_Θ	0.0217 ± 0.0044	0.0198 ± 0.0060	3.32×10^{-57}
IMF_4	BW_k	0.0134 ± 0.0023	0.0127 ± 0.0022	3.97×10^{-41}
	$BW_\wedge$	0.0109 ± 0.0027	0.0112 ± 0.0035	0.0001
	BW_Θ	0.0085 ± 0.0020	0.0085 ± 0.0026	0.5428

continued on following page

Table 1. Continued

IMF	Bivariate Features	X_F Signal	X_{NF} Signal	*p*-value
IMF_5	BW_k	0.0058 ± 0.0012	0.0062 ± 0.0011	3.32×10^{-97}
	$BW_\wedge$	0.0050 ± 0.0013	0.0054 ± 0.0019	3.27×10^{-22}
	BW_Θ	0.0038 ± 0.0010	0.0041 ± 0.0014	1.92×10^{-22}
IMF_6	BW_k	0.0027 ± 0.0007	0.0030 ± 0.0007	1.54×10^{-68}
	$BW_\wedge$	0.0024 ± 0.0007	0.0026 ± 0.0010	2.56×10^{-26}
	BW_Θ	0.0018 ± 0.0005	0.0020 ± 0.0007	5.27×10^{-27}
IMF_7	BW_k	0.0014 ± 0.0004	0.0014 ± 0.0004	2.22×10^{-16}
	$BW_\wedge$	0.0012 ± 0.0004	0.0013 ± 0.0005	2.7478×10^{-13}
	BW_Θ	0.0009 ± 0.0003	0.0010 ± 0.0004	2.2964×10^{-11}
IMF_8	BW_k	0.0008 ± 0.0003	0.0008 ± 0.0003	0.2805
	$BW_\wedge$	0.0007 ± 0.0002	0.0007 ± 0.0003	0.049
	BW_Θ	0.0005 ± 0.0002	0.0005 ± 0.0002	0.0044

Figure 6. IQR of amplitude bandwidth (BW_k) of first eight IMFs extracted from X_F and X_{NF} signals

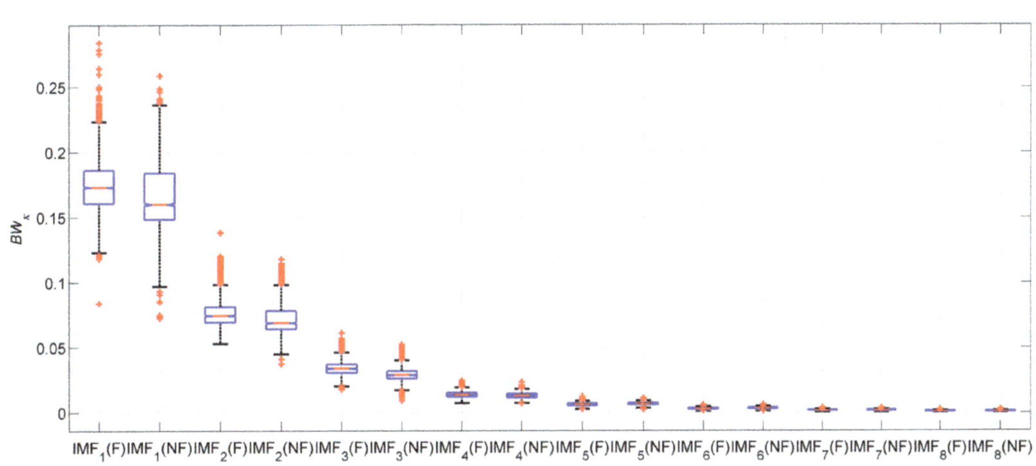

Figure 7. IQR of deformation bandwidth (BW_{Λ}) of first eight IMFs extracted from X_F and X_{NF} signals

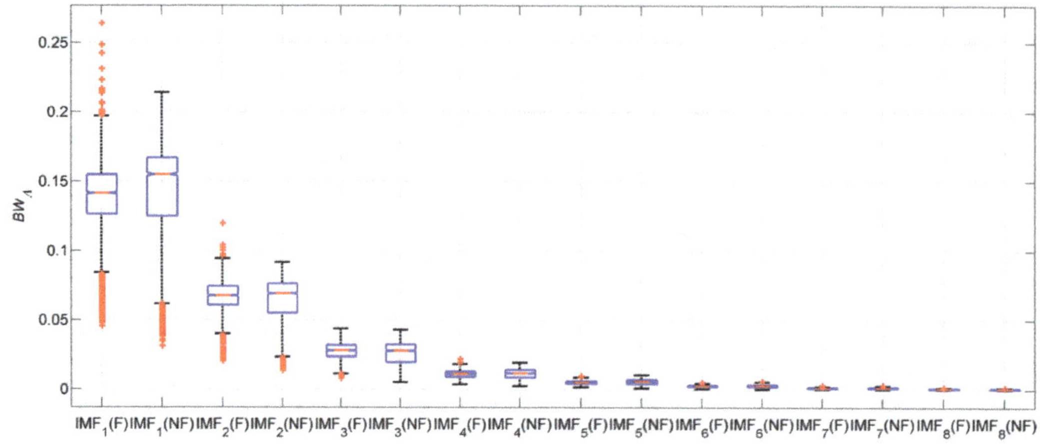

DISCUSSION

The proposed methodology for automated classification is based on the BEMD which is suitable and relevant for efficient representation of bivariate X_F and X_{NF} signals. The nonlinear, non-stationary, and bivariate nature of the X_F and X_{NF} signals makes it suitable to apply BEMD before computation of the bivariate bandwidths. Moreover, the BEMD method decomposes the signal in equal number of IMFs for both time series. These IMFs can be represented by amplitude modulated and frequency modulated (AM-FM) signals. Furthermore, the concept of the instantaneous bandwidth is meaningful for AM-FM signals. In (Amoud et al., 2008), the BEMD method has been applied on center of pressure signals antero-posterior (AP) and mediolateral (ML) signals. The parameters like circular area enclosing 95% of points of the data and average rotation frequency computed from analytic IMFs in complex plane are studied and BEMD method has been compared with EMD and complex-EMD (CEMD). In (Lilly and Gascard, 2006), position time series taken from oceanographic surface float data are decomposed in modulated elliptical signal and a residual using wavelet ridge algorithm. The instantaneous frequency curve is approximated as ridge curve of wavelet transform. In (Dwivedi et al., 2016), the X_F and X_{NF} signals are decomposed using BEMD. The area feature computed from the IMFs is used to perform the discrimination between the focal and non-focal classes. In the our work, for the purpose of classification, bivariate real valued IMFs obtained using BEMD are represented in terms of time-varying ellipse to extract the features. The set of selected significant features using Student's *t*-test maintains the performance of the classifier and reduces overall complexity. The presented study shows a set of only 20 features obtained from the set of 24 features which are sufficient for classification of X_F and X_{NF} signals. The results of the proposed methodology are compared with the existing methods shown in Table 3.

In (Zhu et al., 2013), permutation entropy (PE) and delay permutation entropy (DPE) index features were computed for the 50 and 750 sets of X_F and X_{NF} signals to identify epileptic zone. Only, the recordings of '*x*' signal of bivariate EEG signals were used for study. For 50 and 750 sets they obtained the maximum *ACC* of 84% and 75%, respectively. In (Sharma et al., 2014), the authors used the both '*x*' and '*y*' signals of bivariate EEG signals for classification. The features extracted were average variance of instantaneous frequencies (AVIF) and average sample entropy (ASE) computed from IMFs obtained for

Figure 8. IQR of precession bandwidth (BW_Θ) of first eight IMFs extracted from X_F and X_{NF} signals

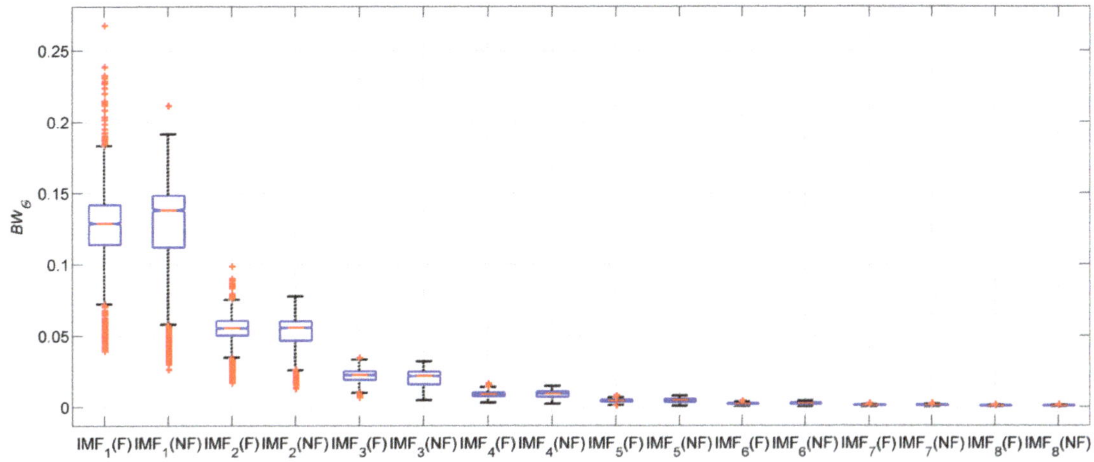

Table 2. Performance of LS-SVM classifier for different kernel functions

Kernel	Kernel Parameters	*ACC*	*SEN*	*SPE*	*PPV*	*NPV*	*MCC*
RBF	$\sigma = 3$	83.60	82.85	84.35	84.13	83.13	0.67
Mexican hat wavelet	a = 12	83.15	82.83	83.47	83.37	82.97	0.66
Morlet wavelet	$\omega = 0.5$, a = 5	84.01	83.47	84.56	84.40	83.68	0.68

Figure 9. Plots of classification accuracies obtained using LS-SVM classifier with varying number of ranked features for different classifier kernels

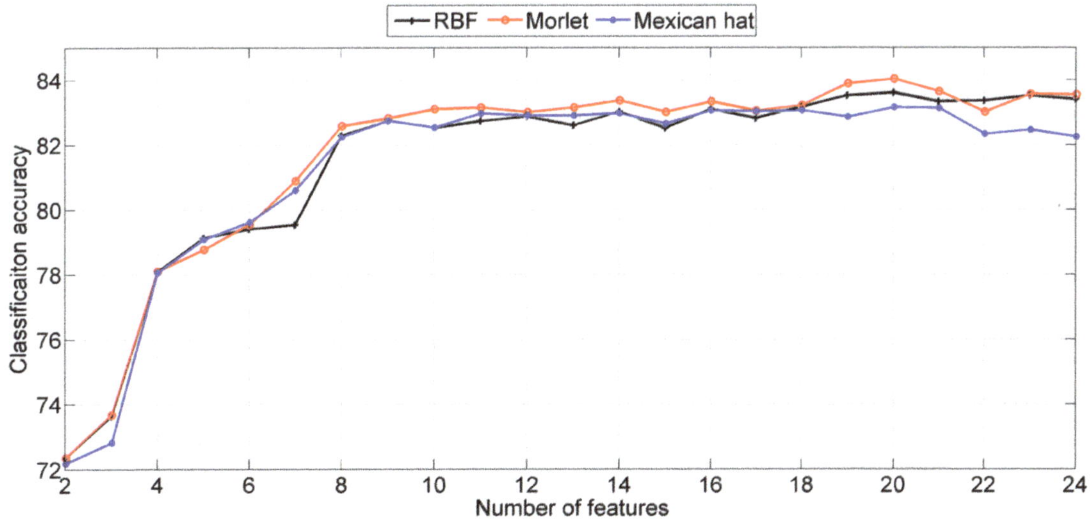

Figure 10. Receiver operating characteristics (ROC) curves for different kernel functions of LS-SVM classifier

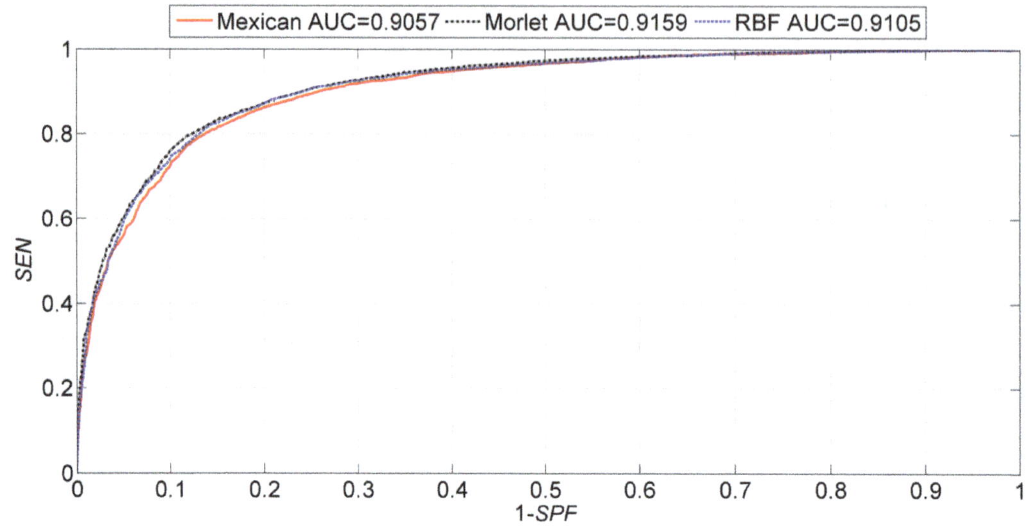

Table 3. Performance comparison of proposed work and other methodologies

Size of Dataset of X_F and X_{NF} Signals	Method and Authors	Classification Accuracy (%)
50 X_F and X_{NF} signals 750 X_F and X_{NF} signals	DPE and SVM (Zhu et al., 2013)	84 75
50 X_F and X_{NF} signals	ASE, AVIF and LS-SVM (Sharma et al., 2014)	85
50 X_F and X_{NF} signals	Entropies computed from IMFs and LS-SVM (Sharma et al., 2015a)	87
50 X_F and X_{NF} signals	DWT based entropies and LS-SVM (Sharma et al., 2015b)	84
50 X_F and X_{NF} signals	EWT, A_{RPS} and LS-SVM (Bhattacharyya et al., 2016)	90
3750 X_F and X_{NF} signals	Time-frequency localized filter banks based wavelets, entropies and LS-SVM (Sharma et al., 2017)	94.25
3750 X_F and X_{NF} signals	EMD-DWT, entropies, and kNN classifier (Das and Bhuiyan, 2016)	89.40
3750 X_F and X_{NF} signals	Multivariate fuzzy entropy computed form TQWT subbands and LS-SVM (Bhattacharyya et al., 2017)	84.67
3750 X_F and X_{NF} signals	Proposed method	84.01

both time-series of these EEG signals. They achieved *ACC* of 85% employing LS-SVM classifier using these features for set of signals comprised of 50 pairs of X_F and X_{NF} signals. In (Sharma et al., 2015a), average sample entropy ($SpEn_{Avg}$), average approximate entropy ($ApEn_{Avg}$), average phase entropies ($S1_{Avg}$ and $S2_{Avg}$), average Shannon entropy ($ShEn_{Avg}$), and average Rényi entropy ($RenEn_{Avg}$) were computed from EEG signals. The dataset used for classification contains is 50 pairs of X_F and X_{NF} signals. The maximum value of *ACC* in this work is 87%. Recently, an integrated index is proposed for discrimination between X_F and X_{NF} signals (Sharma et al., 2015b). Entropy based features were extracted from detailed and approximate sub-band signals resulted from DWT. Finally, employing extracted features: average Rényi wavelet entropy, average Shannon wavelet entropy, average Tsallis wavelet entropy, average permutation entropy, average fuzzy entropy, and average phase entropies with LS-SVM classifier, the reported classification accuracy is 84% for 50 pairs of X_F and X_{NF} signals. The X_F and X_{NF} signals are decomposed using empirical wavelet transform (EWT) in order to obtained rhythms of EEG signals (Bhattacharyya et al., 2016). The area parameter (A_{RPS}) is computed from the 2 dimensional projection of the reconstructed phase space (RPS) of the rhythms. They obtained the classification accuracy of 90% for 50 pairs of X_F and X_{NF} signals with LS-SVM classifier. In (Sharma et al., 2017), X_F and X_{NF} signals are analyzed using wavelets designed by employing a new class of time-frequency localized filter banks. They computed same features as used in (Sharma et al., 2015b) and performed classification using LS-SVM classifier. The maximum classification accuracy reported by presented algorithm is 94.25% for the entire dataset. In the above discussed methods for a pair the features obtained from both the time-series are averaged. In another methodology (Das and Bhuiyan, 2016), the EEG signals are decomposed using EMD. The features are computed form the DWT components of the IMFs obtained from EEG signals. They reported the classification accuracy of 89.40% using k nearest neighbor (kNN) classifier. The time-series in the pair of EEG signals are subtracted as x-y and EMD is applied on the difference time-series. In another study (Bhattacharyya et al., 2017) the X_F and X_{NF} signals are decomposed using TQWT. The TQWT is applied individually on the '*x*' and '*y*' time-series. For a given oscillatory level, the subband signals obtained for '*x*' and '*y*' time-series are used to form a pair of subband signals. The multivariate fuzzy entropy is computed from this pair of subband signals. The reported maximum classification accuracy is 84.67% for the classification of X_F and X_{NF} signals using LS-SVM classifier. In this method, the multivariate fuzzy entropy is used which can quantify the inter-channel information; however, the TQWT is applied on the univariate signals.

As opposed to the previous approaches, the proposed method employs BEMD to decompose the EEG signals which is bivariate in nature. The extracted features are also bivariate in nature, which possibly helps in better representation of underlying dynamics of epileptogenic cortex by exploiting inter-channel relations for both time-series of the pair of EEG signals. In this way, the proposed method is a fully bivariate approach for classification of X_F and X_{NF} signals. The higher values of parameters *ACC, SEN, SPE, PPV, NPV,* and *MCC* (as shown in Table 2) suggest the use of Morlet wavelet kernel with LS-SVM classifier. Furthermore, the AUC for Morlet wavelet is also highest as shown in Figure 10. Results obtained in this study suggest that proposed features, BW_k, $BW_\wedge$, and BW_Θ computed from bivariate IMFs are suitable for classification of X_F and X_{NF} signals. The key attributes of the proposed methodology are as follows:

- The proposed methodology is a new classification scheme and applied on complete dataset of X_F and X_{NF} signals which consists of bivariate EEG recordings.
- Robustness of classification method is ensured by employing ten-fold cross-validation technique.
- The technique can be designed in the form of software for the application of detecting X_F and X_{NF} signals. The knowledge of the electrodes corresponding to X_F signals can be helpful for localizing epileptogenic zone.

CONCLUSION

In this chapter, classification of X_F and X_{NF} signals is performed using bivariate features. The EEG signals in the dataset are available as the pair of time series. The BEMD is found as suitable decomposition method for X_F and X_{NF} signals. New features are derived based on the BEMD for classification of X_F and X_{NF} signals. The BEMD resulted in same number of IMFs for both time series of these bivariate EEG signals, which is useful to extract the bandwidth parameters namely, amplitude bandwidth, deformation bandwidth, and precession bandwidth. The parameters obtained from the IQR of bivariate bandwidths namely, BW_k, BW_Λ, and BW_Θ are found to be significantly useful for classification of X_F and X_{NF} signals. The Morlet wavelet kernel provides most desirable performance for LS-SVM classifier.

Future research may include the development of the new features which can be used along with the proposed features to improve the classification accuracy. In future, an adaptive kernel function and kernel parameters selection strategy can be developed to select the suitable kernel automatically.

ACKNOWLEDGMENT

This work was supported by the Council of Scientific and Industrial Research (CSIR) funded Research Project, Government of India, Grant No. 22/687/15/EMR-II.

REFERENCES

Acharya, U. R., Faust, O., Kadri, N. A., Suri, J. S., & Yu, W. (2013). Automated identification of normal and diabetes heart rate signals using nonlinear measures. *Computers in Biology and Medicine*, *43*(10), 1523–1529. doi:10.1016/j.compbiomed.2013.05.024 PMID:24034744

Adeli, H., Ghosh-Dastidar, S., & Dadmehr, N. (2008). A spatio-temporal wavelet-chaos methodology for EEG-based diagnosis of Alzheimers disease. *Neuroscience Letters*, *444*(2), 190–194. doi:10.1016/j.neulet.2008.08.008 PMID:18706477

Adeli, H., Zhou, Z., & Dadmehr, N. (2003). Analysis of EEG records in an epileptic patient using wavelet transform. *Journal of Neuroscience Methods*, *123*(1), 69–87. doi:10.1016/S0165-0270(02)00340-0 PMID:12581851

Ahmadlou, M., & Adeli, H. (2014). Electroencephalograms in diagnosis of autism. In V. B. Patel, V. R. Preedy, & C. R. Martin (Eds.), *Comprehensive Guide to Autism* (pp. 327–343). doi:10.1007/978-1-4614-4788-7_204

Ahmadlou, M., Adeli, H., & Adeli, A. (2010). Fractality and a wavelet-chaos-neural network methodology for EEG-based diagnosis of autistic spectrum disorder. *Journal of Clinical Neurophysiology*, *27*(5), 328–333. doi:10.1097/WNP.0b013e3181f40dc8 PMID:20844443

Ahrabian, A., Rehman, N. U., & Mandic, D. (2013). Bivariate empirical mode decomposition for unbalanced real-world signals. *IEEE Signal Processing Letters*, *20*(3), 245–248. doi:10.1109/LSP.2013.2242062

Altaf, M. U. B., Gautama, T., Tanaka, T., & Mandic, D. P. (2007). Rotation invariant complex empirical mode decomposition. In *IEEE International Conference on Acoustics, Speech and Signal Processing*, (pp. III–1009–III–1012). Honolulu, HI: IEEE.

Amoud, H., Snoussi, H., Hewson, D., & Duchêne, J. (2008). Univariate and bivariate empirical mode decomposition for postural stability analysis. *EURASIP Journal on Advances in Signal Processing*, *657391*, 1–11.

Andrzejak, R. G., Schindler, K., & Rummel, C. (2012). Nonrandomness, nonlinear dependence, and nonstationarity of electroencephalographic recordings from epilepsy patients. *Physical Review E: Statistical, Nonlinear, and Soft Matter Physics*, *86*(046206), 1–17. PMID:23214662

Azar, A. T., & El-Said, S. A. (2014). Performance analysis of support vector machines classifiers in breast cancer mammography recognition. *Neural Computing & Applications*, *24*(5), 1163–1177. doi:10.1007/s00521-012-1324-4

Badawy, R. A. B., Curatolo, J. M., Newton, M., Berkovic, S. F., & Macdonell, R. A. L. (2007). Changes in cortical excitability differentiate generalized and focal epilepsy. *Annals of Neurology*, *61*(4), 324–331. doi:10.1002/ana.21087 PMID:17358004

Ben-Jacob, E., Doron, I., Gazit, T., Rephaeli, E., Sagher, O., & Towle, V. L. (2007). Mapping and assessment of epileptogenic foci using frequency-entropy templates. *Physical Review E: Statistical, Nonlinear, and Soft Matter Physics*, *76*(051903), 1–8. PMID:18233683

Bhattacharyya, A., Pachori, R. B., & Acharya, U. R. (2017). Tunable-Q wavelet transform based multivariate sub-band fuzzy entropy with application to focal EEG signal analysis. *Entropy*, *19*(3).

Bhattacharyya, A., Sharma, M., Pachori, R. B., Sircar, P., & Acharya, U. R. (2016). A novel approach for automated detection of focal EEG signals using empirical wavelet transform. *Neural Computing & Applications*, 1–11.

Boneau, C. A. (1960). The effects of violations of assumptions underlying the t test. *Psychological Bulletin*, *57*(1), 49–64. doi:10.1037/h0041412 PMID:13802482

Das, A. B., & Bhuiyan, M. I. H. (2016). Discrimination and classification of focal and non-focal EEG signals using entropy-based features in the EMD-DWT domain. *Biomedical Signal Processing and Control*, *29*, 11–21. doi:10.1016/j.bspc.2016.05.004

Dwivedi, A. R., Bari, H., Nath, S., Bajaj, V., Sharma, D., & Kumar, A. (2016). Analysis of focal and non-focal EEG signals using bivariate empirical mode decomposition. *IEEE Students' Conference on Electrical, Electronics and Computer Science*, 1–3. doi:10.1109/SCEECS.2016.7509318

Gutiérrez, J., Alcántara, R., & Medina, V. (2001). Analysis and localization of epileptic events using wavelet packets. *Medical Engineering & Physics*, *23*(9), 623–631. doi:10.1016/S1350-4533(01)00096-0 PMID:11755807

Huang, N. E., Shen, Z., Long, S. R., Wu, M. C., Shih, H. H., Zheng, Q., . . . Liu, H. H. (1998). The empirical mode decomposition and the Hilbert spectrum for nonlinear and non-stationary time series analysis. *Proceedings of the Royal Society of London. Series A: Mathematical, Physical and Engineering Sciences*, *454*(1971), 903–995. doi:10.1098/rspa.1998.0193

Khandoker, A. H., Lai, D. T. H., Begg, R. K., & Palaniswami, M. (2007). Wavelet-based feature extraction for support vector machines for screening balance impairments in the elderly. *IEEE Transactions on Neural Systems and Rehabilitation Engineering*, *15*(4), 587–597. doi:10.1109/TNSRE.2007.906961 PMID:18198717

Kohavi, R. (1995). A study of cross-validation and bootstrap for accuracy estimation and model selection. *Proceedings of the 14th International Joint Conference on Artificial Intelligence*.

Kolekar, M. H., & Dash, D. P. (2015). A nonlinear feature based epileptic seizure detection using least square support vector machine classifier. TENCON 2015 - 2015 IEEE Region 10 Conference, 1–6. doi:10.1109/TENCON.2015.7373164

Kumar, A., & Kolekar, M. H. (2014). Machine learning approach for epileptic seizure detection using wavelet analysis of eeg signals. *International Conference on Medical Imaging, m-Health and Emerging Communication Systems*, 412–416. doi:10.1109/MedCom.2014.7006043

Kumar, T. S., Kanhangad, V., & Pachori, R. B. (2014). Classification of seizure and seizure-free EEG signals using multi-level local patterns. *Proceedings of 19th International Conference on Digital Signal Processing*, 646–650. doi:10.1109/ICDSP.2014.6900745

Lehnertz, K., & Elger, C. E. (1995). Spatio-temporal dynamics of the primary epileptogenic area in temporal lobe epilepsy characterized by neuronal complexity loss. *Electroencephalography and Clinical Neurophysiology*, *95*(2), 108–117. doi:10.1016/0013-4694(95)00071-6 PMID:7649002

Li, S., Zhou, W., Yuan, Q., Geng, S., & Cai, D. (2013). Feature extraction and recognition of ictal EEG using EMD and SVM. *Computers in Biology and Medicine*, *43*(7), 807–816. doi:10.1016/j.compbiomed.2013.04.002 PMID:23746721

Lilly, J. M., & Gascard, J.-C. (2006). Wavelet ridge diagnosis of time-varying elliptical signals with application to an oceanic eddy. *Nonlinear Processes in Geophysics*, *13*(5), 467–483. doi:10.5194/npg-13-467-2006

Lilly, J. M., & Olhede, S. C. (2010). Bivariate instantaneous frequency and bandwidth. *IEEE Transactions on Signal Processing*, *58*(2), 591–603. doi:10.1109/TSP.2009.2031729

Mandic, D. P., Rehman, N. U., Wu, Z., & Huang, N. E. (2013). Empirical mode decomposition–based time–frequency analysis of multivariate signals: The power of adaptive data analysis. *IEEE Signal Processing Magazine*, *30*(6), 74–86. doi:10.1109/MSP.2013.2267931

Manikandan, S. (2011). Measures of dispersion. *Journal of Pharmacology and Pharmacotherapeutics*, *2*(4), 315–316. doi:10.4103/0976-500X.85931 PMID:22025871

Marciani, M. G., Stefanini, F., Stefani, N., Maschio, M. C. E., Gigli, G. L., Roncacci, S., & Bernardi, G. et al. (1992). Lateralization of the epileptogenic focus by computerized EEG study and neuropsychological evaluation. *The International Journal of Neuroscience*, *66*(1–2), 53–60. doi:10.3109/00207459208999789 PMID:1304570

Martis, R. J., Acharya, U. R., Tan, J. H., Petznick, A., Yanti, R., Chua, C. K., Ng, E. Y. K., and Tong, L. (2012). Application of empirical mode decomposition (EMD) for automated detection of epilepsy using EEG signals. *International Journal of Neural Systems*, 22(6), 1–16.

Oweis, R. J., & Abdulhay, E. W. (2011). Seizure classification in EEG signals utilizing Hilbert-Huang transform. *Biomedical Engineering Online*, *10*(38), 1–15. PMID:21609459

Pachori, R. B. (2008). Discrimination between ictal and seizure-free EEG signals using empirical mode decomposition. *Research Letters in Signal Processing*, *293056*, 1–5. doi:10.1155/2008/293056

Pachori, R. B., & Patidar, S. (2014). Epileptic seizure classification in EEG signals using second-order difference plot of intrinsic mode functions. *Computer Methods and Programs in Biomedicine*, *113*(2), 494–502. doi:10.1016/j.cmpb.2013.11.014 PMID:24377902

Panet-Raymond, D., & Gotman, J. (1990). Asymmetry in delta activity in patients with focal epilepsy. *Electroencephalography and Clinical Neurophysiology*, *75*(6), 474–481. doi:10.1016/0013-4694(90)90134-6 PMID:1693892

Park, C., Looney, D., Kidmose, P., Ungstrup, M., & Mandic, D. P. (2011). Time-frequency analysis of EEG asymmetry using bivariate empirical mode decomposition. *IEEE Transactions on Neural Systems and Rehabilitation Engineering*, *19*(4), 366–373. doi:10.1109/TNSRE.2011.2116805 PMID:21342855

Pati, S., & Alexopoulos, A. V. (2010). Pharmacoresistant epilepsy: From pathogenesis to current and emerging therapies. *Cleveland Clinic Journal of Medicine*, *77*(7), 457–467. doi:10.3949/ccjm.77a.09061 PMID:20601619

Patidar, S., & Pachori, R. B. (2014). Classification of cardiac sound signals using constrained tunable-Q wavelet transform. *Expert Systems with Applications*, *41*(16), 7161–7170. doi:10.1016/j.eswa.2014.05.052

Patidar, S., Pachori, R. B., & Garg, N. (2015). Automatic diagnosis of septal defects based on tunable-Q wavelet transform of cardiac sound signals. *Expert Systems with Applications*, *42*(7), 3315–3326. doi:10.1016/j.eswa.2014.11.046

Rilling, G., Flandrin, P., Gonçalves, P., & Lilly, J. M. (2007). Bivariate empirical mode decomposition. *IEEE Signal Processing Letters*, *14*(12), 936–939. doi:10.1109/LSP.2007.904710

Rosenow, F. (2001). Rosenow, F. and Lüders, H. (2001). Presurgical evaluation of epilepsy. *Brain*, *124*(9), 1683–1700. doi:10.1093/brain/124.9.1683 PMID:11522572

Sabesan, S., Good, L. B., Tsakalis, K. S., Spanias, A., Treiman, D. M., & Iasemidis, L. D. (2009). Information flow and application to epileptogenic focus localization from intracranial EEG. *IEEE Transactions on Neural Systems and Rehabilitation Engineering*, *17*(3), 244–253. doi:10.1109/TNSRE.2009.2023291 PMID:19497831

Schevon, C. A., Cappell, J., Emerson, R., Isler, J., Grieve, P., Goodman, R., & Gilliam, F. et al. (2007). Cortical abnormalities in epilepsy revealed by local EEG synchrony. *NeuroImage*, *35*(1), 140–148. doi:10.1016/j.neuroimage.2006.11.009 PMID:17224281

Sharma, M., Dhere, A., Pachori, R. B., & Acharya, U. R. (2017). An automatic detection of focal EEG signals using new class of time-frequency localized orthogonal wavelet filter banks. *Knowledge-Based Systems*, *118*, 217–227. doi:10.1016/j.knosys.2016.11.024

Sharma, R., & Pachori, R. B. (2015). Classification of epileptic seizures in EEG signals based on phase space representation of intrinsic mode functions. *Expert Systems with Applications*, *42*(3), 1106–1117. doi:10.1016/j.eswa.2014.08.030

Sharma, R., Pachori, R. B., & Acharya, U. R. (2015a). Application of entropy measures on intrinsic mode functions for the automated identification of focal electroencephalogram signals. *Entropy*, *17*(2), 669–691. doi:10.3390/e17020669

Sharma, R., Pachori, R. B., & Acharya, U. R. (2015b). An integrated index for the identification of focal electroencephalogram signals using discrete wavelet transform and entropy measures. *Entropy*, *17*(8), 5218–5240. doi:10.3390/e17085218

Sharma, R., Pachori, R. B., & Gautam, S. (2014). Empirical mode decomposition based classification of focal and non-focal EEG signals. In *International Conference on Medical Biometrics*, (pp. 135–140). Shenzhen, China. IEEE. doi:10.1109/ICMB.2014.31

Siuly, L., Li, Y., & Wen, P. P. (2011). Clustering technique-based least square support vector machine for EEG signal classification. *Computer Methods and Programs in Biomedicine*, *104*(3), 358–372. doi:10.1016/j.cmpb.2010.11.014 PMID:21168234

Suykens, J. A. K., & Vandewalle, J. (1999). Least squares support vector machine classifiers. *Neural Processing Letters*, *9*(3), 293–300. doi:10.1023/A:1018628609742

van Mierlo, P., Carrette, E., Hallez, H., Raedt, R., Meurs, A., Vandenberghe, S., & Vonck, K. et al. (2013). Ictal-onset localization through connectivity analysis of intracranial EEG signals in patients with refractory epilepsy. *Epilepsia*, *54*(8), 1409–1418. doi:10.1111/epi.12206 PMID:23647147

van Mierlo, P., Papadopoulou, M., Carrette, E., Boon, P., Vandenberghe, S., Vonck, K., & Marinazzo, D. (2014). Functional brain connectivity from EEG in epilepsy: Seizure prediction and epileptogenic focus localization. *Progress in Neurobiology*, *121*, 19–35. doi:10.1016/j.pneurobio.2014.06.004 PMID:25014528

Vapnik, V. (1995). *The nature of statistical learning theory*. New York: Springer. doi:10.1007/978-1-4757-2440-0

Warren, C. P., Hu, S., Stead, M., Brinkmann, B. H., Bower, M. R., & Worrell, G. A. (2010). Synchrony in normal and focal epileptic brain: The seizure onset zone is functionally disconnected. *Journal of Neurophysiology*, *104*(6), 3530–3539. doi:10.1152/jn.00368.2010 PMID:20926610

Widman, G., Lehnertz, K., Urbach, H., & Elger, C. E. (2000). Spatial distribution of neuronal complexity loss in neocortical lesional epilepsies. *Epilepsia*, *41*(7), 811–817. doi:10.1111/j.1528-1157.2000.tb00247.x PMID:10897151

Worrell, G. A., Parish, L., Cranstoun, S. D., Jonas, R., Baltuch, G., & Litt, B. (2004). High frequency oscillations and seizure generation in neocortical epilepsy. *Brain*, *127*(7), 1496–1506. doi:10.1093/brain/awh149 PMID:15155522

Yuan, Q., Cai, C., Xiao, H., Liu, X., & Wen, Y. (2007). Diagnosis of breast tumours and evaluation of prognostic risk by using machine learning approaches. In D.-S. Huang, L. Heutte, & M. Loog (Eds.), *Advanced Intelligent Computing Theories and Applications. With Aspects of Contemporary Intelligent Computing Techniques* (pp. 1250–1260). Springer. doi:10.1007/978-3-540-74282-1_141

Zavar, M., Rahati, S., Akbarzadeh-T, M.-R., & Ghasemifard, H. (2011). Evolutionary model selection in a wavelet-based support vector machine for automated seizure detection. *Expert Systems with Applications*, *38*(9), 10751–10758. doi:10.1016/j.eswa.2011.01.087

Zhu, G., Li, Y., Wen, P. P., Wang, S., & Xi, M. (2013). Epileptogenic focus detection in intracranial EEG based on delay permutation entropy. *Proceedings of AIP Conference*, 1559, 31–36. doi:10.1063/1.4824993

Chapter 3
A Discrete-Wavelet-Transform- and Hidden-Markov-Model-Based Approach for Epileptic Focus Localization

Deba Prasad Dash
Indian Institute of Technology Patna, India

Maheshkumar H. Kolekar
Indian Institute of Technology Patna, India

ABSTRACT

Epilepsy is the most common neurological disorder with 40-50 million people suffering with it world-wide. Epilepsy is not life threatening but it disables the person to a greater extent due to its uncertainty of occurrences. Epilepsy is detected by repeated occurrences of seizure. Seizure can be generated in brain due to abnormal activity of group of neurons caused by brain tumor, genetic problem, infection, hemorrhage etc. Seizure can be detected by observing the variation in Electroencephalogram (EEG) signal. Focal seizure is defined as seizure localized in one lobe of brain. In this chapter discrete wavelet transform and Hidden Markov Model based focal seizure detection method is proposed for epileptic focus localization. EEG signal was decomposed up to level 5 using dual tree complex wavelet transform and entropy features such as collision entropy, minimum and modified sample entropy were extracted. Hidden Markov model was used for classification purpose. Maximum 80% accuracy was achieved in detecting focal and non-focal EEG signal.

INTRODUCTION

Seizure is defined as sudden surge of synchronous electrical activity of group of neurons. Around 10% of entire population may experience seizure at some point in the life. But repeated seizures indicate epilepsy. Epilepsy may be experienced by person from different age groups. Seizures are not life threatening but

DOI: 10.4018/978-1-5225-2829-6.ch003

may cause injury and disable a person to a great extend. Seizure becomes a burden to a person and also to the care taker. Focal seizures are seizures generated in one lobe of brain and do not spread to other lobes. Generalized or non-focal seizures spread to entire lobes of brain. Frontal and Temporal lobes are mostly affected from seizure. Based on the symptoms seizure can be tonic, clonic, tonic-clonic, myo-clonic, and atonic and absence seizures. Tonic seizure results in muscle stiffness, atonic seizure causes muscles to lose stiffness, absence seizure results in brief loss in consciousness, myoclonic and clonic seizures are indicated by jerky movements. Nearly 20-30% of seizure patient do not respond to available seizure prevention medicine. So surgery is used as an option to treat epilepsy for drug resistant patients by removing the lobe generating seizure. In operative seizure treatment it is important to locate the lobe generating seizure before surgery. An EEG based technique for focal epilepsy detection can be of great use for surgeons for deciding the exact lobe to operate. EEG has the advantage of low cost system and easy to use. Patients with artificial organ implant and small babies cannot go for imaging approach such as functional magnetic resonance imaging. Also there are many seizures which at initial stage cannot be detected by imaging approach. In this chapter a focal epilepsy detection method is proposed. Some of the state-of-art methods are discussed below.

Two most used methods for focal seizure detection are discrete wavelet transform based (DWT) or Empirical mode decomposition based approach. Rajeev Sharma *et.al* (Sharma *et.al* 2014) proposed EMD based classification of focal and non-focal EEG signals. Average sample entropy extracted from each intrinsic mode functions and average variance of instantaneous frequency were used as features along with least square support vector machine classifier (LSSVM) for detecting focal seizure. Only 50 EEG signals are used for classification purpose. EMD along with average Renyi entropy and average negentropy were used for detection of focal seizure by (Dwivedi *et.al* 2016). Artificial neural network are used for classification. Entropy features such as average Shannon entropy, average Renyi entropy, average approximate entropy; average sample entropy and average phase entropy were used for classifying focal and non-focal EEG seizure (Sharma *et.al* 2015). Least square support vector machine classifier was used for classification. Integrated index based focal seizure detection is proposed by Sharma *et.al* (Sharma *et.al* 2015). Various entropy features such as average wavelet, fuzzy, permutation and phase entropy were extracted and least square support vector machine classifier was used for classification purpose. Combined analysis of EMD-DWT based approach was proposed by das *et.al* (Das 2016). Features used were entropy features and classifier used was k nearest neighbor classifier. Duo Chen *et al.* (Chen *et.al* 2015) had proposed discrete wavelet transform based focal and non-focal seizure detection. The best accuracy of epileptic focus localization achieved was 83.07% using sym6 from levels 1 to 7. Piyush Swami *et al.*(Swami *et.al* 2016) had used dual tree complex wavelet transform for seizure classification. All details and last approximation coefficients are used to calculate features such as energy, standard deviation, root-mean-square, Shannon entropy, mean values and maximum peaks. Classification result was high with computation time less than 0.023 sec. Discrete wavelet transforms and support vector machine classifier based focal seizure prediction method was proposed by K. A. Helini Kulasuriya *et al.* (Kulasuriya *et.al* 2015). Statistical features such as maximum, minimum, mean and standard deviation were extracted from approximate and detail coefficients.

Now a days, hidden Markov model (HMM) (Kolekar et. al 2004 Dec) is used for epileptic seizure detection (Dash et. al 2017). Three states HMM for seizure detection is proposed by (Stephen *et.al*, 2007). Stationary wavelet transforms and hidden markov model between Ictal, interictal and seizure EEG signal was used for seizure detection with higher efficiency (Abdullah, 2012).

In this chapter a focal seizure detection method is discussed. Entropy features are extracted from the decomposed bands of wavelet transform and given to hidden markov model for classification. Presented method classifies focal seizure with 80.00% accuracy.

EXPERIMENTAL DATABASE

Dataset for focal and non-focal EEG signal freely available online is used for research purpose (Andrzejak *et.al* 2012). Two set of signals recorded, one from the area generating seizure and other from non focal region. Two sets of data each with two electrode signal x and y are defined in the dataset. The sampling rate of signal is 512 Hz. Total of 3750 EEG signal segments of 20 second duration are included in the dataset with total sample length of 10240. In this chapter total 100 EEG segments were used for research purpose.

PROPOSED APPROACH

Initially 50 Hz power line interference is removed from EEG data using IIR notch filter. EEG data is band pass filtered between 0.2-60 Hz based on the bands representing mental status of the person. Dual tree complex wavelet transform is used to decompose EEG signal into various bands. Complex wavelet transform is used for decomposition of signal up to level 5. Entropy features such as collision entropy, modified sample entropy and minimum entropy are extracted as a marker of focal event. Hidden Markov Model is used for classification purpose. Flowchart of proposed approach is shown in Figure 1.

Figure 1. (a,b) Focal and Non focal x EEG signal, (c,d) Focal and non focal y EEG signal

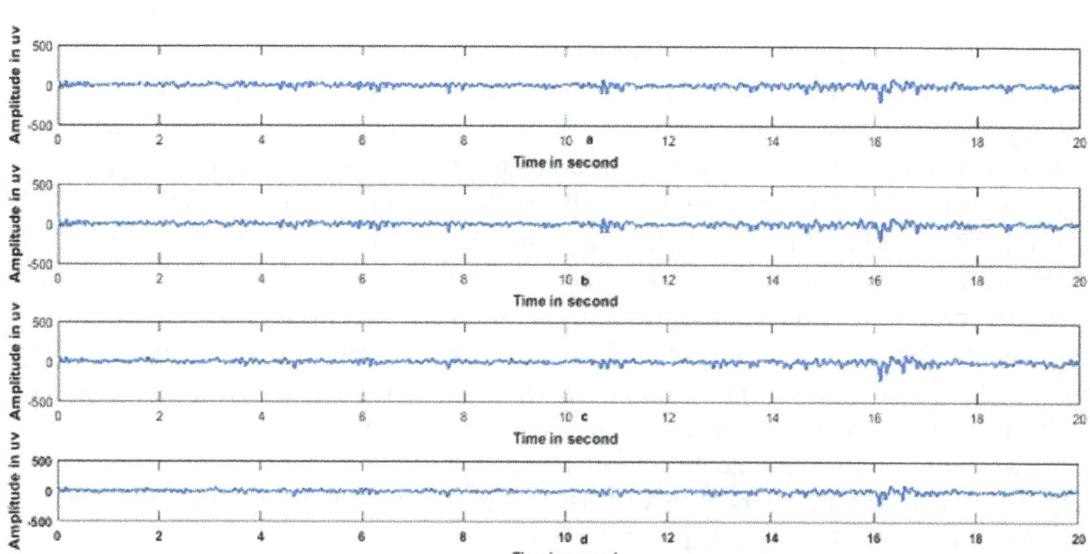

Figure 2. Flowchart of HMM training of focal and non focal seizure

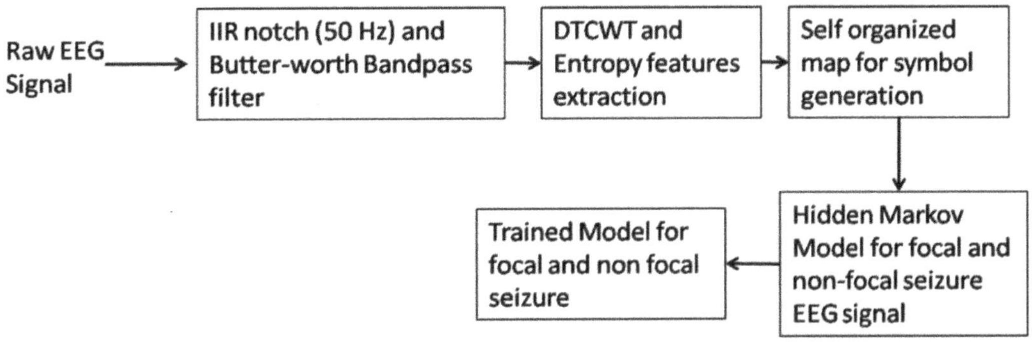

Figure 3. Flowchart of testing approach

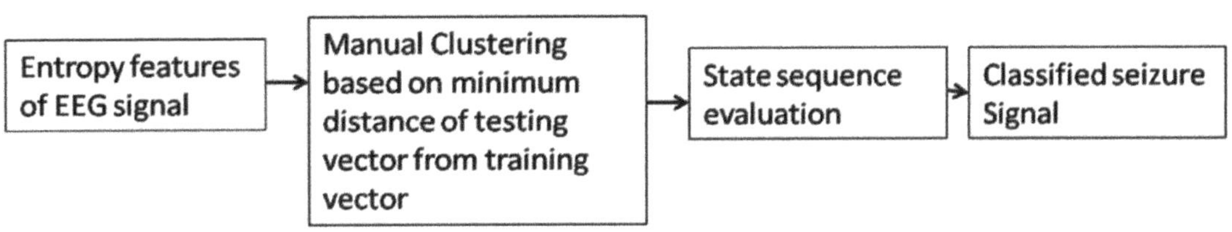

TECHNIQUE USED

Dual Tree Complex Wavelet Transform

Wavelet is a small waveform with average value zero. DWT replaces the sinusoidal basis function to a mother wavelet function for signal decomposition. Every signal can be represented by combination of scaling and wavelet coefficients as presented below.

$$x(t) = \sum_{n=-\infty}^{\infty} c(n) * \varnothing(t-n) + \sum_{j=0}^{\infty} \sum_{n=-\infty}^{\infty} d(j,n) * 2^{\frac{j}{2}} \varphi(2^j t - n) \tag{1}$$

Where c (n) is the scaling coefficient and d (j, n) is the wavelet coefficient. In the above equation n is the shifting coefficient and j is the scaling coefficient. φ is the Bandpass filter and Ø is the low pass filter.

$$c(n) = \int_{-\infty}^{\infty} x(t) * \varnothing(t-n)\, dt \tag{2}$$

$$d(j,n) = 2^{\frac{j}{2}} \int_{-\infty}^{\infty} x(t) * \varphi(2^j t - n)\, dt \tag{3}$$

Dual tree Complex wavelet transforms (DTCWT) (Selesnick *et.al* 2005) concept is same as that of Fourier transform. Fourier transform use an exponential kernel which is combination of sine and cosine kernel. Mathematically it can be expressed as

$$e^{jwt} = \cos\left(wt\right) + j * \sin\left(wt\right) \tag{4}$$

Similarly the complex wavelet transform is expressed as:

$$d_c\left(j,n\right) = d_r\left(j,n\right) + i * d_i\left(j,n\right) \tag{5}$$

Here d_c is the wavelet coefficient with d_r and d_i are the real and imaginary coefficients. DTCWT utilizes two DWT approach. Original signal is reconstructed by average value of two bands. This helps to make the transform rotation invariant.

ENTROPY FEATURES

Modified Sample Entropy

Entropy is defined as the measure of randomness of the signal. Sample entropy calculates the variation among signal in time domain. Each segment of signal is compared with others and based on threshold; variations are counted to get entropy value. Sample entropy is similar to approximate entropy with exception of not considering the self matching count for entropy features. In modified sample entropy (Xie *et.al* 2008) for more faster and correct calculation instead of taking continuous sample, sample at certain interval is considered for entropy calculation. Algorithm is explained below.

1. Begin- Raw EEG Signal
2. Set the threshold value r and signal segment length m
3. Sample gap k is calculated as the first zero crossing point
4. Form a set of vectors from the entire time series data S, $S = \left\{s_i, s_{i+k}, \ldots\ldots s_{i+mk}\right\}$ where i = 1,2,….N-m+1
5. Maximum distance for each segment is found out. $d\left|s_m^i, s_m^j\right| = \max\left(s_{i+mk} - s_{j+mk}\right)$
6. For segments distance is less than r, count c is increased to one. Average of all count is considered.
7. Repeat the above step for segment length m=m+1
8. $Modified\, sample\, entropy = -\ln\left|\dfrac{count\, c\, for\, length\, m+1}{count\, c\, for\, length\, m}\right|$

Collision and Minimum Entropy

Collision entropy (Bosyk *et.al* 2012) is calculated by the logarithm of square of max normalized wavelet approximate coefficients. The probability of occurrence of one element will be more for less random signal compared to random signal. So based on this concept we have another entropy feature called minimum entropy. Both mathematically represented as:

$$Collison\,Entropy = -sum\left(\log\left(\max\left(p_i\right)^2\right)\right) \quad (6)$$

SELF ORGANIZED MAP

Self organized map (Gabor *et.al* 1996) is a type of neural network algorithm used for dimension reduction and classification. It follows three steps to learn the input pattern called competition, co-operation and weight update. In first step based on the minimum Euclidian distance from input feature vector to the weight vector the winning neuron is selected. This mechanism is called winner takes all mechanism. In second step along with winning neuron the nearest neighbor neurons are also selected for updating. In the third step all weights are updates. In this work kohonen self organizing map technique is used for clustering purpose with three cluster and neighbor points. Mathematical explanation of each step is given below.

Let the signal array be $x = \left[x_1,\ x_2,\ldots,x_m\right]^t$, and the weight vector $w = \left[w_{j1}, w_{j2}, ..w_{jm}\quad\right]^t$

The winning neuron can be found by maximizing $||x-w_j||$. Once the winning neuron is selected next step is to find the neighbor neuron for updating. Gaussian function is selected for such purpose. Mathematically expressed as:

$$h_{j,i} = \exp\left(\frac{-d_{j,i}^{\ 2}}{2\sigma^2}\right) \quad (8)$$

σ is the width of the Gaussian function which decreases with lateral distance.

HIDDEN MARKOV MODEL

In this work HMM (Kolekar *et.al* 2004) (Kolekar *et.al* 2005) is used for classification. HMM model is based on markov chain rule. According to Markov chain rule the probability of future state depends on only present state and not on past states. Mathematically it can be defined as:

$$p\left(X_{n+1} = x | X_1 = x_1, \ldots\ldots X_n = x_n\right) = p\left(X_{n+1} = x | X_n = x_n\right) \quad (9)$$

Here focal and non focal EEG signal are used as states and features extracted from each states as observation. Here two states are used for classification with observation as average modified sample features extracted from each signal. Initial state transition matrix is given in Table 1.

Baum Welch algorithm is used for training purpose. Baum Welch algorithm is also called forward-backward probability calculation both used in training algorithm. Total of 200 iterations are used for

Table 1. State transition model

State	1	2
1	0.6	0.4
2	0.4	0.6

training focal and non focal event HMM model. In testing purpose manual clustering is used to generate symbol sequence which is used to calculate present state of the system. Baum Welch algorithm is explained below.

Step 1: Take arbitrary state transition probability a_{ij} and emission probability b_{jk}. Take any initial probability value pi. Define the sequence for which model has to be trained.

Step 2: The forward probability of the given sequence is calculated using the below formulae.

$$\propto_j(t) = \begin{cases} 0, & t = 0 \, and \, j \neq initial \, state \\ 1, & t = 0 \, and \, j = initial \, state \\ \sum_j [\propto_i (t-1) * a_{ij}] * b_{jkv(t)} \, Otherwise \end{cases} \tag{10}$$

V- Sequence for which model is to be trained, I=row, J=column

Step 3: Backward probability is calculated using the below formulae.

$$\beta_i(t) = \begin{cases} 0, \, if \, w_i(t) \neq w_0 \, and \, t \neq T \\ 1, \, if \, w_i(t) \neq w_0 \, and \, t = T \\ \sum_j \beta_j(t+1) * a_{ij} * b_{jkv(t+1)} \, otherwise \end{cases} \tag{11}$$

Step 4: The probability of being in state s_i at time t, and state s_j at time t+1, given the model (θ) and observation sequence (O) $p(q_t = s_i, q_{t+1} = s_j \mid O, \theta)$ is calculated by –

$$\vartheta_{i,j}(t) = \frac{\propto_i (t-1) * a_{ij} * b_{jkv(t)} * \beta_{i+1}(t)}{p(O \mid \theta)} \tag{12}$$

Step 5: The state transition probability and emission probability are updated.

$$a_{ij} = \frac{\sum_{t=1}^{T} \vartheta_{i,j}\left(t\right)}{\sum_{t=1}^{T} \sum_{k} \vartheta_{i,k}\left(t\right)}$$

$$b_{jk} = \frac{\underset{\vartheta\left(t\right) = \vartheta\left(k\right)}{\sum_{t=1}^{T} \sum_{l} \vartheta_{jl}\left(t\right)}}{\sum_{t=1}^{T} \sum_{l} \vartheta_{j.l}\left(t\right)} \tag{13}$$

Step 6: Repeat step 2 to 5 till convergence.
Step 7: Output obtained is the trained state transition probability and emission probability.

VITERBI ALGORITHM

Hidden markov model output is evaluated based on the present state of the system. Distance of test feature vector with that of training feature vector was evaluated. Index of training feature vector having minimum distance with test feature vector was selected to be the test symbol sequence. The detailed algorithm is explained below.

Viterbi Algorithm:

1. Initialization:

$$\Delta_1\left(i\right) = \pi_i * b_i\left(O_1\right)$$

$$1 \leq i \leq N$$

$$\varphi_1\left(i\right) = 0$$

2. Recursion:

$$\Delta_t\left(j\right) = max_{1 \leq i \leq N}\left[\Delta_{t-1}\left(i\right) * a_{ij}\right] * b_j\left(O_t\right)\ 2 \leq t \leq T$$

3. Termination:

$$P = max_{1 \leq i \leq N}\left[\Delta_t\left(i\right)\right]$$

4. Path (State sequence) is calculated backward

Here b (o) is defined as probability of emission of symbol, a_{ij} is the state transition probability and p is the final probability of symbol sequence in each state.

RESULTS AND DISCUSSION

Focal and Non focal seizure signals available online has two x and y signal component. Features are extracted from individual x, y, and difference x and y EEG signal and classification ability of features are evaluated. Detail results are shown in table below.

As shown in table above, the features extracted are significant. The value shown in bold indicates the highest F value for defined feature. The difference value was selected as it has maximum variation in all features. Signal x-y has highest feature differentiation for focal and non focal EEG signal but for other features result achieved is low. Signal x has significant entropy features but not more than x-y signal. The total AVOVA test is also considered. AVOVA result Table 3 and box plot is shown in Figure 4.

Feature variation between both focal and non focal is very important as the classification accuracy increases with more variation. In this technique, feature clustering is an important step as HMM is trained using the symbol sequence generated after clustering approach. As per the ANOVA test three entropy features are significant in signal classification. Maximum differentiation was achieved by modified sample entropy approach. Table 3 shows ANOVA table for x-y signal entropy features. F value obtained was 17.14 with p value less than 0.05. The f value obtained for average modified sample entropy was higher as compared to total feature F vales. So initial 3 bands modified sample entropy feature was averaged and used for symbol sequence generation. Self organized map is used for clustering. Cluster obtained for both focal and non focal EEG signal is unique for modified sample entropy. Symbol sequence generated was used for training HMM model. The trained model is used for classifying focal and non focal EEG signal. Total of 100 EEG signals were used for training purpose and 100 EEG signal was used for testing purpose. Average accuracy achieved was 80.00%. HMM model obtained for each signal is given in Table 4.

Table 2. ANOVA comparison for different features

EEG Signal	Modified Sample Entropy		Collision Entropy		Minimum Entropy	
	F	P	F	P	F	P
x	22.41	$4.18*10^{-6}$	14.42	$2.0*10^{-4}$	13.56	$3.0*10^{-4}$
y	19.3	$1.8*10^{-5}$	1.71	$1.9*10^{-1}$	1.29	$2.5*10^{-1}$
(x-y)	**35.78**	$1.01*10^{-8}$	**26.96**	$5.12*10^{-7}$	**24.66**	$1.47*10^{-6}$

Table 3. ANOVA Table of x-y signal entropy features

Source	SS	df	MS	F	Prob>F
Groups	57.79	1	57.7857	17.14	$3.9*10^{-5}$
Error	2015.6	598	3.370		
Total	2073.39	599			

Figure 4. ANOVA Box plot for entropy features

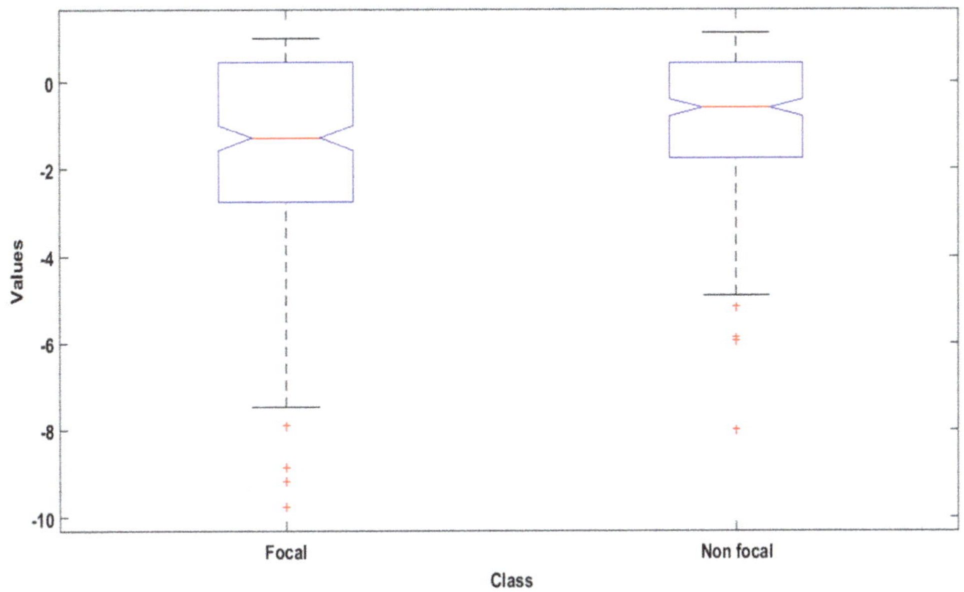

Table 4. State transition matrix for focal and non focal EEG signal

Focal EEG HMM		
State	**Focal**	**Non Focal**
Focal	0.9	0.1
Non Focal	0.1	0.9

As shown in the transition matrix above system has higher probability to remain in same state for HMM model. Accuracy obtained by HMM is also compared with least square support vector machine classifier (LSSVM). Maximum accuracy achieved was 66.00% for modified sample entropy. Radial basis function was used as kernel for feature modification. Accuracy obtained by other features is shown in Table 5. HMM is found to give better result as compared to LSSVM.

As observed in this work single level decomposition does not give good accuracy in classifying seizure and non seizure EEG signal. Entropy features are significant in classification but the accuracy achieved in HMM is low. Focal seizure was classified with 100% accuracy. Similar features can also be used in

Table 5. LSSVM Classification Accuracy Comparison

EEG Signal	Modified Sample Entropy (%)	Collision Entropy (%)	Minimum Entropy (%)
X	66.00	60.00	68.00
Y	67.50	65.50	65.50
X-Y	66.00	63.00	60.50

dual decomposition approach for achieving better accuracy. Dual decomposition can be with wavelet or with empirical mode decomposition. Others spectral features such as spectral skewness, spectral kurtosis, spectral crest factor and spectral entropy features were also extracted from focal and non focal EEG signal but features were not significant indicating there is less spectral variation in both signal. Higuchi fractal dimension (Kolekar et. al, 2000) was also extracted but system achieved less accuracy.

CONCLUSION AND FUTURE SCOPE

The proposed system uses DTCWT to decompose signal to various sub-bands. Good difference in entropy features are observed in higher bands. Beta and alpha bands are found more effective in classification. Entropy features such as minimum, collision and modified sample entropy are evaluated for focal and non focal seizure classification. Highest accuracy of 80.00% is achieved by HMM classifier. In future author will recommend dual decomposition of signal to find efficient features. In future other probabilistic classifier such as Bayesian Belief Network classifier (Kolekar, 2011; Kolekar et al., 2015) will be used to achieve good accuracy.

REFERENCES

Abdullah, M. H., Abdullah, J. M., & Abdullah, M. Z. (2012). Seizure detection by means of hidden Markov model and stationary wavelet transform of electroencephalograph signals. *International Conference on Biomedical and Health Informatics*, 62-65. doi:10.1109/BHI.2012.6211506

Andrzejak, R. G., Schindler, K., & Rummel, C. (2012). Nonrandomness, nonlinear dependence, and nonstationarity of electroencephalographic recordings from epilepsy patients. *Physical Review E, 86*(4).

Baldassano, S., Wulsin, D., Ung, H., Blevins, T., Brown, M. G., Fox, E., & Litt, B. (2016). A novel seizure detection algorithm informed by hidden Markov model event states. *Journal of Neural Engineering, 13*(3).

Bosyk, G. M., Portesi, M., & Plastino, A. (2012). Collision entropy and optimal uncertainty. *Physical Review A, 85*(1).

Chen, D., Wan, S., & Bao, F. S. (2015) Epileptic focus localization using EEG based on discrete wavelet transform through full-level decomposition. *IEEE International Workshop on Machine Learning for Signal Processing*, 1–6. doi:10.1109/MLSP.2015.7324317

Das A B & Bhuiyan M I H (2016), Discrimination and classification of focal and non-focal EEG signals using entropy-based features in the EMD-DWT domain, Biomedical Signal Proceesing and control, 29, 11-21.

Dash, D. P., & Kolekar, M. H. (2017), EEG based Epileptic Seizure Detection using Empirical Mode Decomposition and Hidden Markov Model, Int conf Symhealth, Pune.

Dwivedi, A. R., Bari, H., Nath, S., Bajaj, V., Sharma, D., & Kumar, A. (2016). Analysis of focal and non-focal EEG signals using bivariate empirical mode decomposition. *IEEE Students' Conference on Electrical, Electronics and Computer Science*, 1-3. doi:10.1109/SCEECS.2016.7509318

Gabor, A. J., Leach, R. R., & Dowla, F. U. (1996). Automated seizure detection using a self-organizing neural network. *Electroencephalography and Clinical Neurophysiology, 99*(3), 257-266.

Kolekar, M. H. (2011). Bayesian Belief Network Based Broadcast Sports Video Indexing. *Int. Springer Journal of Multimedia Tools and Applications, 54*, 27–54.

Kolekar, M. H., & Sengupta, S. (2004). Hidden Markov Model Based Structuring of Cricket Video Sequences Using Motion and Color Features. *Indian Conference on Computer Vision, Graphics and Image Processing*, 632-637.

Kolekar, M. H., & Sengupta, S. (2004 Dec), Hidden Markov Model based Video Indexing with Discrete Cosine Transform as a Likelihood Function, *IEEE INDICON Conference*, India.

Kolekar, M. H., & Sengupta, S. (2005). *Semantic Indexing of News Video Sequences: A Multimodal Hierarchical Approach Based on Hidden Markov Model, IEEE Int. Region 10 Conference*. Melbourne, Australia: TENCON.

Kolekar, M. H., & Sengupta, S. (2015). Bayesian Network-Based Customized Highlight Generation for Broadcast Soccer Videos. *IEEE Transactions on Broadcasting, 61*(2), 195–209.

Kolekar, M. H., Talbar, S. N., & Sontakke, T. R. (2000). Texture Segmentation using Fractal Signature. *IETE Journal of Research, India, 46*(5), 319–323.

Kulasuriya, K. H., & Perera, M. (2011) Focal epileptic seizure forecasting in EEG signals using wavelet transform and artificial neural networks. *IEEE International Conference on Control System, Computing and Engineering*, 296–301. doi:10.1109/ICCSCE.2011.6190540

Selesnick, I. W., Baraniuk, R. G., & Kingsbury, N. C. (2005). The dual-tree complex wavelet transforms. *IEEE Signal Processing Magazine, 22*(6), 123-151.

Sharma, R., Pachori, R. B., & Acharya, U. R. (2015). Application of entropy measures on intrinsic mode functions for the automated identification of focal electroencephalogram signals. *Entropy, 17*(2), 669–691. doi:10.3390/e17020669

Sharma, R., Pachori, R. B., & Acharya, U. R. (2015). An integrated index for the identification of focal electroencephalogram signals using discrete wavelet transform and entropy measures. *Entropy, 17*(8), 5218-5240.

Sharma, R., Pachori, R. B., & Gautam, S. (2014, May). Empirical mode decomposition based classification of focal and non-focal EEG signals. *International Conference on Medical Biometrics*, (pp. 135-140). IEEE. doi:10.1109/ICMB.2014.31

Swami, P., Gandhi, T.K., Panigrahi, B.K., Tripathi, M., & Anand, S. (2016). A novel robust diagnostic model to detect seizures in electroencephalography. *Expert Systems With Applications, 56*, 116–130.

Xie, H. B., He, W. X., & Liu, H. (2008). Measuring time series regularity using nonlinear similarity-based sample entropy. *Physics Letters A, 372*(48), 7140-7146.

Chapter 4
Classification and Compression of ECG Signal for Holter Device

Chandan Kumar Jha
Indian Institute of Technology Patna, India

Maheshkumar H. Kolekar
Indian Institute of Technology Patna, India

ABSTRACT

ECG signal processing for holter monitoring of heart patients is still exploratory. Many signal processing techniques have been evolved for classification and compression of ECG signal. Despite an increase in research in this area, many challenges remain in designing an efficient classification and compression algorithm for ECG signal. These challenges include classification accuracy, good compression ratio with acceptable diagnostic quality etc. This chapter addresses a classification and a compression algorithm based on discrete wavelet transform. Classification algorithm uses discrete wavelet transform based feature to classify abnormal heart beat from ECG signal. Support vector machine is used as a classifier to detect abnormal heartbeat. The compression algorithm utilizes discrete wavelet transform and run-length encoding as a compression tool. Proposed classification and compression algorithms can be employed in monitoring of cardiac patients using holter device.

INTRODUCTION

Heart muscles generate tiny electrical impulses which can be recorded by electrodes by placing it on patient's body surface. This recording is called electrocardiogram (ECG) which is a non-invasive clinical tool in the field of cardiology. It is widely used by cardiologists for diagnosis of heart diseases. ECG waveform of a normal cardiac cycle is depicted in Figure 1 which consist P-wave, QRS-complex and T-wave (Chen *et. al*, 2014). Depolarization of atrium produces P-wave. Depolarization of right atrium reflects first half of the P-wave while latter half of the P-wave indicates depolarization of left atrium. Q-wave, R-wave and S- wave are collectively known as QRS-complex.

DOI: 10.4018/978-1-5225-2829-6.ch004

Figure 1. ECG waveform of normal cardiac cycle

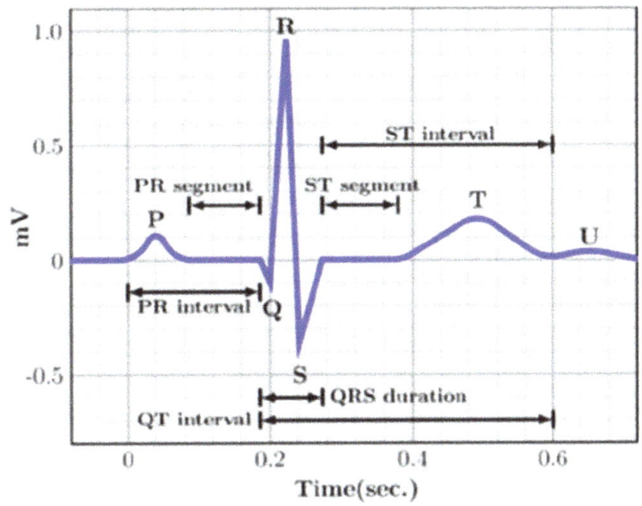

It is generated by left and right ventricular depolarization. Ventricular re-polarization generates T-wave. Cardiologists diagnose heart diseases on the basis of different features of ECG waveform which includes amplitudes of PQRST waves and time intervals between different segments. ECG signal is recorded for several hours in holter monitoring of cardiac patients.

Holter Monitor

In pathological ECG test, ECG is recorded for very short duration. For a cardiac patient, it is possible that abnormal heart rhythm may come and go. In general, cardiologist cannot detect abnormal behavior of heart by observing short duration of pathological ECG record. Therefore long time monitoring of cardiac patient is necessary. Holter monitor provides this facility to cardiologist using which observation of heart function is possible on long-term basis. It also helps the cardiologist to determine medicine is working properly or not on cardiac patients. Holter monitor is a battery operated, small device which is used to record ECG signal for 12 hours to 48 hours continuously during normal daily routine of a cardiac patient. Holter monitoring is also called ambulatory ECG monitoring.

Classification of Heartbeats

Classification of heartbeats plays a major role to detect abnormal heartbeat during monitoring of heart patients. Many heartbeat classification techniques have been developed based on its features. These features include morphological features (De Chazal *et. al*, 2004), segmentation based features (De Chazal *et. al*, 2004) and frequency domain features (Romero *et. al*, 2001, De Chazal *et. al*, 2004). The technique of classification of heartbeats started two decades before using artificial neural network as a classifier (Hu *et. al*, 1992). At present classifier such as support vector machine (SVM) (Osowski *et. al*, 2004), hidden Markov model (HMM) (Coast *et. al*, 1990, Kolekar *et. al* 2004), artificial neural network (Hu *et. al*, 1992, Hu et. al, 1997, Barro *et. al*, 1998), self organizing maps (Lagerholm *et. al*, 2000) are widely used for classification of ECG heartbeats. A classification technique based on discrete wavelet transform and HMM is proposed in (Andreão *et. al*, 2006) using which a premature ventricular contraction (PVC) beat can be classified. In this technique Mexican hat mother wavelet is used for feature extraction of ECG heartbeats. A patient specific classification technique based on discrete wavelet transform (DWT) and artificial neural network (ANN) is proposed in (Ince *et.al*, 2009) which can be used for detection of ventricular ectopic beats (VEBs) and supra-VEBs. For personalized ECG classification, a block based neural network classifier is proposed in (Jiang *et. al,* 2007). To classify different class of heartbeats, a technique based on SVM and particle swarm optimization (PSO) is proposed in (Melgani *et. al*, 2008) which can classify 5 classes of heartbeat. Ye et.al, 2012 proposed a classification algorithm using discrete wavelet transform and SVM. He used morphological features as well as dynamic features (R-R interval) of heart-beats to classify 16 class of ECG signal. Despite an increase in research in classification techniques of ECG heartbeats, good classification accuracy in practical scenario is still a challenge for a classifier.

Compression of ECG Signal

For Holter monitoring of heart patients ECG signal is recorded for 24 hours to 48 hours. Due to this long time of recording, recorded ECG signal occupies large memory space. Compression of ECG signal provides less memory requirement for storage. It also provides less bandwidth requirement in case of transmission of ECG signal in a healthcare system for telemedicine or remote monitoring. Many ECG signal compression techniques have been proposed in literature which uses signal processing approaches including Walsh transform (Kuklinski *et. al*, 1983), Karhunen- Loeve transform (KLT) (Olmos *et. al*, 1996), discrete Fourier transform (Reddy et. al, 1986), discrete cosine transform (Allen et. al 1992, Jha et. al 2017) and discrete wavelet transform (Rajoub *et. al*, 2002, Tai *et. al*, 2005, Lu et. al, 2000, Jha *et. al,* 2016). Compression algorithms developed by employing DCT uses energy compaction property of DCT. Lee (Lee *et. al*, 2008) proposed a real time ECG data compression algorithm based on DCT. He further improves the compression performance in (Lee *et. al*, 2011) using DCT and Huffman encoding. Lee (Lee *et.al*, 1999) proposed a compression method based on cut and align beats (CAB) and 2D-DCT. To apply 2D-DCT, a 2D-array was formed using CAB technique on ECG signal. A compression technique using image coder (JPEG 2000) on 2-D ECG array is proposed in (Bilgin *et. al*, 2003). Since last decade, DWT has been widely used for ECG data compression. DWT preserves the local features of the signal very well. Hence it is useful for ECG signal compression where to preserves the main information of the signal is a vital point. Kim (Kim *et.al*, 2006) proposed a wavelet based low delay ECG compression algorithm for continuous ECG transmission. An ECG compression algorithm based on two dimensional DWT and vector quantization is proposed in (Wang *et. al*, 2008). Mitra (Mitra *et.al*, 2012) proposed an ECG data compression technique for global service of mobile (GSM) based offline Tele-cardiology which was based on downsampling, single side difference generation, encoding and zero sequence compression. This technique is not suitable for prolonged ECG recording. A new ECG signal compression algorithm based on mother wavelet parameterization and best threshold selection is proposed in (Abo-Zahhad *et. al*, 2013). Increased computational complexity is the main drawback of this algorithm. Kumar (Kumar *et.al*, 2013) proposed an ECG data compression algorithm based on a new wavelet called beta wavelet and run length encoding. Despite many compression techniques have been developed in past but good compression ratio with less reconstruction error is still a problem in compression techniques.

In this chapter a classification algorithm based on DWT and SVM has been addressed. An ECG compression algorithm is also presented which employs DWT. These algorithms are implemented with ECG records which are taken from MIT-BIH arrhythmia database (Moody *et. al*, 2001). Organization of this chapter is as follows: section 2 describes the methodology of classification algorithm and experimental results. Section 3 elaborates compression algorithm and experimental results using different records of ECG signals. Section 4 concludes this chapter.

DISCRETE WAVELET TRANSFORM

DWT is used for analysis of the signal in time domain and frequency domain both. It preserves the local features of the signal very well. Hence it is widely used in biomedical signal processing. According to (Kumar *et.al*, 2013), wavelet transform decomposes a signal into many functions by using translation and dilation parameter of mother wavelet $\psi(t)$ which can be defined as

$$\Psi^{p,q}(t) = \frac{1}{\sqrt{p}}\Psi\left(\frac{t-q}{p}\right) \tag{1}$$

where, p and q are dilation and translation parameter respectively which can consists any real values. Using this mother wavelet, continuous wavelet transform of a signal $x(t)$ can be defined as

$$X_W\left(p,\ q\right) = \frac{1}{\sqrt{p}}\int_{-\infty}^{+\infty} x\left(t\right)\ \psi^*\left(\frac{t-q}{p}\right)dt \tag{2}$$

where, asterisk denotes complex conjugate of mother wavelet function. Continuous wavelet transform for discrete values of translation and dilation parameter is called discrete wavelet transform. Discrete values of p and q are chosen as $p = 2^{-m}$ and $q = n.2^{-m}$, where m and n are integer values. Discrete wavelet transform is implemented using filter banks which decomposes the input digital signal $x(n)$. The filter bank uses following two equations at each decomposition level

$$c\left(n\right) = \sum_{i=1}^{2n} x\left(n\right).h\left(2n-i\right) \tag{3}$$

$$d\left(n\right) = \sum_{i=1}^{2n} x\left(n\right).g\left(2n-i\right) \tag{4}$$

where $c(n)$ and $d(n)$ are called approximate and detail coefficients respectively. Approximate and detail coefficients are found after passing the signal from low pass filter $g(n)$ and high pass filter $h(n)$ respectively. Figure 2 depicts the filter bank implementation of DWT for input digital signal $x(n)$.

SUPPORT VECTOR MACHINE

Support vector machine (SVM) (Kampouraki et. al, 2009; Scholkopf et. al, 1997; Kolekar et. al 2015) is a powerful mathematical tool which is widely used in classification applications. This is a machine learning approach which uses a training set of examples belonging to two classes with associated output values. Examples of training set are in the form of attribute vector and SVM finds a hyper plane to separate the examples according to their class.

Linear SVM Classifier

If the training examples are linearly separable, there exists a linear function *f(x)* which can be represented by

$$f\left(x\right) = w^T x + b \quad \ldots \tag{5}$$

where $f\left(x\right) \geq 0 \, for \, y_i = +1$ and $f\left(x\right) \leq 0 \, or \, y_i = -1$.

Vector w and b represents the hyper plane represented by Eq. (2). It separates the two classes linearly.

$$w^T x + b = 0 \tag{6}$$

The linear SVM classifier can be represented by:

$$f\left(x\right) = sign\left(\sum_{i=1}^{l} \alpha_i y_i x x_i + b\right) \tag{7}$$

where, α_i are constraints

$$\alpha_i > 0 \text{ and} \sum_{i=1}^{l} \alpha_i y_i = 0$$

Figure 2. DWT filter bank

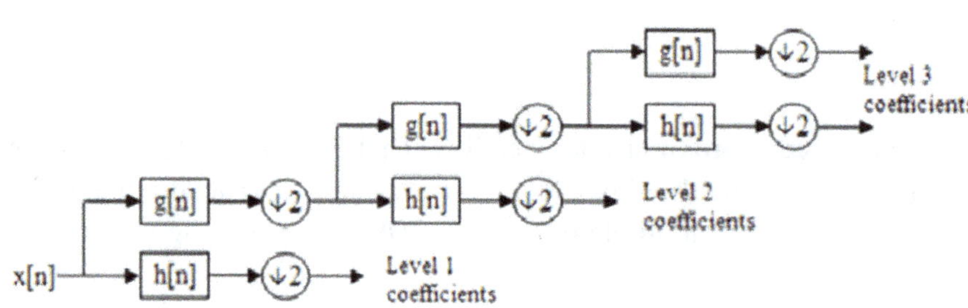

Kernel Based SVM Classifier

Kernel based SVM classifiers are used to separate training examples which involves complex geometry of hyper plane. These classifiers can be defined by

$$f(x) = sign\left(\sum_{i=1}^{l} \alpha_i y_i K(x, x_i) + b\right) \tag{8}$$

where, K (x, x_i) is Kernel function. There are many types of Kernel function such as polynomial, sigmoid, Gaussian radial basis function etc. In the proposed work, Gaussian radial basis function (rbf) is used which decreases monotonically and can be defined as-

$$K(x, x_i) = e^{\left(-\frac{x - x_i^2}{2\sigma^2}\right)}, \quad \sigma > 0 \tag{9}$$

where, x and x_i are two feature vectors and $x - x_i^2$ indicates square of Euclidean distance between them. σ denotes variance.

METHODOLOGY

Abnormal Heartbeat Classification Using DWT and SVM

This chapter elaborates an abnormal heartbeat classification algorithm based on DWT and SVM. Figure 3 depicts the stepwise flow of the algorithm. At first, R-peak is detected from the input ECG signal using Pan-Tompkins algorithm (Pan *et. al*, 1985) and verified with annotations mentioned in MIT-BIH arrhythmia database. After detection of R-peak, 103 samples before the R-peak and 153 samples after the R-peak is selected i.e, total 256 samples are taken for one heartbeat. Total number of R-peaks gives the total number of heartbeats. To extract the features of heartbeats DWT has been used. DWT is performed for each heartbeat up to 4 levels of decomposition with mother wavelet db2 whose shape is most likely to heartbeat. At fourth level of decomposition, approximate coefficients are preserved as a feature of heartbeat and based on this feature classification is performed using SVM (Melgani *et. al*, 2008). The SVM classifier is trained with 650 heartbeats out of which 250 heartbeats are normal and other are abnormal suffered with different heart diseases. The classifier is tested with 1100 heartbeats.

Performance Metrics of Classification Algorithm

Following performance metrics are used for evaluation of classifier results:

1. **Accuracy (Acc)**: Defined as the total number of true events detected by the classifier.

Figure 3. Block diagram for heartbeat classification

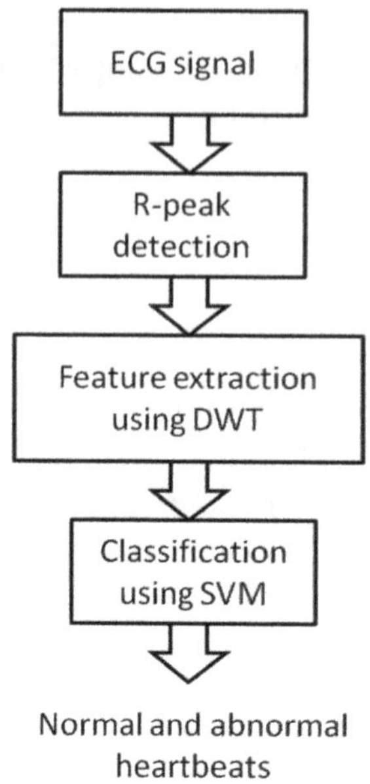

$$Acc = \frac{TP + TN}{P + N} \times 100\% \tag{10}$$

2. **Sensitivity (Se):** Also called true positive rate. It is defined as the ability of the classifier to detect true positive events.

$$Se = \frac{TP}{TP + FN} \times 100\% \tag{11}$$

3. **Specificity (Sc):** Also called true negative rate. It is defined as the ability of the classifier to detect true negative events.

$$Sc = \frac{TN}{TN + FP} \times 100\% \tag{12}$$

4. **Positive Predictive Value or Precision (Ppv):** Defined as the ability of the classifier to predict true positive events.

$$Ppv = \frac{TP}{TP + FP} \times 100\% \tag{13}$$

where P, N, TP, TN, FP and FN indicates total positive, total negative, true positive, true negative, false positive and false negative events respectively.

DWT Based ECG Signal Compression

This chapter includes a compression algorithm based on DWT and run length encoding. Figure 4 describes the methodology of the compression algorithm. Since raw ECG signal is suffered from many high frequency noises, hence to remove this noise Savitzky-Golay filtering has been performed. Savitzky-Golay filter (SGF) smoothes the ECG signal by removing insignificant high frequency component. Order and window dimension of SGF have been selected empirically which are 3 and 19 respectively. Difference between waveforms of raw ECG and filtered ECG using SGF is shown in Figure 5 and Figure 6. After performing SGF, DWT is applied to ECG signal which decomposes the signal to 3 levels with mother wavelet 'bior4.4'. Shape of the mother wavelet 'bior4.4' is similar to QRS-complex of ECG heartbeat which contains vital information of heartbeat. Hence it is chosen for compression algorithm where to remove the redundant information of the signal is main focus. To remove the redundant DWT coefficients, thresholding operation have been performed which produces many zero values. After performing thresholding, rounding operation has been performed. It increases the repetition of data points. To exploit this repetition, run-length encoding is used. It is a lossless encoding technique which gives the compressed form of ECG signal. This compressed ECG signal can be stored or transmitted in case of remote monitoring of heart patients. At the receiver side, inverse process of compression is followed to decompress the ECG signal which includes inverse run-length encoding and inverse DWT.

Performance Metrics of ECG Compression Algorithm

According to [Lee et. al, 2011], performance of the ECG compression algorithm is evaluated using following metrics:

1. **Compression Ratio (CR):**

$$CR = \frac{size\ of\ \ the\ original\ signal}{Size\ of\ the\ reconstructed\ signal} \tag{14}$$

Figure 4. Block diagram of ECG signal compression

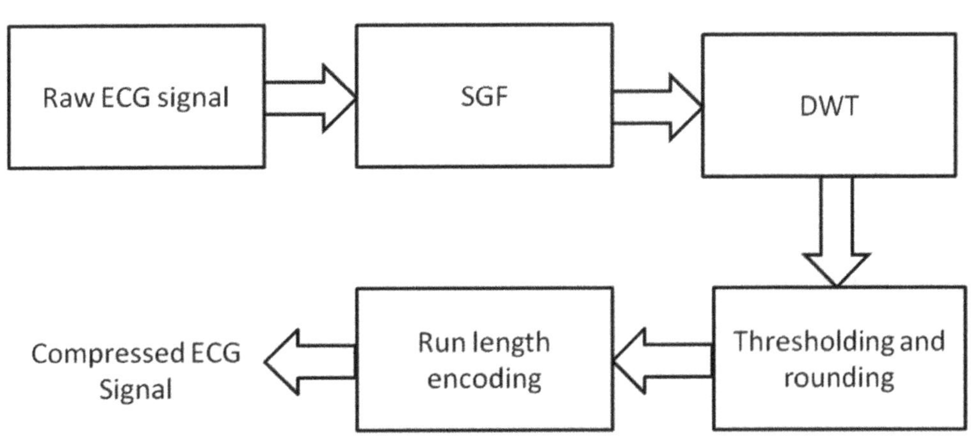

Figure 5. Raw ECG signal

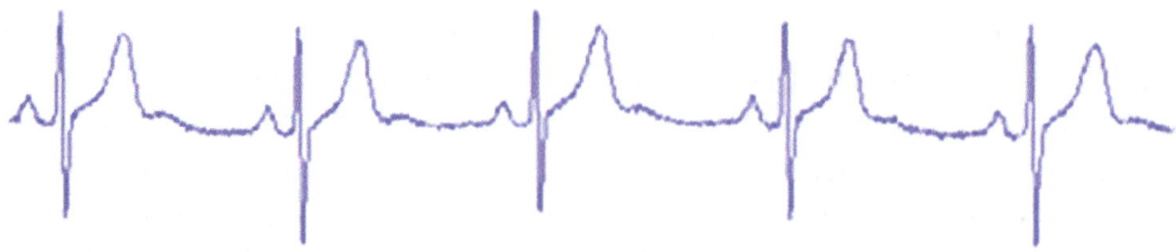

Figure 6. Savitzky-Golay filtered ECG signal

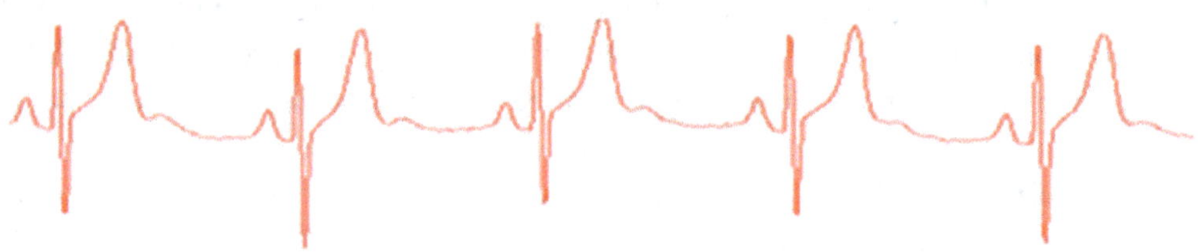

High value of CR indicates good compression performance.

2. **Percent Root Mean Square Difference (PRD):**

$$PRD = \sqrt{\frac{\sum_{0}^{N-1}\left(x\left(n\right)-r\left(n\right)\right)^{2}}{\sum_{0}^{N-1}\left(x\left(n\right)\right)^{2}}} \times 100\ \% \tag{15}$$

Low value of CR indicates less reconstruction error which is desirable.

3. **Quality Score (QS):**

$$QS = \frac{CR}{PRD} \tag{16}$$

It shows the trade-off between CR and PRD. For a good compression algorithm QS value should be high.

4. **Normalized PRD (PRDN):**

$$PRDN = \sqrt{\frac{\sum_{0}^{N-1}\left(x\left(n\right)-r\left(n\right)\right)^{2}}{\sum_{0}^{N-1}\left(x\left(n\right)-\overline{x\left(n\right)}\right)^{2}}} \times 100\% \tag{17}$$

It is another parameter to measure reconstruction error. For a good compression performance value of PRDN should be low.

5. **RMS Error:**

$$RMS = \sqrt{\frac{\sum_{0}^{N-1}\left(x\left(n\right)-r\left(n\right)\right)^{2}}{N-1}} \tag{18}$$

Low RMS error indicates good compression performance.

6. **Signal to Noise Ratio (SNR):**

$$SNR = 10 \times log\left(\frac{\sum_{0}^{N-1}\left(x\left(n\right)-\overline{x\left(n\right)}\right)^{2}}{\sum_{0}^{N-1}\left(x\left(n\right)-r\left(n\right)\right)^{2}}\right) \tag{19}$$

where $x(n)$, $\overline{\boldsymbol{x}\left(\boldsymbol{n}\right)}$ and $r(n)$ are original signal, mean of original signal and reconstructed signal respectively.

RESULTS AND DISCUSSION

The classification algorithm presented in this chapter uses 1100 heartbeats for testing purpose. These heartbeats are taken from ECG signals of MIT-BIH arrhythmia database (Moody *et. al,* 2001). ECG signals with record number 105, 109, 111, 113,115, 118, 122, 124, 202, 207, 208, 210, 212, 214, 217, 221 and 231 have been used for selection of training and testing heartbeats. Testing results of the classification algorithm over 1100 heartbeats is tabulated in Table1. From this table it is clear that the classification algorithm offers good classification results.

The proposed compression algorithm is also tested with 11 records of ECG signal which are taken from MIT-BIH arrhythmia database. Average value for of CR, PRD, QS, PRDN, RMS and SNR offered by the proposed algorithm for 11 records are 8.43, 0.26, 34.30, 5.0, 2.53 and 60.96 respectively. Figures 7-9 show CR, PRD and QS values for 11 records of ECG signal respectively. Figures 10-12 show PRDN, RMS and SNR values for 11 records of ECG signal respectively and it clear that variations these of parameters from average values are very less. This shows the working ability of the presented compression algorithm on different morphology of ECG signal. Original signal and reconstructed signal for record no. 111 are shown in Figure 13 which shows that reconstructed signal is very much similar to original signal. It ensures the medical acceptability of reconstructed signal.

CONCLUSION

This chapter addresses a classification and compression algorithm for ECG signal. The classification algorithm utilizes DWT and SVM Classifier (Abhishek et. al 2014) to detect abnormal heartbeats. For validation of the classification algorithm 1100 heartbeats are tested with this. Accuracy, sensitivity, specificity and positive predictive value offered by the classification algorithm are 97.2%, 94.2%, 98.5% and 96.8% respectively which are in good agreement. The compression algorithm is based on DWT and run length encoding. It offers good compression results over 11 records of ECG signal which are taken from MIT-BIH arrhythmia database. In the future, Bayesian Belief network based classifier (Kolekar et. al.) will be tested to improve classification accuracy of holter monitoring devices.

Table 1. Classification results

Accuracy	Sensitivity	Specificity	Positive Predictive Value
97.2%	94.2%	98.5%	96.8%

Figure 7. CR for 11 records of ECG signal

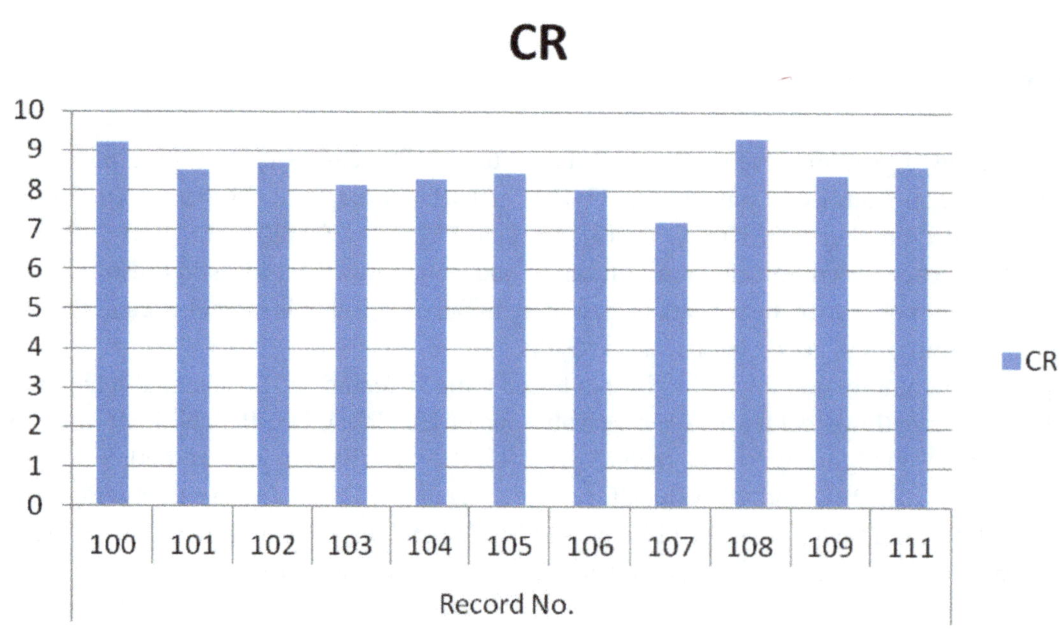

Figure 8. PRD for 11 records of ECG signal

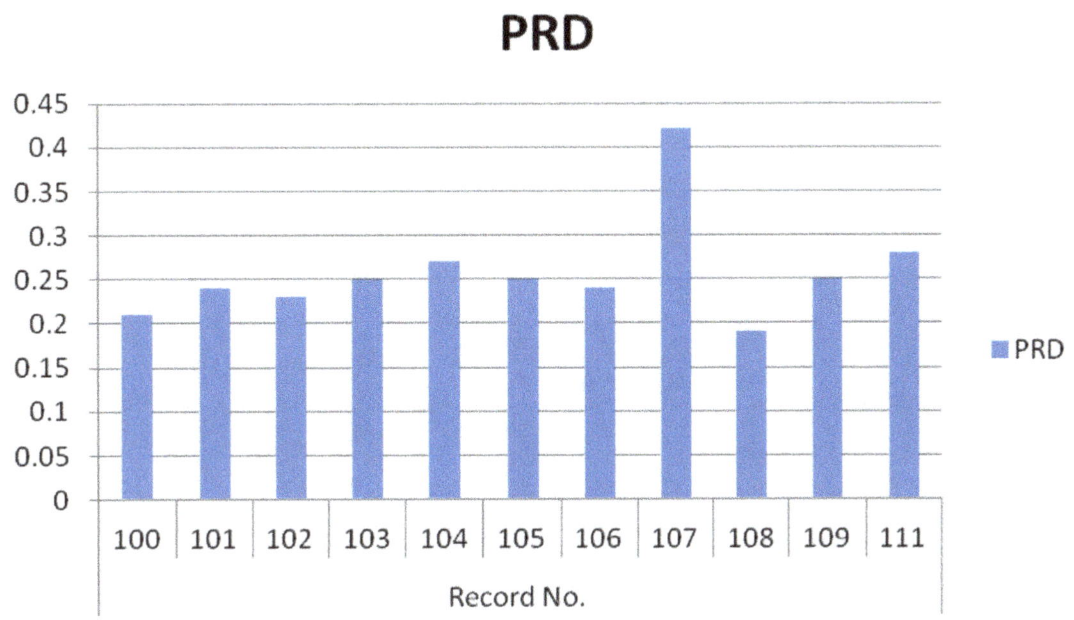

Figure 9. QS for 11 records of ECG signal

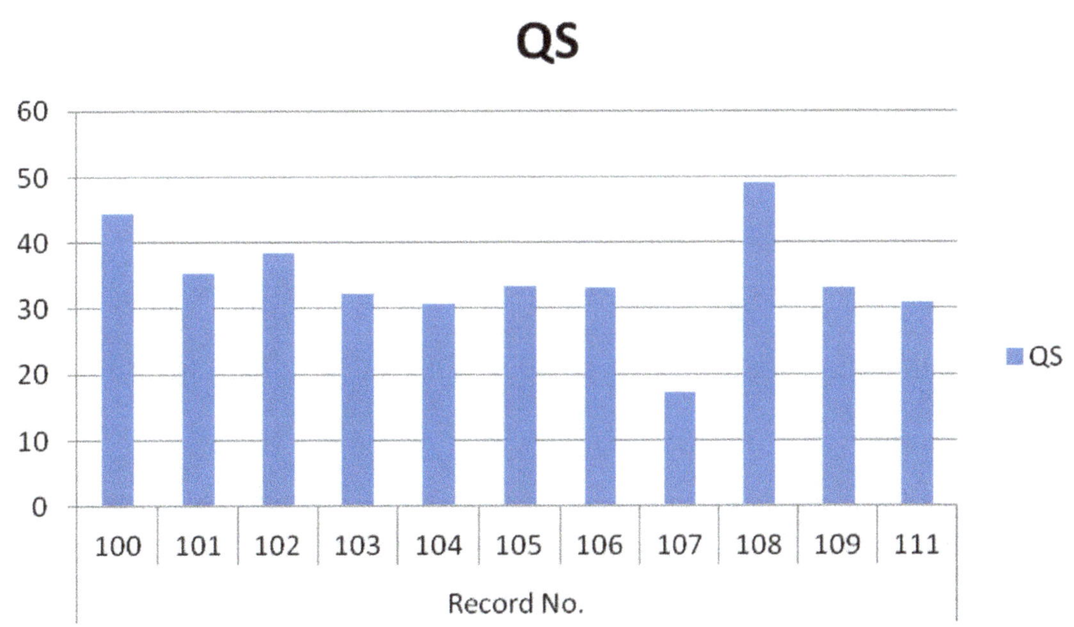

Figure 10. PRDN for 11 records of ECG signal

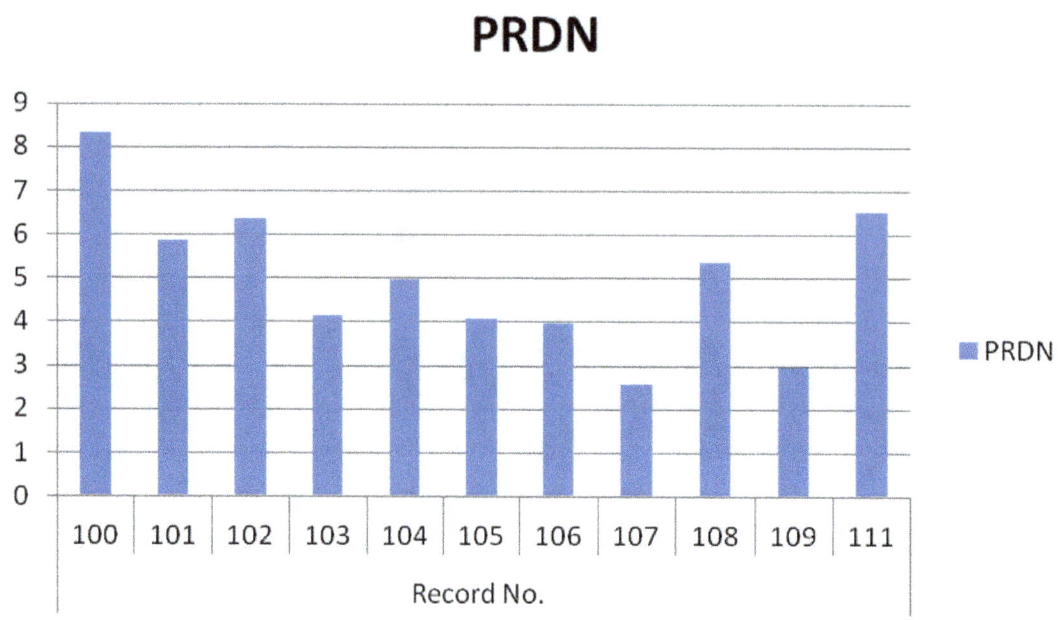

Figure 11. RMS for 11 records of ECG signal

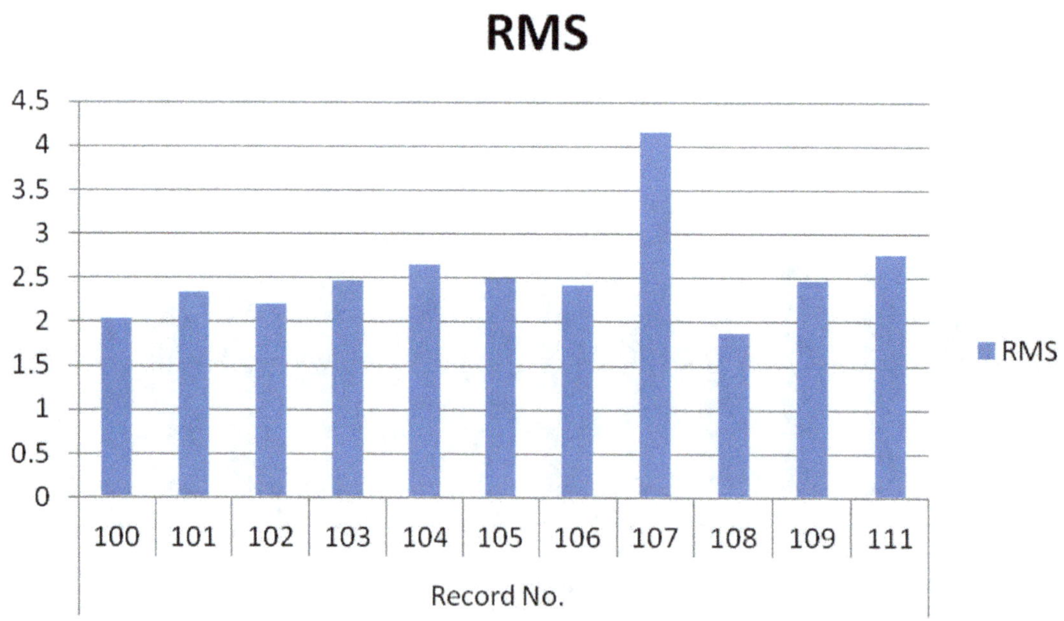

Figure 12. SNR for 11 records of ECG signal

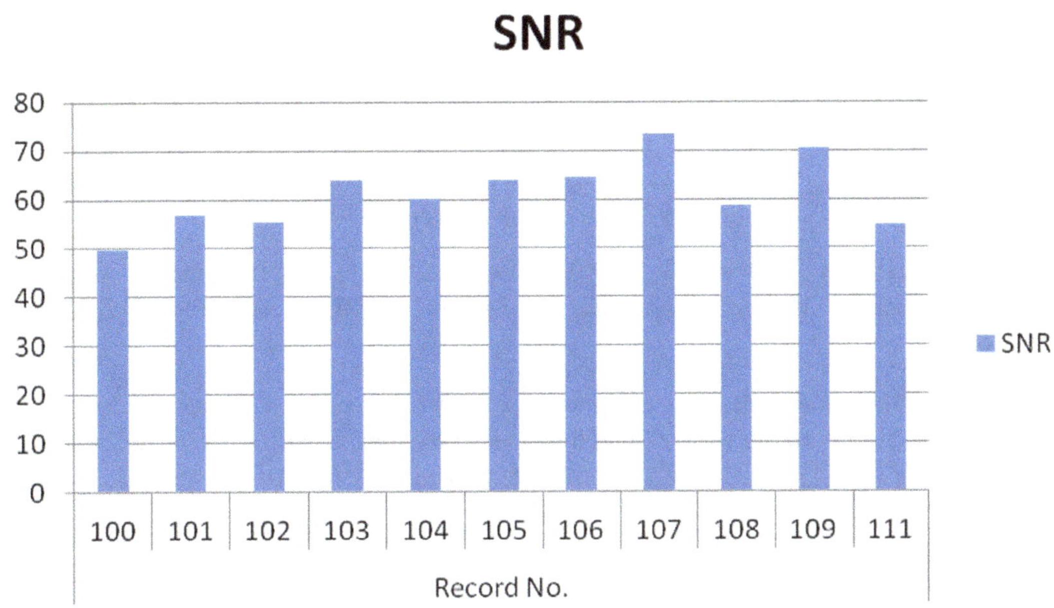

Figure 13. (a) Original signal and (b) reconstructed signal for record no. 111

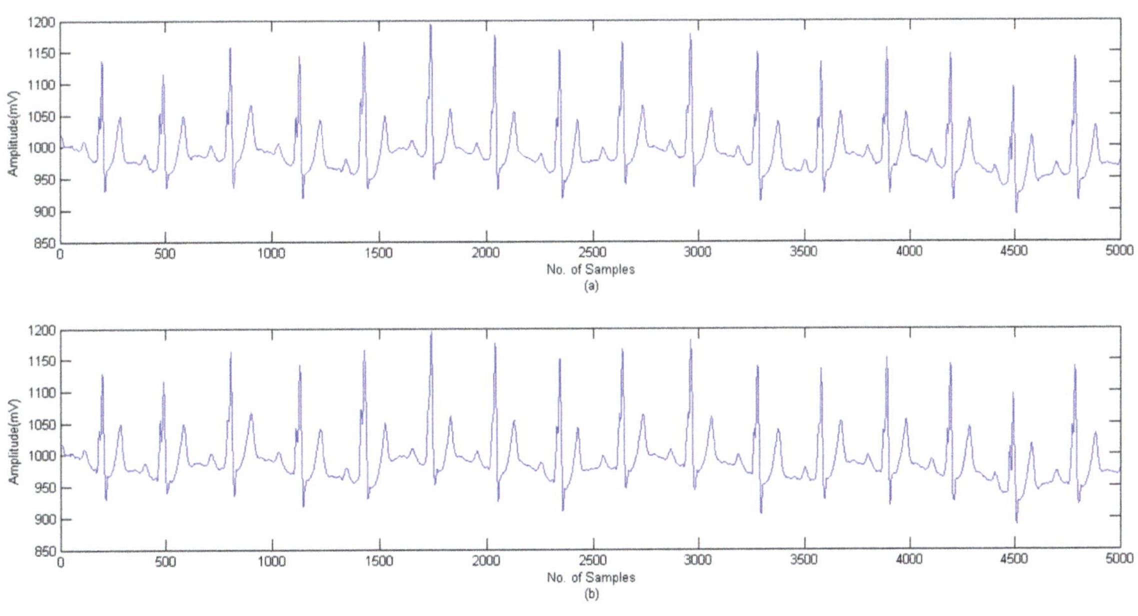

REFERENCES

Abo-Zahhad, M., Al-Ajlouni, A. F., Ahmed, S. M., & Schilling, R. J. (2013). A new algorithm for the compression of ECG signals based on mother wavelet parameterization and best-threshold levels selection. *Digital Signal Processing*, *23*(3), 1002–1011. doi:10.1016/j.dsp.2012.11.005

Allen, V. A., & Belina, J. (1992, October). ECG data compression using the discrete cosine transform (DCT). In Computers in Cardiology 1992, Proceedings of (pp. 687-690). IEEE.

Andreão, R. V., Dorizzi, B., & Boudy, J. (2006). ECG signal analysis through hidden Markov models. *IEEE Transactions on Bio-Medical Engineering*, *53*(8), 1541–1549. doi:10.1109/TBME.2006.877103 PMID:16916088

Barro, S., Fernandez-Delgado, M., Vila-Sobrino, J. A., Regueiro, C. V., & Sanchez, E. (1998). Classifying multichannel ECG patterns with an adaptive neural network. *IEEE Engineering in Medicine and Biology Magazine*, *17*(1), 45–55. doi:10.1109/51.646221 PMID:9460620

Bilgin, A., Marcellin, M. W., & Altbach, M. I. (2003). Compression of electrocardiogram signals using JPEG2000. *IEEE Transactions on Consumer Electronics*, *49*(4), 833–840. doi:10.1109/TCE.2003.1261162

Chen, S. T., Guo, Y. J., Huang, H. N., Kung, W. M., Tseng, K. K., & Tu, S. Y. (2014). Hiding Patients Confidential Datainthe ECG Signal viaa Transform-Domain Quantization Scheme. *Journal of Medical Systems*, *38*(6), 54. doi:10.1007/s10916-014-0054-9 PMID:24832688

Coast, D. A., Stern, R. M., Cano, G. G., & Briller, S. A. (1990). An approach to cardiac arrhythmia analysis using hidden Markov models. *IEEE Transactions on Bio-Medical Engineering*, *37*(9), 826–836. doi:10.1109/10.58593 PMID:2227969

De Chazal, P., O Dwyer, M., & Reilly, R. B. (2004). Automatic classification of heartbeats using ECG morphology and heartbeat interval features. *IEEE Transactions on Bio-Medical Engineering*, *51*(7), 1196–1206. doi:10.1109/TBME.2004.827359 PMID:15248536

De Chazel, P., & Reilly, R. B. (2000). A comparison of the ECG classification performance of different feature sets. *Computers in Cardiology*, *2000*, 327–330.

Hu, Y. H., Palreddy, S., & Tompkins, W. J. (1997). A patient-adaptable ECG beat classifier using a mixture of experts approach. *IEEE Transactions on Bio-Medical Engineering*, *44*(9), 891–900. doi:10.1109/10.623058 PMID:9282481

Hu, Y. H., Tompkins, W. J., Urrusti, J. L., & Afonso, V. X. (1992). Applications of artificial neural networks for ECG signal detection and classification. *Journal of Electrocardiology*, *26*, 66–73. PMID:8189150

Ince, T., Kiranyaz, S., & Gabbouj, M. (2009). A generic and robust system for automated patient-specific classification of ECG signals. *IEEE Transactions on Bio-Medical Engineering*, *56*(5), 1415–1426. doi:10.1109/TBME.2009.2013934 PMID:19203885

Jha, C. K., & Kolekar, M. H. (2016, January). Efficient ECG data compression and transmission algorithm for telemedicine. In *2016 8th International Conference on Communication Systems and Networks (COMSNETS)* (pp. 1-6). IEEE. doi:10.1109/COMSNETS.2016.7439988

Jiang, W., & Kong, S. G. (2007). Block-based neural networks for personalized ECG signal classification. *IEEE Transactions on Neural Networks*, *18*(6), 1750–1761. doi:10.1109/TNN.2007.900239 PMID:18051190

Kampouraki, A., Manis, G., & Nikou, C. (2009). Heartbeat time series classification with support vector machines. *IEEE Transactions on Information Technology in Biomedicine*, *13*(4), 512–518. doi:10.1109/TITB.2008.2003323 PMID:19273030

Kim, B. S., Yoo, S. K., & Lee, M. H. (2006). Wavelet-based low-delay ECG compression algorithm for continuous ECG transmission. *IEEE Transactions on Information Technology in Biomedicine*, *10*(1), 77–83. doi:10.1109/TITB.2005.856854 PMID:16445252

Kolekar, M. H., & Dash, D. P. 2015, November. A nonlinear feature based epileptic seizure detection using least square support vector machine classifier. In TENCON 2015-2015 IEEE Region 10 Conference (pp. 1-6). IEEE.

Kolekar, M. H., & Sengupta, S. 2004, December. Hidden markov model based video indexing with discrete cosine transform as a likelihood function. In India Annual Conference, 2004. Proceedings of the IEEE INDICON 2004. First (pp. 157-159). IEEE.

Kolekar, M. H., & Sengupta, S. (2015). Bayesian Network-Based Customized Highlight Generation for Broadcast Soccer Videos. *IEEE Transactions on Broadcasting*, *61*(2), 195–209.

Kuklinski, W. S. (1983). Fast Walsh transform data-compression algorithm: ECG applications. *Medical & Biological Engineering & Computing*, *21*(4), 465–472. doi:10.1007/BF02442635 PMID:6888014

Kumar, A., & Kolekar, M. H. (2014), Machine Learning Approach for Epileptic Seizure Detection Using Wavelet Analysis of EEG Signals, *Int. Conf. on Medical Imaging, M-health and Emerging Communication Systems.*

Kumar, R., Kumar, A., & Pandey, R. K. (2013). Beta wavelet based ECG signal compression using lossless encoding with modified thresholding. *Computers & Electrical Engineering*, *39*(1), 130–140. doi:10.1016/j.compeleceng.2012.04.008

Lagerholm, M., Peterson, C., Braccini, G., Edenbrandt, L., & Sornmo, L. (2000). Clustering ECG complexes using Hermite functions and self-organizing maps. *IEEE Transactions on Bio-Medical Engineering*, *47*(7), 838–848. doi:10.1109/10.846677 PMID:10916254

Lee, H., & Buckley, K. M. (1999). ECG data compression using cut and align beats approach and 2-D transforms. *IEEE Transactions on Bio-Medical Engineering*, *46*(5), 556–564. doi:10.1109/10.759056 PMID:10230134

Lee, S., Kim, J., & Lee, M. (2011). A real-time ECG data compression and transmission algorithm for an e-health device. *IEEE Transactions on Bio-Medical Engineering*, *58*(9), 2448–2455. doi:10.1109/TBME.2011.2156794 PMID:21606020

Lee, S., & Lee, M. (2008, August). A real-time ECG data compression algorithm for a digital holter system. In *2008 30th Annual International Conference of the IEEE Engineering in Medicine and Biology Society* (pp. 4736-4739). IEEE. doi:10.1109/IEMBS.2008.4650271

Lu, Z., Kim, D. Y., & Pearlman, W. A. (2000). Wavelet compression of ECG signals by the set partitioning in hierarchical trees algorithm. *IEEE Transactions on Bio-Medical Engineering*, *47*(7), 849–856. doi:10.1109/10.846678 PMID:10916255

Melgani, F., & Bazi, Y. (2008). Classification of electrocardiogram signals with support vector machines and particle swarm optimization. *IEEE Transactions on Information Technology in Biomedicine*, *12*(5), 667–677. doi:10.1109/TITB.2008.923147 PMID:18779082

Mitra, M., Bera, J. N., & Gupta, R. (2012). Electrocardiogram compression technique for global system of mobile-based offline telecardiology application for rural clinics in India. *IET Science. Measurement Techniques*, *6*(6), 412–419.

Moody, G. B., & Mark, R. G. (2001). The impact of the MIT-BIH arrhythmia database. *IEEE Engineering in Medicine and Biology Magazine*, *20*(3), 45–50. doi:10.1109/51.932724 PMID:11446209

Olmos, S., Millan, M., Garcia, J., & Laguna, P. (1996, September). ECG data compression with the Karhunen-Loeve transform. In Computers in Cardiology, 1996 (pp. 253-256). IEEE.

Osowski, S., Hoai, L. T., & Markiewicz, T. (2004). Support vector machine-based expert system for reliable heartbeat recognition. *IEEE Transactions on Bio-Medical Engineering*, *51*(4), 582–589. doi:10.1109/TBME.2004.824138 PMID:15072212

Pan, J., & Tompkins, W. J. (1985). A real-time QRS detection algorithm. *IEEE Transactions on Bio-Medical Engineering*, *BME-32*(3), 230–236. doi:10.1109/TBME.1985.325532 PMID:3997178

Rajoub, B. A. (2002). An efficient coding algorithm for the compression of ECG signals using the wavelet transform. *IEEE Transactions on Bio-Medical Engineering*, *49*(4), 355–362. doi:10.1109/10.991163 PMID:11942727

Reddy, B. S., & Murthy, I. S. N. (1986). ECG data compression using Fourier descriptors. *IEEE Transactions on Bio-Medical Engineering*, *BME-33*(4), 428–434. doi:10.1109/TBME.1986.325799 PMID:3957398

Romero, I., & Serrano, L. (2001). ECG frequency domain features extraction: a new characteristic for arrhythmias classification. In *Engineering in Medicine and Biology Society, 2001. Proceedings of the 23rd Annual International Conference of the IEEE* (*Vol. 2*, pp. 2006-2008). IEEE. doi:10.1109/IEMBS.2001.1020624

Scholkopf, B., Sung, K. K., Burges, C. J., Girosi, F., Niyogi, P., Poggio, T., & Vapnik, V. (1997). Comparing support vector machines with Gaussian kernels to radial basis function classifiers. *IEEE Transactions on Signal Processing*, *45*(11), 2758–2765. doi:10.1109/78.650102

Tai, S. C., Sun, C., & Yan, W. C. (2005). A 2-D ECG compression method based on wavelet transform and modified SPIHT. *IEEE Transactions on Bio-Medical Engineering*, *52*(6), 999–1008. doi:10.1109/TBME.2005.846727 PMID:15977730

Wang, X., & Meng, J. (2008). A 2-D ECG compression algorithm based on wavelet transform and vector quantization. *Digital Signal Processing*, *18*(2), 179–188. doi:10.1016/j.dsp.2007.03.003

Section 2
Biomedical Image Processing

This section includes different topics of medical image processing which are MRI denoising, medical image and text report retrieval system, image registration in ultrasound assisted brain surgery, retinal, blood cell, and smear tuberculosis image analysis.

Chapter 5
MRI Denoising for Healthcare

Kalyani Rajiv Joshi
PES Modern College of Engineering, India

Shraddha Dinesh Oza
Army Institute of Technology, India

ABSTRACT

Biomedical Image processing is an important research domain which contributes to the human health care. Magnetic resonance imaging (MRI) is the most popularly used medical imaging modality for its ability to scan any organ or tissue of a body without causing health risk to patient. Because of immense potential of MRI in health care it is very popular with the researchers. Along with improvisations in MR machines, the researchers are exploring different de noising filters, implementation techniques, and platforms so as to improve the MR image quality and enhance accuracy of diagnosis. The chapter discusses all the aspects of MRI - its physics, image attributes, rician noise pdf, different denoising filters and their implementation aspects. The performance analysis being significant in evaluating image quality, different quality measures used are discussed in details. The chapter also briefs about possible opportunities of research in the said domain.

MAGNETIC RESONANCE IMAGING (MRI)

Medical Images are images of internal body organs, tissues and thus an extremely powerful means to diagnose a disease or injury. There exist many imaging modalities such as Computer Tomography, X ray, Ultrasound and Magnetic Resonance Imaging. Out of these, MRI is a technique extensively used and preferred by doctors for its ability to capture every possible body organ and tissue which otherwise could not be seen by any other imaging technique. The main advantage of MRI technique is it can acquire scans in different planes such as coronal, axial, sagittal without altering position of the object. This helps the medical practitioner to diagnose a disease or deformity with more accuracy. MR imaging has clinical advantage as it does not involve any invasion, surgery to patient. The next section elaborates significance of MRI for patient healthcare.

DOI: 10.4018/978-1-5225-2829-6.ch005

MRI and Patient Healthcare

Due to the unique ability to generate images of soft tissues, MR imaging is specially used for scanning body parts such as brain, spine, and joints. Neurosurgeons use this technique to identify swelling or bleeding in patient's brain. MRI of head can detect brain tumors as well as brain aneurysms, strokes, etc. The MR image can identify abnormality of tissue which may occur due to multiple sclerosis. Thus, the disease can be treated in its early stages and help restore patient's health. The orthopedic doctors use MR scans to analyse proper functioning of spinal cord and knee joints. The MR scans show important information about soft tissues, bones, glands and organs inside abdomen. The MR scans also help to inspect structure of heart, aorta or any other defects/tears that are present. MRI has a unique advantage of being painless and does not use any form of radiation.

There are no known dangers to MRI scan itself. The procedure can be repeated without problems. MR scans are not performed on pregnant woman for the risk to fetus. Patients with artificial valves in heart, metallic ear implants, bullet fragments, insulin pumps cannot undergo MRI procedure.

The next sections discuss different aspects of MRI such as its physics, the evolution of MRI systems, technical specifications of MR image and noise in MR image (Catherine W. 2008; E. Mohammed et al 2012; H.Yoshioka, H. Gudbjartsson et al 2008; K. Ineiewski,2009; IMAIOS: Medical websites and e-learning for healthcare professionals www.imaios.com/en, Xiaoping Hu, 2004).

Physics of MRI

MRI technique is based on the operating principle of nuclear magnetic resonance. The human body mainly consists of hydrogen atoms in the form of water. The proton in the hydrogen atom spins at a fast rate and produces a small magnetic field. The spinning proton when placed near a large magnetic field aligns itself with the same. This principle forms basis of MRI scanner.

The MRI scanner is a tube which is surrounded by a circular large magnet. The patient to be scanned is placed on a bed which is inserted inside this circular magnet (Figure 1). This causes the hydrogen atoms wihin the body to spin. The magnetic vector of spinning protons is split in two components –longitudinal or Z component and transverse component which lies in the XY plane. These two components are orthogonal to each other. The atoms while spinning get aligned either in parallel or anti parallel to the large external magnetic field. To these aligned hydrogen atoms, RF signal is applied which makes them tilt from their position as shown in Figure 2.

On removal of RF pulse sequence three events occur:

1. The RF signal is retransmitted by hydrogen atoms as they return to their initial state from state of excitation. This is NMR signal which is proportional to proton density.
2. The spinning hydrogen atoms return to the initial orientation i.e. parallel or antiparallel to the external magnetic field. The time required for 63.2% of magnetization to align back to the external magnetic field is known as relaxation time constant T1. This is also called Spin-lattice relaxation or Longitudinal relaxation. (Figure 3)
3. The in phase, spinning excited protons while returning to initial state dephase resulting in signal decay (Figure 4). This is also known as transverse or spin-spin relaxation time denoted as T2 and is the time when signal decays to 36.8% of its original value.

Figure 1. The MRI operating principle

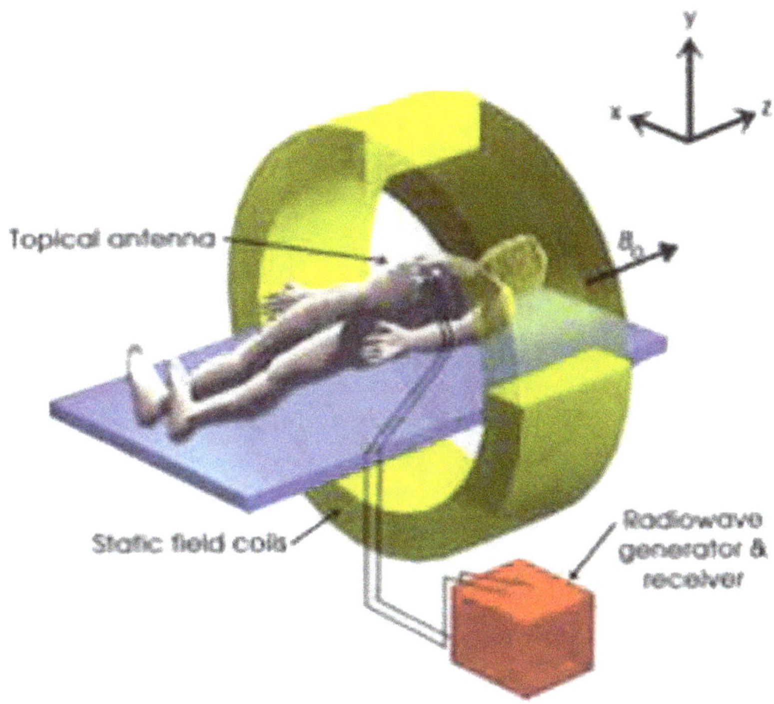

Figure 2.
a. Net magnetization vector is parallel to external magnetic field B0 (before application of RF pulse)
b. The net magnetization vector tilts away from Z axis.
c. Effect of 90⁰ RF pulse
d. M0: longitudinal component along Z axis, Mxy: transverse component in XY plane

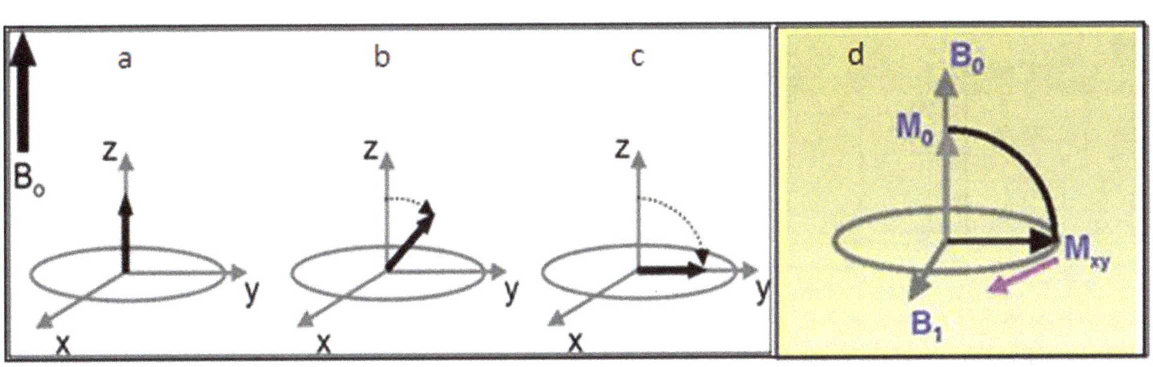

The signal density of MR image is governed by parameters:

1. Proton Density
2. T1 relaxation time
3. T2 relaxation time

Figure 3. T1 Recovery curve

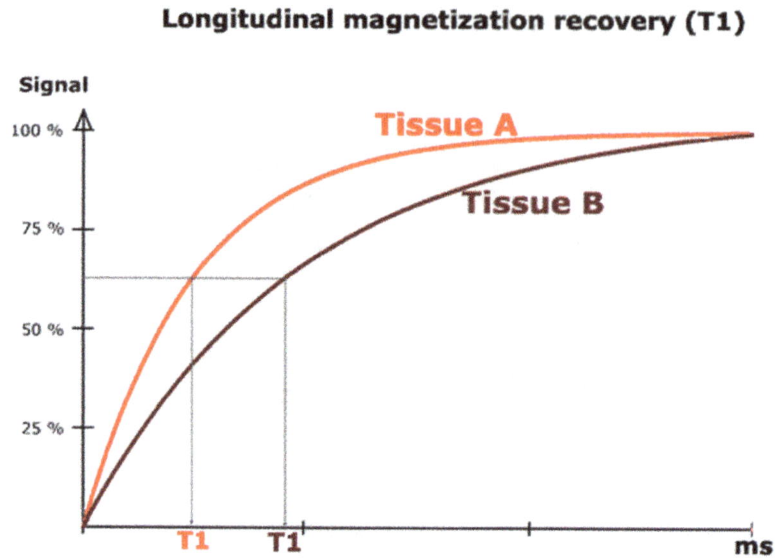

Figure 4. T2 Decay curve

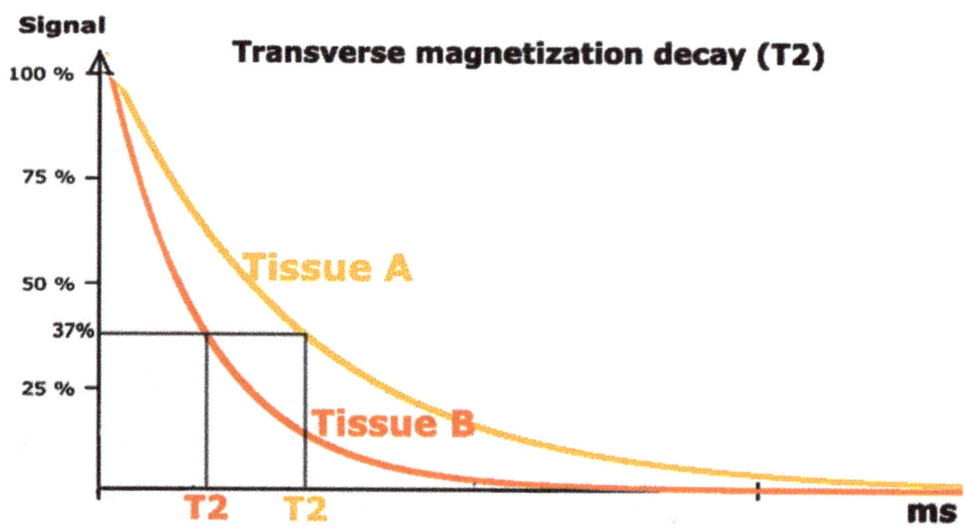

Value of T1 and T2 time constants are unique to every tissue and thus are instrumental in generating MR images of almost all the body tissues.

The generated MR scan depends on number of RF pulses, strength of the RF pulse and timing between consecutive pulses. Repetition time TR and Echo time TE are the two important pulse sequence parameters which affect quality and type of MR image. The first parameter TR is the time period between two consecutive 90 degree RF pulses while the second parameter TE is the time which is lapsed between application of RF pulse and receiving of MR signal. The MR image contrast can be controlled by controlling these two parameters. Most commonly used pulses sequences are T1 weighted (characterized by short TR and TE time intervals) and T2 weighted (characterized by long TR and TE time interval).

During TR interval, tissues with short T1 are able to regain back their original longitudinal magnetization and thus appear bright. The rate at which longitudinal magnetization grows (T1) back is different for protons associated with different tissues and is the main source of contrast in T1-weighted images. For example, white matter has very short T1 time and relaxes rapidly contributing to lighter pixels in image while cerebrospinal fluid CSF has long T1 and contributes to darker pixels in image.

In case of T2 weighted image, echo time is kept long. Thus tissues with short T2 loose most of the signal and appear dark in the final image while CSF with long T2 appears brighter in T2 weighted image. (Figure 5, http://www.svuhradiology.ie/diagnostic-imaging/mri/)

The quality of MR image is attributed with spatial resolution, image contrast, signal to noise ratio and artifacts. The image voxel volume is defined by matrix size, field of view and slice thickness.

MRI System: Past, Present

It took almost 100 years for MRI scanner to become a reality since the invention of rotating magnetic field by Nikol Tesla. In 1977, Raymond Damadian build the first MRI scanner by hand and generated successfully MRI scan of a healthy human body. MRI scan of a human body diseased with cancer was achieved only the year next i.e.1978. Peter Mansfield developed echo-planar technique, which could produce the MR images in seconds. In the year 2000, Cardiac MRI, MRI of whole body, fetal image scanning, and functional MRI were further developed and are being used in many radiology centers.

An MRI system consists of a large magnet to generate magnetic field. Shim coils are used to make the magnetic field homogeneous. The system includes Radio frequency coil to transmit RF pulses into the body part to be scanned. A receiver coil is used to detect the returning RF signal. The gradient coils provide the spatial localization of the signals. A computer based system with dedicated hardware and software is used to reconstruct the RF signals into MR image. (Figure 6)

Figure 5.
a: axial T1 weighted image of brain slice(short TR, TE, bright)
b: axial T2 weighted image of brain slice (long TR, TE, dark)

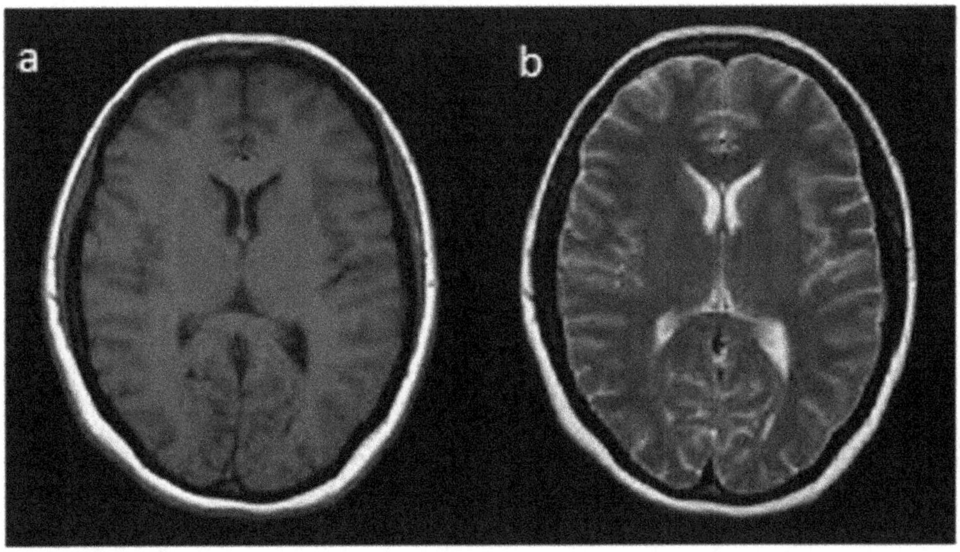

Figure 6. MRI system components

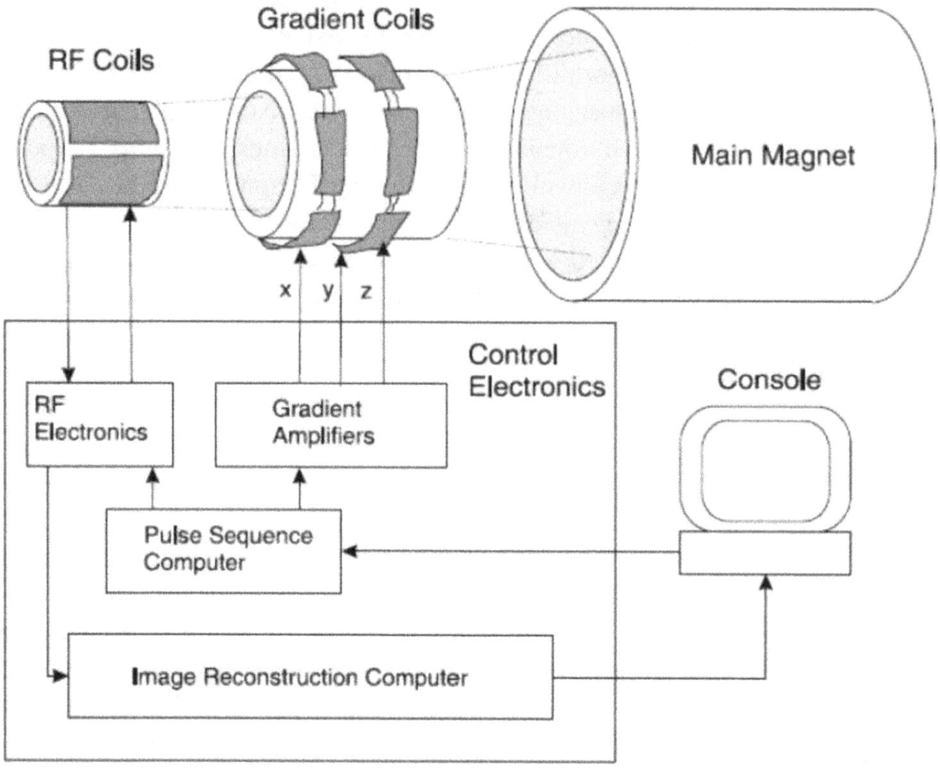

The legacy MRI systems have been tremendously improvised in the last 10 years. In November 2004, the Siemens Medical Solutions (SMS) launched a 1.5T tunnel magnet with very large bore of 70 cm diameter. For examination of inpatient who have several devices attached or implanted such as catheters, monitoring sensors, IV lines, or equipment of anesthesia, MRI systems with wide bore were found to be extremely useful. In conditions when the patients are non-cooperative or unconscious, large bore magnet systems efficiently provide ease of close monitoring.

The design of RF subsystem is under an evolution process. Their design, and the way they are operated is under major changes. The RF or MRI receiver coil in this system is an RF resonator (or an antenna) known as "phased array" (PA). SMS broke traditional phased array RF systems and introduced Magnetom Avanto in December 2003, which is based on the concept of the *Total Imaging Matrix* (TIM). As against their original implementation, the new TIM systems were improvised to allow group of multiple coils, plugged into respective receiver channels, at the same time. This was a breakthrough as it provided flexibility to the user for combining several elements to plug in the system as per requirement of the imaging and then to build the coil.

In the old MRI systems, the analog interface between RF coils and the bank of analog to digital converters was long in length due to which added noisy to the MR signal. In later versions of MRI systems, this distance was reduced so as to improve SNR. The ADC circuitry is located within the magnet enclosure itself in majority of wide bore systems which is most advantageous.

Parallel MR Imaging (pMRI) is state of art technology (Nathan et al, 2015) in which MR images are acquired and reconstructed with a parallel mechanism. Thus, the images produced are much more in number as compared to the conventional MR system. With decrease in the total examination time, these systems provide comfort and ease to patient. Presently, researchers are taking efforts to accelerate acquisition time of 3D images and to increase number of receiver channels for better speed up.

MRI technology is continuously evolving and is introducing new methods of scanning to make the diagnostic process more accurate and simpler. The state of art MRI systems are designed to produce better throughput and scans of better image quality.

Specifications of MR Image

The MRI machine has the capability to generate scan of every body part in mainly three planes: a side view (sagittal), a front view (coronal), and bottom-up view (axial). MR scan is a collection of sequential multi-slice series of images taken typically at intervals of 3-5 mm with scanning direction of left to right. The scanning technique makes it possible to capture even minutest detail of the body part.

The generated MR image is composed of pixels whose intensity values represent the content of volume elements or *voxels.* A voxel is a smallest picture unit point or a pixel in three dimensional space defined by X, Y and Z dimension. The three dimensions indicate position of the voxel, color of the voxel and its density in the 3D image space.

The quality of image is affected by Field of View and Slice thickness. Field Of View (FOV) is size of the area that the matrix of phase (y gradient) and frequency encoding (x gradient) cover. Resolution of MR image is determined by the number of pixels in a specified FOV. Decreasing FOV increases spatial resolution. The higher the image resolution, the better the small pathologies which can be diagnosed. Size of each pixel in the image can be calculated by the formula – FOV/matrix size. Say for e.g. for FOV 320, the pixel size is 160X160==> 320/160=2mm. 2D MR image has two resolution parameters – basic and phase. Basic resolution decides size of image matrix. Phase resolution is the number of pixels in the phase direction. Phase resolution when decreased increases pixel size in one direction i.e. a square pixel becomes rectangular. Basic resolution is inversely proportional to size of pixel. Voxel volume is determined by the matrix size, FOV and slice thickness.

Noise in MRI: Rician Noise Model

Random variation of brightness or color content in an image is defined as noise. It is an electronic noise which is introduced because of different electronic devices, sensors used for capturing image. The noise can be broadly classified as being additive or multiplicative. There exist different noise models under these two categories wherein Gaussian, Poisson noise distributions are examples of additive noise model while Speckle, Rayleigh follow multiplicative noise model.

In case of MRI, the process of capturing MR signal introduces signal dependent noise in the image which identifies with two different noise models viz Gaussian (additive) and Rayleigh (Multiplicative). This noise was modeled as Rician distributed by Hákon Gudbjartsson and Samuel Patz. The Rician distribution for an image with magnitude M is represented as (H. Gudbjartsson et al, 2008)

$$pM\left(M\right)=\left(\frac{M}{\sigma 2}\right)e^{\frac{-\left(M^2+A^2\right)}{\left(2\sigma 2\right)}}I0\left(\frac{AM}{\sigma 2}\right) \qquad (1)$$

Here A is the original signal level, σ is the standard deviation of Gaussian noise and I0 is the modified zeroeth order Bessel function of the first kind. It is shown in Figure 7.

The probability density function of rician noise follows Gaussian distribution for SNR > 2 and approximates Rayleigh curve for low SNR < 2. Noise being signal dependent is extremely critical to remove. Special denoising techniques need to be used to improve image quality of MRI and to make the process of diagnosis more accurate.

For long, researchers are working on different denoising algorithms so as to effectively remove rician noise from MR image. The challenge is to retain tissue structures and edges in the image during noise removal process, as they define accuracy of diagnosis. The next section gives details of denoising filters which have been proved to be effective for rician noise model.

Figure 7. Rician distribution of Magnitude Vs Signal to noise ratio A/ σ
(H. Gudbjartsson et al, 2008)

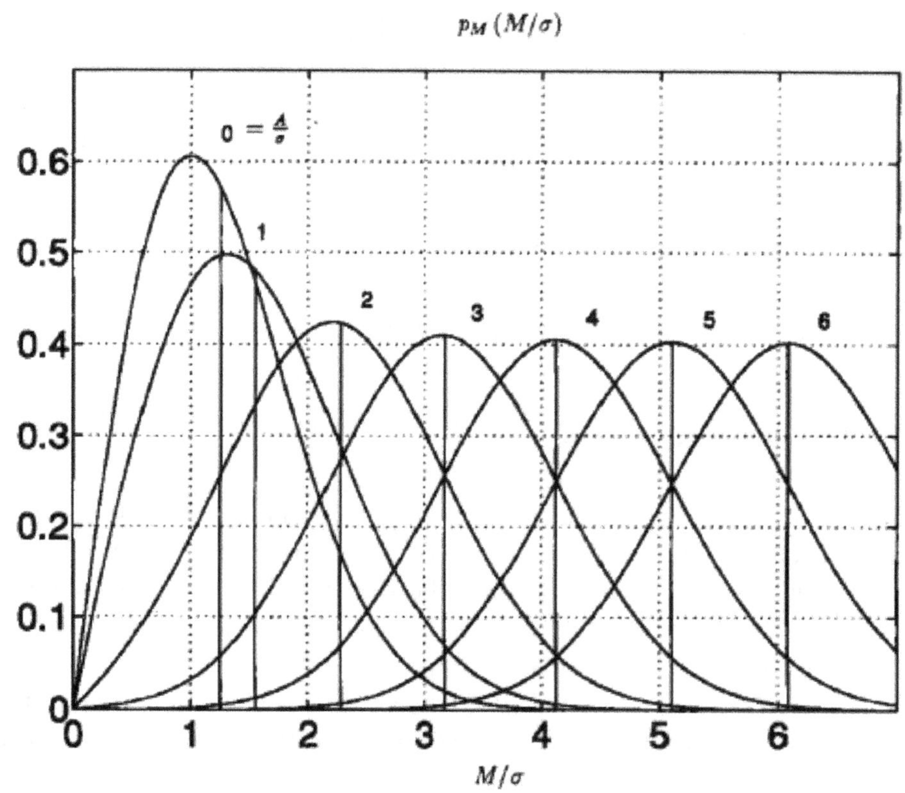

DENOISING FILTERS

Quality of MR image cannot be compromised as it may affect diagnosis of a disease and in turn patient healthcare. The noise in MR image can be reduced either during its acquisition process or by applying a denoising filter post acquisition. Implementing noise reduction methods during MR acquisition time would prolong the acquisition process itself thereby compromising patients comfort. Also, reduction in image acquisition time may lead to spatially varying image noise in the MR image. Thus, post acquisition filtering approach is generally preferred.

The main purpose of denoising filter is to remove rician noise from MR image in the post acquisition phase and alongside most importantly, to retain the original features and tissue structures in the original image. Selection of proper filter for efficient noise removal is extremely important, as this would improve accuracy of medical diagnosis. The following section discusses different filters proposed by researchers specially for MR image denoising.

Filters Used for MR Denoising

The denoising filters can broadly be classified on basis of their implementation domain or the functional approach. A third category of filters are the ones which are implemented with a statistical approach. The classification is as shown in Figure 8.

Gaussian Filter

Gaussian filter is a linear filter which uses a Gaussian or bell shaped kernel for convolving noisy MR image. The 2D Gaussian kernel is circularly symmetric and is given by

$$GF\left(If\right)=\frac{1}{2\pi\sigma^2}e^{\frac{-\left(m^2+n^2\right)}{2\sigma^2}} \tag{2}$$

Here, σ represents standard deviation in the image I_f with zero mean. McVeigh et al. (1985) discussed a spatial filter to reduce Gaussian noise in MR images. But this technique could not handle Rayleigh noise present in MR image with low SNR. Also, this filter has a disadvantage of blurring edges. With Gaussian filter there exists a compromise between de noising and loss of soft tissue structures.

Bilateral Filter

Bilateral Filter was initially presented as nonlinear neighborhood form of Gaussian filter (Aurich & Weule, 1995) which was later rediscovered as "Bilateral" (Tomasi & Manduchi,1998). Its biggest advantage is it removes noise alongside retaining sharp edges in the image. The filter can be looked at as a combination of domain Gaussian $G\sigma s$ and range Gaussian $G\sigma r$ filter and is given by the equation

Figure 8. Classification of MRI Denoising Filters

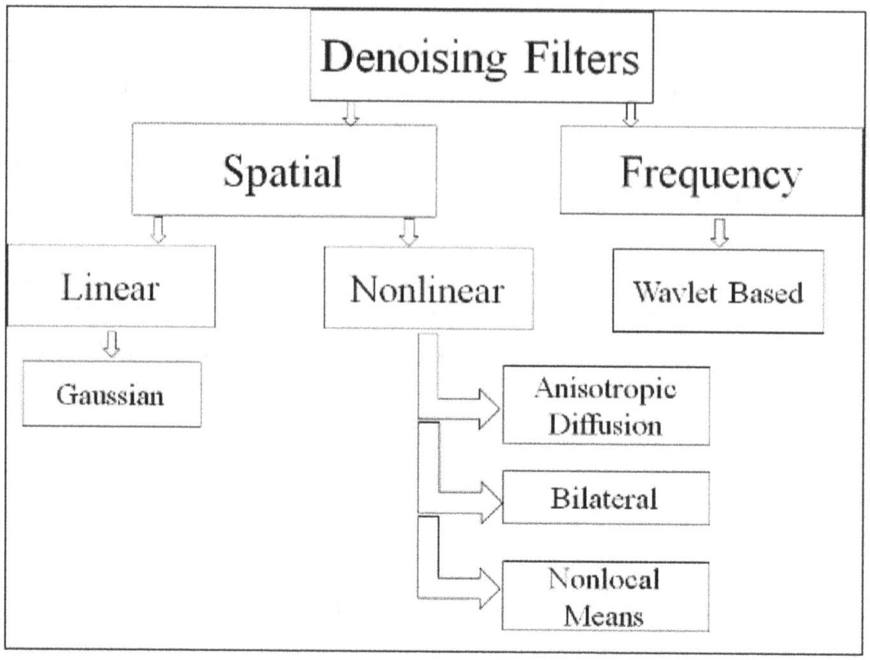

$$BF\left[I_f\right] = \frac{1}{Wm} \sum_{n \in S} G\sigma s\left(m - n\right) \, G\sigma r\left(\left|Im - In\right|\right) \, In \tag{3}$$

Here, *In* is the noisy image and Wm is the normalization factor. The noisy pixel 'm' in the image is replaced by weighted average of all the pixels in the search window s. The weighted average takes into account gaussian as well as range weight of pixel. Maximum range weight of unity is assigned to most similar pixels and it reduces as the difference increases. Similarly the domain weight assigned is minimum for the most distant pixel in the search window. Definition of search window size value is a compromise between accuracy and computation time over head. The filter performance is controlled by mainly value of σ_r and σ_s i.e. standard deviation in range and spatial domain respectively. With increase in σ_r the filter distribution moves closer to being Gaussian Blur while increasing σ_d even the larger features in the image smooth out.

Bilateral has grown popular over the years with researchers in different domains such as gaming, photography, computer vision, and medical imaging (E. Eisemann & F. Durand, 2002; S. Paris et al 2008). M Elad et al (2002) has discussed different techniques to enhance filter performance of bilateral filter. It was Wong et al (2004) who improvised the filter to preserve structures in biomedical images. Walker et al. (2006) and Xie et al. (2008)applied bilateral filter for MR image for better denoising results while Hamarneh and Hradsky (2007) applied the filter to denoise diffusion tensor MRI. Wong et al. (2004) proposed the trilateral filter for reduction of noise in medical images which works along similar lines to bilateral filtering. R. Riji et al displayed iterative feature of bilateral filter to nullify Rician noise from MR images (2015). In terms of PSNR and MSSIM quality measure, the results show that iterative bilateral filter performs better than UNLM and NLM filter. S. Oza & K R Joshi (2017) have demonstrated with experimentation on T2 weighted brain slice MR image that Bilateral filter outperforms NLM and Linear filter in terms of PSNR as well as SSIM.

Non Local Means Filter

The non-local means algorithm is based on the assumption that every image contains lot of redundant or self similar information. The filter uses the basis of self similarity to remove noise in the image. It was Efros and Leung (1999) who presented their work on texture synthesis using the concept of self-similarity. In 2005, Buades et al. first introduced Non Local Means Filter which was an extension of Yaroslavasky Filter. For a noisy image I_n, NLM filter looks for a pixel with similar neighborhood in the whole image. It replaces each pixel m by computing weighted average of all the pixels in the image with similar neighborhood. The weight w(m,n) is measure of the similarity between the pixel neighborhoods Nm and Nn. The filter is given by the equation -

$$NLM\left[I_f\right]=\sum w\left(m,n\right)In \tag{4}$$

For very large image such as a medical image, the huge search area may lead to huge computation and time overhead. The computation area can be restricted to a search window S which is a subset of the whole image. The similarity w(m,n) is then calculated for the search window as

$$w\left(m,n\right)=\frac{1}{Zp}e^{\frac{d(m,n)}{h^2}} \tag{5}$$

Zp is the normalizing constant, h is the exponential decay control parameter, d is a Gaussian weighted Euclidian distance of all the pixels of each neighborhood.

Performance of NLM filter is controlled by three parameters - the exponential decay parameter 'h', the radius 'r' of the neighborhood and the search window size S. A very high value of 'h' may blur the image while too low a value may not be able to remove all the noise. If the neighborhood size for a pixel is set too high, possibility of finding a similar neighborhood reduces. With a very small sized neighborhoods the disadvantage is too many similar neighborhoods may be identified which would reduce accuracy of denoising. For better denoising performance, r may be set to 3 or 4 pixels which further would define neighborhood matrix size as 7X7 or 9X9 respectively. The search window size S which is centered around the pixel to be replaced will define the computation overhead. For search window size of 15X15, the computations required to calculate weighted average will be 15^2 as compared to that of N^2 for an image with size NXN. (Manjon et al, 2008).

For its ability to retain edges in the image, it has been used for MR image denoising. To remove rician noise especially in the multispectral MRI, Manjon et al. (2007) proposed an improvised form of the original NLM algorithm. To improve SNR, Liu et al. (2006) proposed weight computation based on Gaussian filtered image. In the proposed work, the image is first denoised using NLM filter. To this preprocessed image, unbiased correction is applied to remove the bias deviation if any. The results confirm the filter performance being better than the original NLM as well as unbiased NLM filter. To denoise diffusion tensor MRI, Wiest-Daessle et al. (2007) modified the original NLM algorithm for better performance than UNLM filter. To denoise MR images with spatially varying noise levels, an adaptive NLM filter was proposed by Manjon et al. (2010). In this method, the denoising index is computed by estimating noise in local neighborhood.

In case of 3D MR data, computational complexity of NLM algorithm increases there by discouraging its use. To overcome this problem, Coupe et al. (2006) proposed an optimized and parallelized (multi-threading) implementation of the NLM filter. This filter considerably decreases the computational time up to the factor of 50.

Anisotropic Diffusion Filter

Anistropic Diffusion filter (ADF) is a multi-scale image smoothing iterative technique based on process of diffusion. The ADF was proposed by Perona and Malik (1990) as a solution to overcome the unwanted blurring effect produced by linear filtering. The filter applies a process, non-homogeneous in nature, which reduces the diffusivity at edges or contours in the image. ADF has become a powerful technique in denoising as it respects the boundaries and edges in an image to be denoised. The ADF process is given by

$$\frac{\partial}{\partial m} I\left(m,n,t\right) = \mathrm{div}\left(\left(c\left|\nabla\ \mathrm{I}\left(m,\mathrm{n},\mathrm{t}\right)\right|\right)\left(\bar{m},t\right)\nabla \mathrm{I}\left(m,n,t\right)\right) \tag{6}$$

Here, defines the MR image obtained after diffusion time t while is called the *diffusion function* or edge stopping function. It decreases monotonically with the image gradient magnitude:

The behavior of the filter and the extent of diffusion are governed by the gradient threshold parameter and the edge stopping parameter. Overestimating one of the parameters may lead to an over blurred image while under estimating them may not remove all the noise from the image. The values need to be determined for every iteration of the diffusion process for optimum filter performance.

The anisotropic diffusion filter has proved to be an efficient preprocessing technique for segmentation and edge detection in MR image, and for correcting inhomogeneity in MR image. It has the advantage of being simple in implementation and gives good computation speed. The filter gives good results for images with unvarying noise (Perona & Malik, 1990). Gerig et al (1992) successfully applied this technique for denoising 2D and 3D MR images. But in this technique, the edge sharpening causes a region with a constant gray value slope as the underlying image model is piecewise constant. The other disadvantage of the filter is it presumes noise to be Gaussian distributed thus may not be useful for MR image with SNR < 3. As an extension this work Tang et al. (2007) presented improved version of the filter with better denoising performance. For catering to the requirements of rician noise model, the work suggested gradient computation to be done by averaging gradients is all the four directions. Also the threshold was defined adaptively with local noise level. Samsonov and Johnson (2004) proposed an adaptive model of ADF for MR images with spatially varying noise levels.

Discrete Wavelet Transform Based Denoising Filter

Temporal filter must be chosen in appropriate relation to the sampling interval in order to avoid the aliasing artifacts. This filter at best would work only on spin echo images. A temporal filter with too narrow a frequency response diminishes the signal at the edges of the image, too broad a frequency response introduces additional noise through aliasing.

Discrete Wavelet transforms is a multi resolution method which decomposes an image signal in coarsest to finest scale and represents the local features either spatially or in terms of spectral value. Nowak (1999) proposed a denoising filter based on wavelet transform for MR images as it was found to be suitable for rician noise model. Wood and Johnson (1999) proposed an improved technique which was based on the wavelet packet rather than single basis wavelet denoising method. This method comprised of three stages viz wavelet packet trans-formation, best-basis selection, and coefficient thresholding. This technique proved to be more suitable for MR images with low SNR.

Over the years researchers have proposed many wavelet transform based denoising techniquesfor MR Image (Wood & Jhonson, 1999; ME Alexander et al 2000; Anand & Shahambi, 2010). They prove to have advantage of preserving the edges and fine details of the body tissue alongside rician noise removal. The image can be iteratively processed for multiple transform scales each on representing a unique degree of image decomposition or details. The filter performance depends on the value of wavelet coefficients and the threshold. The only disadvantage of this technique is it may add artifacts to existing image matrix which would affect image quality.

Statistical Based Filtering Approach: Maximum Likelihood Filter

In the statistical denoising approach, noise vaiance is estimated from the noisy MR image and SNR is computed from the same. H Gudbjartsson (2008) estimated noise from magnitude MR image for the first time and modeled the noise as rician distributed. The work also proposed a noise correction technique based on image intensity data.

It was McGibney and Smith (1999)who proposed a conventional approach by utilizing the noise properties of the second order moment. Sijbers et al. (1998, 2004) performed signal reconstruction using maximum likelihood (ML) approach based on rician noise estimation from the image. In case of cardiac or lung images, no background information is generally available. For such cases, Rajan et al. (2011) proposed the ML based estimation of the local variance for each pixel of the image using a local neighborhood. Based on ML estimation using restricted local neighborhoods, Rajan et al. (2010) also proposed denoising for spatially varying noise levels in MR images. Recently, Rajan et al. (2012) presented the nonlocal maximum likelihood estimation for denoising multiple coil MR images.

SUMMARY

Following table summarizes the strengths and weaknesses of the filters specifically for rician noise model of MR data with reference to quantified results from referred research work.

Quantitative analysis of MR image quality is extremely critical for correct interpretation of the clinical data in the image. The next section elaborates significance of different quality measures in assessment of MR image.

Table 1. Advantages and Disadvantages of Denoising Filters for MRI

Filter	Advantage	Disadvantage
Gaussian	Simple to implement, effective for MR image with high SNR	Blurs edges, structures
Bilateral	Simple to implement, retains edges and soft tissue structures	Execution time more than Gaussian
NLM	Retains edges and soft tissue structures	High computational complexity and time overhead
Anisotropic Diffusion	Good computational speed and simple to implement. Retains edges	Not suitable for image with varying noise level
Wavelet based	Fast, Retains edges	Adds artifacts to image
Maximum Likelihood	Suitable for spatially varying noise levels	Complex to implement

IMAGE QUALITY ASSESSMENT

The purpose of image quality assessment is to achieve accuracy in analysis of MR image data and thus support medical diagnostics. Quality assessment can be done broadly in two ways viz subjectively or using objective techniques. Subjective assessment is an ideal technique as it is based on data from human observers. But, main disadvantage of the subjective assessment is that the accuracy of results is based on large number of human observers as well as mental and physical state of the human observer. These techniques are costly in terms of time and practically difficult to realize. They cannot be used for real time applications. Also, observations of the human observer are greatly affected by the quality of display equipment as well as available light.

Classification

The objective quality assessment techniques are algorithms or methods which can analyse the image and evaluate its quality without any human intervention. The classification of quality measures is shown in Figure 9. Based on the availability of noise free original image, the objective image quality metrics can be further classified into three categories viz No reference, Full reference, and Reduced reference technique. In the full reference method, the filtered image is analysed by comparing it with available reference image while in the reduced reference technique only some features or parameters of the ideal quality reference image is available. The "no reference" technique does not have any ideal image for comparison with the filtered image. As this being a real world practical situation, these techniques are extremely popular in practice.

It is necessary to assess quality of the denoised MR image using different types of objective quality measures which compute on the basis of edges, pixel intensity, structural content, contrast, spectral distance and human vision system (M A Joshi et al, 2015). A major emphasis in recent research has been given to a deeper analysis of the Human Visual System (HVS) features. Researchers assume that incorporating knowledge of the human visual system and human perception into objective quality assessment algorithms could increase their accuracy. The underlying premise is that humans do not perceive images as signals in a high-dimensional space, but are interested in various attributes of those images, such as brightness, contrast, shape and texture of objects, orientations, smoothness, etc. The next section defines statistical quality measures popularly used for MR image quality assessment.

Figure 9. Classification of Image Quality Assessment

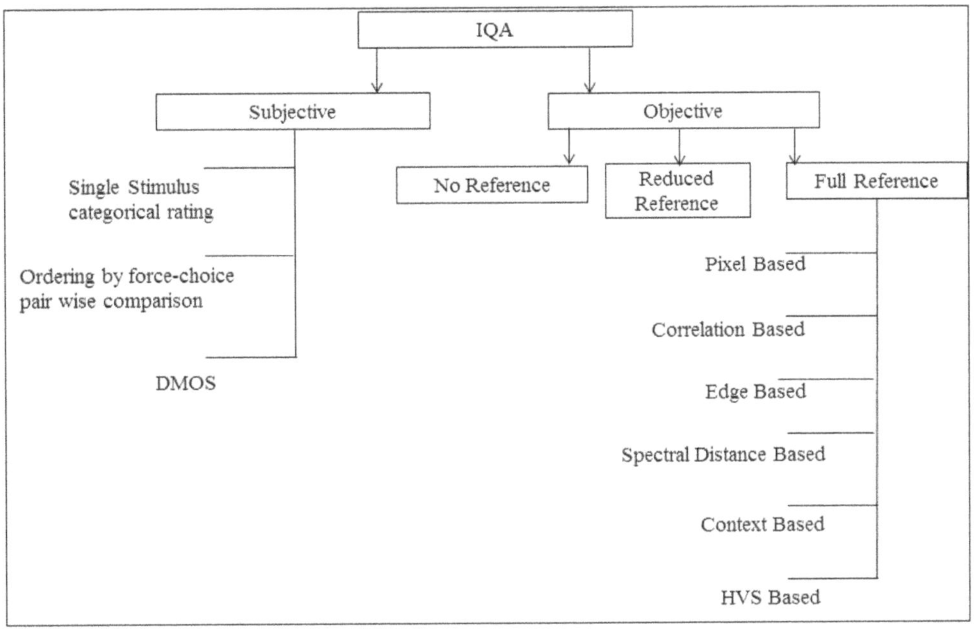

Quality Measures Used for MR Image IQA

Mean Squared Error (MSE)

One obvious way of measuring this similarity is to compute an error signal by subtracting the test signal from the reference, and then computing the average energy of the error signal. The mean-squared-error (MSE) is the simplest, and the most widely used, full-reference image quality measurement. This metric is frequently used in signal processing and is defined as follows:

$$\mathrm{MSE} = \frac{1}{mn}\sum_{i=0}^{m-1}\sum_{j=0}^{n-1}\left[\mathrm{I}(i,j) - \mathrm{K}(i,j)\right]^2 \tag{9}$$

where $I(i, j)$ represents the original (reference) image and $K(i, j)$ represents the distorted (modified) image and i and j are the pixel position of the m×n image.

MSE is zero when $I(i, j) = K(i, j)$.

Peak Signal to Noise Ratio (PSNR)

PSNR is inversely proportional the Mean Squared Error and is evaluated in decibels. It is given by the equation (M A Joshi et al, 2015):-

$$\text{PSNR} = 20\log 10\left(\text{MAX I}\right) - 10\log 10\left(\text{MSE}\right) \tag{10}$$

Universal Image Quality Index (UIQI)

Wang and Bovik proposed a technique in 2002, which compares the test image with a reference image on the basis of three parameters viz contrast, luminance and structures. The three equations are given as

$$l\left(i,j\right) = \frac{\mu_i \mu_j}{\mu_i^2 + \mu_j^2} \tag{11}$$

$$c\left(i,j\right) = \frac{2\sigma_i \sigma_j}{\sigma_i^2 + \sigma_j^2} \tag{12}$$

$$s\left(i,j\right) = \frac{2\sigma_{ij}}{\sigma_i + \sigma_j} \tag{13}$$

Here, covariance is represented by $\mu_i \mu_j$ .and $\sigma_i \sigma_j$ indicate the mean value and standard deviation of the original orreferenceimage and noisy image respectively. Based on the above equations, UIQI is defined by equation

$$\text{UIQI(i,j)} = \frac{4\mu_i \mu_j \mu_{ij}}{\left(\mu_i^2 + \mu_j^2\right)\left(\sigma_i^2 + \sigma_j^2\right)} \tag{14}$$

Unfortunately, UIQI does not correlate well with subjective assessment and does not compute close to human perception. Also, the metric is unstable for values of $\left(\mu_i^2 + \mu_j^2\right) and \ (\sigma_i^2 + \sigma_j^2)$ close to zero. Thus Wang et al improvised the metric and proposed structural similarity index.

Structural Similarity Index Metric (SSIM)

UIQI was modified and presented as SSIM by Wang et al in 2004. SSIM identifies similarity in structures of two images tries to quantify the same in SSIM index. It is a model which presumes that degradation or noise in an image is a perceived change in structural content of the image. The computation algorithm applies luminance and contrast mask to the entire image. The SSIM index is calculated for a local neighborhood. Mean SSIM index is computed by averaging SSIM over all the neighborhoods in the entire image. The equations for SSIM and MSSIM are given as

$$SSIM\left(i,j\right) = \frac{\left(2\mu i\ \mu j + c1\right)\left(\sigma ij + c2\right)}{\left(\mu_i^2 + \mu_j^2 + C1\right)\left(\sigma_i^2 + \sigma_j^2 + C2\right)} \tag{15}$$

Pratt's Figure of Merit (Pratt Measure)

This measure introduced by Pratt (Amiya Halder et al, 2011) considers both edge location accuracy and missing / false alarm edge elements. This measure is based on the knowledge of an ideal reference edge map, where the reference edges should have preferably a width of one pixel. The figure of merit is defined as:

$$E1 = \frac{1}{max\left\{n_d, n_t\right\}} \sum_{i=1}^{n_d} \frac{1}{1 + ad_i^2} \tag{17}$$

where *nd* and *nt* are the number of detected and ground-truth edge points, respectively, and *di* is the distance to the closest edge candidate for the *i*th detected edge pixel.

Edge-Based Structural Similarity (ESSIM)

This measure indicates edge quality of the filtered image. It compares the edge information between the distorted image block and the original one, and replaces the structure comparison s(**i,j**) in equation (1) by the edge-based structure comparison e(i,j). (G. Chen et al., 2006)

The edge based SSIM is defined as

$$\mathrm{ESSIM}\left(\mathrm{i, j}\right) = \left[\mathrm{l}\left(\mathrm{i, j}\right)\right]^{\propto} \cdot \left[\mathrm{c}\left(\mathrm{i, j}\right)\right]^{2} \cdot \left[\mathrm{e}\left(\mathrm{i, j}\right)\right]^{3} \tag{18}$$

The edge comparison e(i,j) is computed by calculating the correlation coefficient of the director vectors Di and Dj of the reference image. The overall image structure similarity is calculated as the mean of all the sub images *ESSIM.*

Significance of IQA for Healthcare

The various types of quality measures quantify degradation in the features of MR image and its statistical attributes. This can be helpful to radiologist to assess the extent of disease or abnormality in the body organs and tissue structures. These assessment measures can also be used to adjust quality of image dynamically in an application like telemedicine where patient to be treated and the medical expert are at different geographical locations. The IQA techniques can be further used to optimize image processing, and image denoising algorithms. Also, these measures can be of great use in designing and modeling the adaptive filters. The IQA metrics can be used to benchmark MR image denoising algorithms and systems which would be useful for medical diagnosis and patient healthcare.

REFERENCES

Alexander, M. E., Baumgartner, R., Summers, A. R., Windischberger, C., Klarhoefer, M., Moser, E., & Somorjai, R. L. (2000). A wavelet-based method for improving signal-to-noise ratio and contrast in MR images. *Magnetic Resonance Imaging*, *18*(2), 169–180. doi:10.1016/S0730-725X(99)00128-9 PMID:10722977

Amiya Halder et al. (2011). *Edge Detection: A Statistical Approach*. IEEE.

Anand, C. S., & Sahambi, J. S. (2010). Wavelet domain non-linear filtering for MRI denoising. *Magnetic Resonance Imaging*, *28*(6), 842–861. doi:10.1016/j.mri.2010.03.013 PMID:20418039

Aurich, V., & Weule, J. (*1995*). Nonlinear Gaussian Filters Performing Edge preserving Diffusion. *Mutererkennung 17, DAGM-Symposium*, 538-545.

Buades, . (2005). A Non Local Algorithm For Image Denoising. *IEEE International Conference on Computer Vision and Pattern Recognition*, 2, s60-65. doi:10.1109/CVPR.2005.38

Chen, G. (2006). *International Conf. on Acoustic, Speech and Signal processing*. IEEE Xplore Digital Library.

Coupe, P., Yger, P., & Barillot, C. (2006). Fast non local means denoising for MR images. *Proceedings at the 9th International Conference on Medical Image Computing and Computer assisted Intervention (MICCAI)*, 33–40. doi:10.1007/11866763_5

Efros & Leung. (1999). Texture synthesis by non-parametric sampling. *International Conference on Computer Vision*, 2(9), 1033–1038.

Eisemann, E., & Durand, F. (2002). Flash Photography Enhancement via Intrinsic Relighting. *ACM Transactions on Graphics*, *23*(3), 673–678. doi:10.1145/1015706.1015778

Elad, M. (2002, October). On the Bilateral Filter and Ways To Improve It. *IEEE Transactions on Image Processing*, *11*(10), 1141–1151. doi:10.1109/TIP.2002.801126 PMID:18249686

Elmaoğlu, M., & Çelik, A. (2012). *MR Physics, Patient Positioning, and Protocols*. Springer.

Gerig, G., Kubler, O., Kikinis, R., & Jolesz, F. A. (1992). Nonlinear anisotropic filtering of MRI data. *IEEE Transactions on Medical Imaging*, *11*(2), 221–232. doi:10.1109/42.141646 PMID:18218376

Gudbjartsson & Partz. (2008). *The Rician Distribution of Noisy MRI data*. HHS Public Access Manuscript, PMC.

Hamarneh, G., & Hradsky, J. (2007). Bilateral filtering of diffusion tensor magnetic resonance images. *IEEE Transactions on Image Processing*, *16*(10), 1723–1730. doi:10.1109/TIP.2007.904964 PMID:17926929

Hu, X. (2004). The Past, Present And Future Of Magnetic Resonance Imaging. Frontiers in Biomedical Engineering, 283-294. DOI doi:10.1007/978-1-4419-8967-3_18

IMAIOS. (n.d.). *Medical websites and e learning for medical professionals*. Retrieved from www.imaios.com

Iniewski, K. (2009). *Medical Imaging Principles, Detectors & Electronics*. John Wiley & Sons, Inc.

Joshi, M. A., & Joshi, K. R. (2015). Quantitative analysis of MR image quality is extremely critical for correct interpretation of the clinical data in the image. CRC Press.

Manjon, Robles, & Thacker. (2007). Multispectral MRI de-noising using non-local means. *Med. Image Understand. Anal. (MIUA)*, 41–46.

Manjón, J. V., Carbonell-Caballero, J., Lull, J. J., García-Martí, G., Martí-Bonmatí, L., & Robles, M. (2008). MRI denoising using non-local means. *Medical Image Analysis*, *12*(4), 514–523. doi:10.1016/j.media.2008.02.004 PMID:18381247

Manjón, J. V., Coupe, P., Martí-Bonmatí, L., Collins, D. L., & Robles, M. (2010). Adaptive non-local means denoising of MR images with spatially varying noise levels. *Magnetic Resonance Imaging*, *31*(1), 192–203. doi:10.1002/jmri.22003 PMID:20027588

McGibney, G., & Smith, M. (1993). Unbiased signal-to-noise ratio measure for magnetic resonance images. *Medical Physics*, *20*(4), 1077–1078. doi:10.1118/1.597004 PMID:8413015

McVeigh, E. R., Henkelman, R. M., & Bronskill, M. J. (1985). Noise and filtration in magnetic resonance imaging. *Medical Physics*, *12*(5), 586–591. doi:10.1118/1.595679 PMID:4046992

Nowak, R. D. (1999). Wavelet-based Rician noise removal for magnetic resonance imaging. *IEEE Transactions on Image Processing*, *8*(10), 1408–1419. doi:10.1109/83.791966 PMID:18267412

Oza & Joshi. (2017). Performance Analysis of Denoising Filters for MR Images. Advances in Computing Applications, 87-96.

Paris, S., Kornprobst, P., Tumblin, J. T., & Durand, F. (2008). Bilateral Filtering: Theory and Applications. *Computer Graphics and Vision*, *4*(1), 1–73. doi:10.1561/0600000020

Perona, P., & Malik, J. (1990). Scale-space and edge detection using anisotropic diffusion. *IEEE Transactions on Pattern Analysis and Machine Intelligence*, *12*(7), 629–639. doi:10.1109/34.56205

Rajan, J., Jeurissen, B., Verhoye, M., Audekerke, J. V., & Sijbers, J. (2011). Maximum like-lihood estimation-based denoising of magnetic resonance images using restriced local neighborhoods. *Physics in Medicine and Biology*, *56*(16), 5221–5234. doi:10.1088/0031-9155/56/16/009 PMID:21791732

Rajan, J., Poot, D., Juntu, J., & Sijbers, J. (2010). Noise measurement from magnitude MRI using local estimates of variance and skewness. *Physics in Medicine and Biology*, *55*(16), 441–449. doi:10.1088/0031-9155/55/16/N02 PMID:20679694

Rajan, J., Veraat, J., Audekerke, J. V., Verhoye, M., & Sijbers, J. (2012). Nonlocal maximum likelihood estimation method for denoising multiple-coil magnetic resonance images. *Magnetic Resonance Imaging*, *30*(10), 1512–1518. doi:10.1016/j.mri.2012.04.021 PMID:22819583

Riji, R., Rajan, J., Sijbers, J., & Nair, M. S. (2015). Iterative Bilateral Filter for Rician Noise Reduction in MR Images, *Signal. Image and Video Processing*, *9*(7), 1543–1548. doi:10.1007/s11760-013-0611-6

Samsonov, A., & Johnson, C. (2004). Noise-adaptive nonlinear diffusion filtering of MR images with spatially varying noise levels. *Magnetic Resonance in Medicine*, *52*(4), 798–806. doi:10.1002/mrm.20207 PMID:15389962

Sijbers, J., & den Dekker, A. J. (2004). Maximum likelihood estimation of signal amplitude and noise variance form MR data. *Magnetic Resonance Imaging*, *51*, 586–594. PMID:15004801

Sijbers, J., den Dekker, A. J., Scheunders, P., & Van Dyck, D. (1998). Maximum likelihood destimation of Rician distribution parameters. *IEEE Transactions on Medical Imaging*, *17*(3), 357–361. doi:10.1109/42.712125 PMID:9735899

Sijbers, J., den Dekker, A. J., Van Audekerke, J., Verhoye, M., & Van Dyck, D. (1998). Estimation of the noise in magnitude MR images. *Magnetic Resonance Imaging*, *16*(1), 87–90. doi:10.1016/S0730-725X(97)00199-9 PMID:9436952

Tang, J., Sun, Q., Liu, J., & Cao, Y. (2007). An adaptive anisotropic diffusion filter for noise reduction in MR images. *Proceedings of IEEE International Conference on Mechatronics and Automation*, 1299–1304. doi:10.1109/ICMA.2007.4303737

Tomasi, C., & Manduchi, R. (1998). Bilateral Filtering for Gray and Color Images. *Proc. Int. Conf. Computer Vision*, 839-846. doi:10.1109/ICCV.1998.710815

Walker, S. A., Miller, D., & Tanabe, J. (2006). Bilateral spatial filtering: Refining methods for localizing brain activation in the presence of parenchymal abnormalities. *NeuroImage*, *33*(2), 564–569. doi:10.1016/j.neuroimage.2006.06.051 PMID:16942890

Wang, Z. (2002). A Universal Image Quality Index. *IEEE Signal Processing Letters*, *20*.

Wang, Z., Bovik, A. C., Sheikh, H. R., & Simoncelli, E. P. (2004). Image Quality Assessment: From Error Visibility to Structural Similarity. *IEEE Transactions on Image Processing*, *13*(4), 600–612. doi:10.1109/TIP.2003.819861 PMID:15376593

Westbrook, C. (2008). Handbook of MRI Technique. John Wiley & Sons, Ltd.

Wiest-Daesslé, N., Prima, S., Coupé, P., Morrissey, S. P., & Barillot, C. (2007). *Nonlocal means variants for denoising of diffusion-weighted and diffusion tensor MRI*. Med. Image Comput. Comput. Assist. Interv.

Wong, W. C. K., & Chung, A. C. S. (2004). A nonlinear and non-iterative noise reduction technique for medical images: Concept and methods comparison. *Elsevier International Congress Series*, *1268*, 171–176. doi:10.1016/j.ics.2004.03.143

Wong, W. C. K., Chung, A. C. S., & Yu, S. C. H. (2004). Trilateral filter for biomedical images. *Proceedings of ISBI*, 820–823.

Wood, J. C., & Johnson, K. M. (1999). Wavelet packet denoising of magnetic resonance images: Importance of Rician noise at low SNR. *Magnetic Resonance in Medicine*, *41*(3), 631–635. doi:10.1002/(SICI)1522-2594(199903)41:3<631::AID-MRM29>3.0.CO;2-Q PMID:10204890

Xie, J., Heng, P. A., & Shah, M. (2008). Image diffusion using saliency bilateral filter. *IEEE Transactions on Information Technology in Biomedicine*, *12*(6), 768–771. doi:10.1109/TITB.2008.926462 PMID:19000957

Yanasak et al. (2015). *Parallel Imaging in MRI: Technology, Applications, and Quality Control.* American Association of Physicists in Medicine.

Yoshika, H. (n.d.). *Magnetic resonance imaging.* Retrieved from www.intl.elsevierhealth.com/media/us/samplechapters

Chapter 6
Framework for Integration of Medical Image and Text-Based Report Retrieval to Support Radiological Diagnosis

Siddhivinayak Kulkarni
MAEER's MIT College of Engineering, India

Amit Savyanavar
MAEER's MIT College of Engineering, India

Pradnya Kulkarni
Federation University, Australia & MAEER's MIT College of Engineering, India

Andrew Stranieri
Federation University, Australia

Vijay Ghorpade
Dr. D. Y. Patil College of Engineering and Technology, India

ABSTRACT

Medical images are vital part of diagnostics and patient treatment. With the advent of technology, there is a rapid increase in the number of radiological images produced every day. Attempts have been made to use a Content Based Image Retrieval (CBIR) approach for assisting in radiological diagnosis. However, this approach suffers from the semantic gap problem. Few text retrieval systems are in place for assisting the radiologist to retrieve similar past cases. However, for the least experienced radiologist it is hard to describe the unknown case using text query. Therefore, the aim of this chapter is integrating the radiological CBIR and text based reports retrieval in order to support radiological diagnosis. The proposed technique is described in three stages: a) retrieval by image similarity, b) retrieval by text, and c) fusion of image and text retrieval for better diagnosis. Number of experiments are demonstrated along with their evaluation techniques on mammogram image database.

DOI: 10.4018/978-1-5225-2829-6.ch006

INTRODUCTION

Background and Motivation

Imaging of body parts by using different techniques such as X-ray, MRI, Ultrasound, and Computed tomography (CT) is helpful in diagnosing serious diseases such as cancer. Due to advancement in technology and growth in population, there is a vast increase in the number of radiological images. For instance about 200,000 images were generated per day in one of the hospitals in Geneva in 2011 (http://medgift.hevs.ch/silverstripe/index.php/). Radiology images are used for many applications including diagnostics, therapy and teaching.

It has been observed that diagnostic radiologists struggle to maintain high interpretation accuracy while trying to fulfil efficiency targets (Rubin, 2000). Misdiagnosis by radiologists due to non-medical reasons are reported to be in the range of 2% to 4% (Siegle et al., 1998; Soffa et al, 2004). The misinterpretation of cancer lesions increases patients' anxiety, health-care costs and also results in death in rare cases. According to (Muramatsu et al., 2005), radiological image interpretation consists of three tasks; perception of image findings, interpretation of these findings to render a differential diagnosis and recommendations for clinical management. The perception of image findings and their interpretation requires two types of knowledge. One is formalized domain knowledge which is present in texts and other written documentation. Second is implicit or tacit knowledge consisting of radiologists' individual expertise, organisational practices and past cases (Montani and Bellazzi, 2002).

In the diagnostic scenario if a radiologist fails to express the unknown abnormality in text query, then the text retrieval for a similar case would naturally fail. And so, Query by image content has been more successful in retrieving similar past cases to help diagnosis (Shyu et al., 1999; Aisen et al., 2003; Xue et al., 2009; Fischer et al., 2012; Zhou et al., 2012).

The proposed system will be designed to handle following two scenarios:

- Search for images with lesions that look similar and query text describing what the radiologist thinks is present as a clinical feature/finding.
- Search for images with lesions that look similar and text query text describing the diagnosis the radiologist is thinking about.

According to radiologists, there could be more than one clinical features or findings that look the same on mammograms. For example a Cyst and a Mass would look very similar on a mammographic image. Also, the clinical feature/finding present could possibly be because of more than one disease. Table 1 below shows some of the examples.

Radiologist Delineated Regions of Interest (ROI)

While looking for similarity the radiologists are often interested in the abnormalities in an image. The region occupied by the abnormality is called a Region of Interest (ROI). Figure 1 shows example ROI containing a circumscribed mass. The region of interest will be marked by expert radiologists.

A medical case is composed of an image and its associated radiology report. A Query composed of an example ROI and free text is given for retrieval purposes. An idea of calculating cross-media relevance for multimedia objects called pseudo-relevance feedback has shown to work better than lin-

Table 1. Different diagnosis for same clinical findings in mammograms

Finding	Possible Diagnosis	Example
Speculated lesion	Cancer Post operative scar Breast abcess Fat necrosis	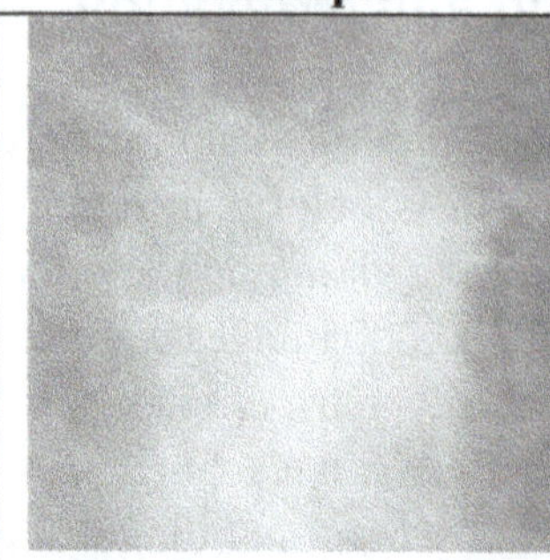
Round or oval circumscribed mass	Cysts Cancer Galactocele Dilated duct Papilloma Phylloides tumor Fibroadenoma	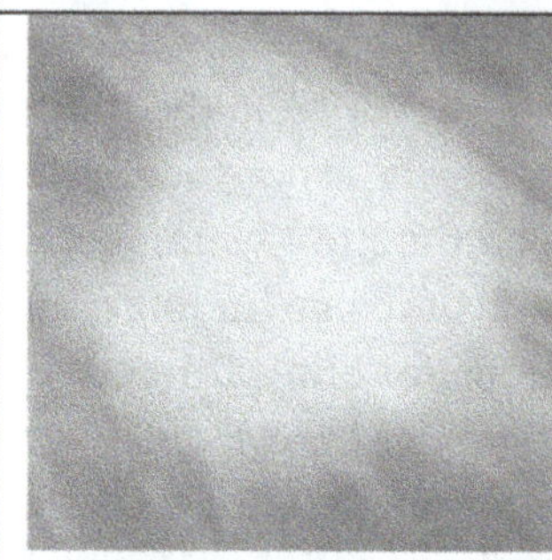
Calcification	Co-ductal carcinoma Oil cyst Fibroadenoma Oil cysts Post operative	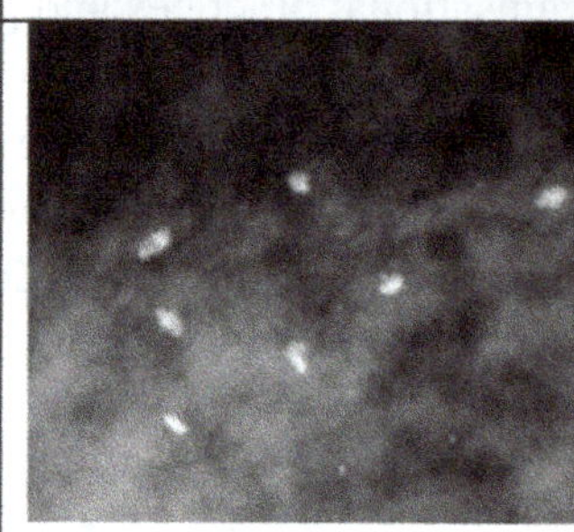

Figure 1. Example ROI

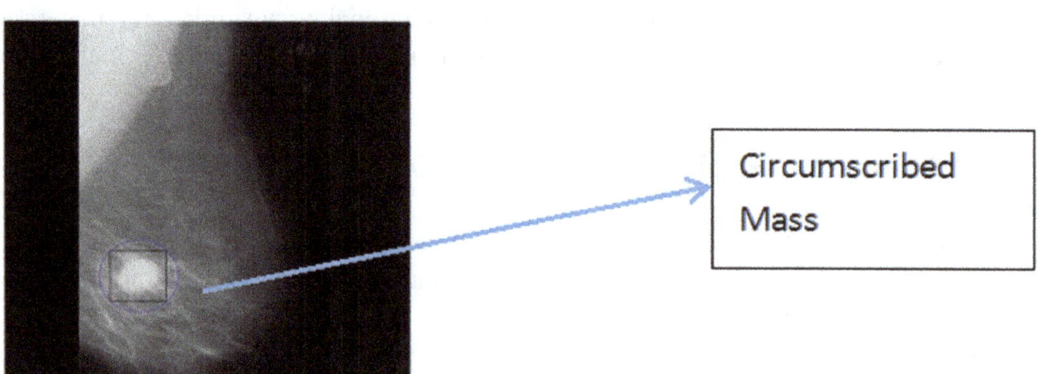

ear summing of monomedia similarity scores (Clinchant et al., 2007). The pseudo-relevance feedback mechanism works as follows: From the image query the visual similarity can be computed and the first set of relevant cases is retrieved. As each image also has associated text, this text can be used as feedback for text retrieval. Thus the modality of data is switched from image to text and text to image. In our case this pseudo-relevance feedback would actually be achieved by handling the monomedia similarity scores (visual similarity/textual similarity). Csurka et al. (2014) shows how a graph based technique can successfully be used for implementing the idea of pseudo-relevance feedback just by manipulating the monomedia similarity scores. It is therefore intended to use similar graph-based transmedia pseudo-relevance feedback technique for case similarity score computation.

LITERATURE REVIEW

This section is mainly divided into three sections: The first section overviews CBIR along with medical CBIR systems discussing various techniques of image retrieval, and of use of Medical CBIR for diagnostic purposes, Section two details various techniques used for Text-based report retrieval and section three confers combination of image and Text-based retrieval systems.

Content Based Image Retrieval (CBIR)

Advancements in computer and multimedia technologies produce large repositories of digital images for various applications such as medicine, art, security and meteorology. The retrieval of images according to user's needs from large databases is a challenging problem. To solve this problem, traditional way (proposed in 1970s) is to manually annotate the images with keywords and use the text query to search through the manual annotations associated with the images. One of the drawbacks of this method is that manual annotation is a time consuming and labour intensive process; the second drawback is the subjectivity of human perception and interpretation from various perspectives (Liu et al., 2007) and third is the language dependency. To overcome these drawbacks of text based image retrieval, content based image retrieval (CBIR) was originated in early 1980s. Content based Image Retrieval (CBIR) is based on retrieving similar images by using visual features such as colours, textures, shapes. Some of the early commercial CBIR systems and experimental prototypes are IBM's Query By Image Content (QBIC) (Flickner et al., 1995; Niblack et al., 1993), Virage (Bach et al., 1996), Photobook (Pentland et al., 1996), Candid (Kelly et al., 1995), and Netra (Ma et al., 1997). Successful application of CBIR techniques in various real world applications can be seen in (Hermitage Museum, 2003) and ALIPR (Li and Wang, 2006). The detailed survey of general CBIR systems can be found in Long et al. (2003) and Datta et al. (2008). Although, CBIR systems try to find visually similar images by automated feature extraction, users are interested in underlying semantic meanings of an image. A user's notion of similarity is based on high level abstractions, such as objects, events or activities. Therefore, there is always a gap between the information modelled by low level features of an image and the user's information needs. This is called as *semantic gap* problem. In order to narrow the semantic gap, various approaches have been proposed. Five major categories of the state-of-the-art approaches are: (1) Using object ontologies to define high level concepts, (2) Automatic annotation using machine learning, (3) Using relevance feedback to learn user's intentions, (4) Generating semantic template and (5) Fusion of evidences from the visual content and associated text are mentioned in a review article by Liu et al. (2007).

Medical CBIR for Diagnosis

The first prototype system for diagnostic purpose ASSERT (Automated Search and Selection Engine with Retrieval Tools) is designed with physician-in-the-loop approach in which the human delineates the pathology bearing region (PBR) or Region of Interest. This system is used for High Resolution Computed Tomography (HRCT) images of lung (Shyu et al., 1999). The HRCT images of lung do not possess sharp edges and contours. It employs features such as Texture (GLCM), Shape features (longer axis, shorter axis Fourier descriptors and moments) and the position of ROI with respect to certain anatomical landmarks. Indexing is based on hashing function based on feature grouping. Advantage is due to multidimensional hashing the system is quite fast. However, weakness of this system is the computer algorithms used for extraction of features and generating indexes are quite complex and the ROIs have to be delineated by the experts. Moreover, the accuracy of delineation is subjective. Aisen et al. (2003) studied the use of ASSERT system as diagnostic aid and he observed that the diagnostic accuracy of the radiologists increased from 29% to 62% showing that this system is useful for computer-assisted diagnosis. But the limitation of this study is the small number of test images used (29).

An effort to reduce the PBR delineation time (Semi- automatic segmentation) can be seen in the work of Huang et al. (2005). They designed a diagnostic support tool using image-matching for brain disease of children. This system uses a database containing brain magnetic resonance (MR) images of 2500 paediatric patients aged between 0 and 18 with known brain lesions. In the registration phase the images are registered to a common global coordinate system. The seed pixel is selected by the expert clinician and the ROI is extracted automatically by the software reducing the time required for delineation. Image features used include location, size, shape, texture, denseness. Similarity is calculated using Euclidean distance. Similarity measurement is robust to slight misalignments even after image registration. It has been observed that between 10% and 60% of the search results either produced the known, true diagnosis, or diagnoses that were judged by the expert neuroradiologist to represent possible alternative. Although, the results of their experiment show that image-matching could be useful to assist the physician in surveying possible differential diagnoses for a range of diseases, the accuracy of the search results is different for different diseases and for some diseases it is very low (10%).

Another such system for chest computed tomography for solitary pulmonary nodules is described in (Endo et al., 2012). The database consists of CT images, diagnosis reports, and confirmed diagnoses from 439 patients with 461 solitary pulmonary nodules. Here the user clicks on the pulmonary nodule and the border is automatically detected. The mean, standard deviation, maximum and minimum circularity values on the extracted border area are used as feature indices. Furthermore, the proportions of low-density areas and each area to the entire nodule area are used as feature indices of the cavity region of internal property based on threshold processing and labelling processing. From the retrieved cases, when the user selects the most similar case then the lesion size, affected area of the lung in the report gets filled out automatically and all other fields get selected as the reference case thus helping in semiautomatic report generation. Evaluation is done by looking at the number of diagnostic matches (benign/malignant) between the queries and four presented cases. Results show that percentage of correct diagnoses for the radiologist improved from 80% to 93% by using the system. Moreover only one click was required to extract the region of interest. Limitation of this system is that the similarity is determined only by image analysis; a case with a different diagnosis may also be retrieved.

More detailed review about other medical CBIR systems can be found in Müller et al. (2004), Akgül et al. (2011), Ghosh et al. (2011), Hwang et al. (2012), and Müller et al. (2013). It can be concluded from these reviews that for improved semantic case retrieval, image retrieval techniques should be effectively integrated with external knowledge present in associated text such as reports, annotations and clinical parameters.

To summarize, in order to use CBIR as a diagnostic aid three things are vital: 1) Accuracy of retrieval needs to be high, 2) Time required for retrieval needs to be less, 3) Query by region of interest should be allowed. It is evident from the literature that for medical images it is often impractical to accurately extract the regions of interest by automatic image segmentation techniques. Therefore, we have decided to use radiologist delineated regions of interest for our study. Using radiologist delineated regions of interest would ensure getting higher segmentation accuracy, thereby guaranteeing better retrieval accuracy as compared to automatic segmentation techniques. Furthermore, very promising results are obtained in our preliminary work using Visual Character N-gram features of ROI for mammographic classification. We intend to improve it by trying N-gram features in various directions and combining different length N-gram features in the future work. While we decided to use the mammographic database for our work, the character N-gram features are general and can be extended easily for any other domains. Moreover, the N-gram feature extraction algorithm is simple and computationally less expensive reducing the time and resources required for retrieval process.

As pointed out earlier there is a semantic gap problem with the CBIR approach. This gap represents a major opportunity to develop diagnostic decision support systems that integrates image features and the associated text features. Thus design of diagnostic decision support system would have to incorporate use of textual descriptions in the form of metadata, reports, clinical history, broadening the system from "image based search" to "case-based" reasoning. We therefore take the opportunity to bridge the semantic gap by integrating the N-gram based CBIR with the ontology based radiology reports retrieval in order to find similar past cases for radiological diagnosis. Our approach allows free text query to enhance the usability of the system.

Text Based Reports Retrieval

Medical records are always stored in free text and the forms of these records are different from one health care system to another. Information Retrieval (IR) is one of the significant techniques applied for retrieving similar text data. There are different well known IR techniques for document indexing and retrieval in general. Index terms are normally the content words. The terms used are normally stems instead of full words. This ensures that the matches are not missed through word variations with singular/plural forms. Stemming algorithms such as Porter (1980) are commonly used in information retrieval context. One simple way to rank the output is to rank based on number of matching terms. For example, for a request with 4 terms first by documents with all 4, then by documents with any 3, etc.

Relevance Weighting / Term Weighting

Raw frequency of a term is the number of times the term appears in a document. Boolean frequency is another way to represent rank documents whose value would be 1 if the term exists in a document and 0 if it does not exist. Using Raw or Boolean frequency suffers from a critical problem. All terms are considered equally important. Usually, some of the terms have a little discriminating power in determining relevance. Therefore, choosing a term capable of retrieving few relevant documents from many non-relevant ones definitely increases the retrieval performance. This is achieved by term weighting also called as relevance weighting.

Main sources to be considered for weighting are: 1) Inverse Document Frequency (IDF), 2) Term Frequency (TF), and 3) Document Length. Terms that occur in few documents are usually more important than the ones occurring in many documents. IDF measures whether the term is common or rare across all documents. The Inverse Document Frequency can be calculated as $IDF = \log \frac{N}{n}$ where, N = number of documents in the collection and n = number of documents the term appears.

The more often a term appears in a document, the more likely that it is important for that document. Therefore, TF is the number of occurrence of term in a document. A term that appears same number of times in short and long document is most likely to be important for the short document. Hence, length of document could be considered for weighting of terms. The most commonly used weighting scheme is $TF \times IDF$.

- **Natural Language Processing:** The most critical issue for information retrieval performance is the term mismatch. Natural language processing (NLP) is making computers understand the natural language using syntactic and semantic analysis. Use of NLP reduces the semantic gap between the users query and the retrieval system and hence increases the retrieval performance. In clinical scenario, for example radiology, some of the information is implicit; many short forms are used and also different clinicians use different words to mention the same concept. NLP systems are therefore been widely used in clinical scenarios to: 1) index or categorize reports, 2) extract, structure, and codify clinical information in the reports so that the information can be used by other computerized applications, 3) generate text to produce patient profiles or summaries, and 4) improve interfaces to health care systems (Friedman, 2005). Comprehensive reviews about NLP in biomedicine can be seen in (Demner-Fushman et al., 2009; Nadkami et al., 2011; Friedman et al., 2011). The RadMiner (Gerstmair et al., 2012) system makes use of NLP techniques to parse the free text radiology reports.

Following are some of the techniques used for IR using NLP.

- **Query Expansion:** Different users often use different words to refer to same or similar meaning. This is called synonymy. Synonymy decreases the recall. Query expansion comprises finding out synonyms of the query terms using thesaurus. The original query term along with the additional synonym terms are then used for judging the relevance of the documents. Therefore query expansion improves the recall of the information retrieval system. Please refer to Carpineto et al. (2012) for detailed review of query expansion techniques.
- **Word Sense Disambiguation (WSD):** A word can have different meanings depending on the context it is used. This is called as polysemy. Polysemy decreases the precision of the retrieval system. Identifying the meaning of words in context is called as Word Sense Disambiguation (WSD). Schütze and Pedersen (1995) shows one of the earliest successful use of WSD for information retrieval. Metamap is another example of recent WSD feature (Aronson, 2006).

- **Word N-Grams:** Instead of using words, combination of words (phrases) is more useful in determining the underlying semantic meanings. Document representation using Bag-of-Phrases model also called as Word N-grams have worked better than the Bag-of-Words model.
- **Conceptual Retrieval:** Ontology is a hierarchical grouping of the entities based on similarities and differences. For example SNOMED-CT is a standardised healthcare terminology including comprehensive coverage of diseases, clinical findings, therapies, procedures and outcomes. It has been demonstrated by the work of many researchers that concept based information retrieval works better in clinical context (Hersh et al., 1995; Chu et al., 2001; Houston et al., 2000; Li and Wu, 2006; Dang et al., 2009). Chu and Cesnik (2001) use conceptual graphs to capture the structure and semantic information contained in the medical documents. Mao and Chu (2007) proposed a phrase-vector space model for medical documents retrieving. MetaMap (Aronson, 2006) identifies UMLS concepts in text and returns them in a ranked list. Nassif (2009) developed a mammographic text retrieval system based on BI-RADS lexicon.

Combination of Image and Text Based Systems

It is often necessary to retrieve information based on textual and image queries for different appliications. Image and textual queries are expressed at different semantic levels. It is a challenging task to correlate both representations in order to satisfy the information need of a user (Clinchant et al., 2011). The fusion of text and visual content has been found to be more effective than using purely text or visual content separately (Kludas et al., 2008; Zha et al., 2012; Weyand and Deselaers, 2005; Ferecatu and Sahbi, 2008). Information fusion has the potential of improving retrieval performance because the heterogeneity of multiple information sources allows cross-correction of some of the errors (Depeursinge and Müller, 2010). On top of that the fusion tries to reduce the semantic gap (Smeulders et al, 2000). Text based search is more efficient than the content based image search; firstly, because it is more difficult to extract semantics of an image compared to text and secondly, image feature extraction techniques are computationally very expensive. Moreover, it has been observed that the textual retrieval performs better than the content based image retrieval in terms of recall, but content based image retrieval achieves higher early precision (Müller et al., 2010). Most of the fusion techniques developed so far fall in three categories: Low level fusion/Early fusion, High level fusion/Late fusion and Transmedia fusion.

Low Level Fusion or Early Fusion (Feature Level Fusion)

In Low level fusion, low level image features and the text features are concatenated into one feature vector to create a unique feature space (Snoek et al., 2005; Depeursinge et al., 2010). One of the best automatic mixed run of medical task in imageCLEF2009 (Müller et al., 2010) competition used low level fusion approach (Berber and Alpkocak, 2009). The simplest early fusion method involves concatenating both image and text feature representations (Ferecatu and Sahbi, 2008). However, more elaborated joint models such as Canonical Correlation Analysis have been investigated (Mori et al., 1999; Lavrenko et al., 2003; Vinokourov et al., 2003; Rasiwasia et al., 2010).

Feature level fusion can utilize correlation between multiple features from different modalities at an early stage which helps in better information retrieval (Atrey et al., 2010). The other advantage is it requires only one learning phase on the combined feature vector (Snoek et al., 2005; Depeursinge et al.,

Figure 2. Fusion approaches for combining Image and Text

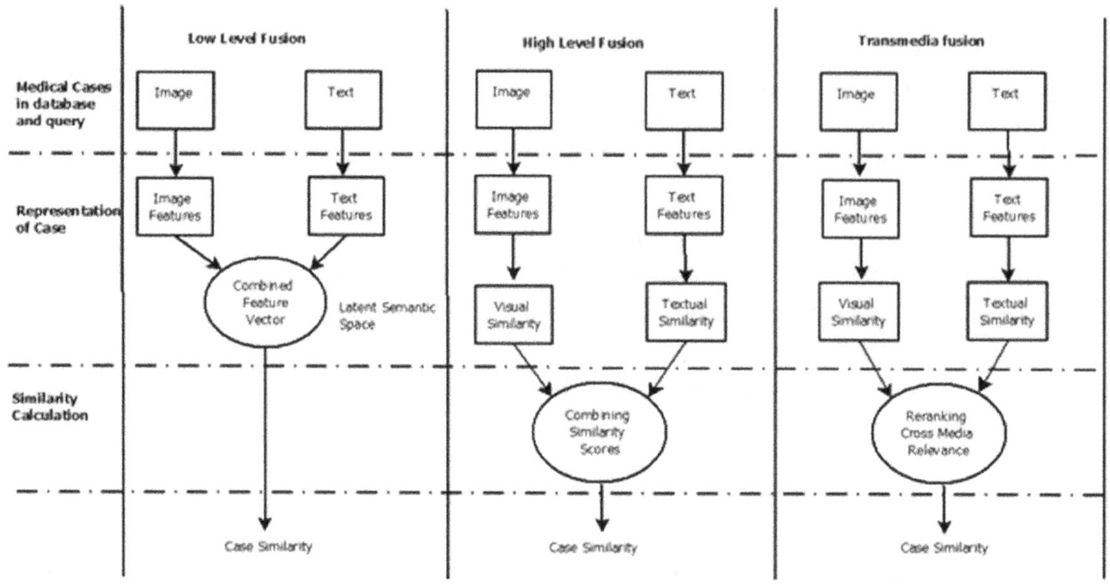

2010). Early fusion offers potentially high flexibility for promoting relevant modalities in the context of a particular query.

A major drawback of this fusion strategy is that it suffers from the curse of dimensionality as the high dimensional spaces tend to scatter the homogeneous clusters of instances belonging to same concepts (Depeursinge and Müller, 2010). Moreover, negative interactions among features can occur. The problem of dimensionality can be handled using a weighted combination of features (van Zaanen et al., 2005) which is usually difficult to achieve because majority of features are important to predict one class but introduce noise for other classes. In fact there are some cases where the fusion of image and text features has degraded performance with text only retrieval (Moulin et al., 2009). Various feature weighting methods have been investigated for medical information fusion in (van Zaanen and de Croon, 2005; Deselaers et al., 2005; Cheng et al., 2005; Deselaers et al., 2006, 2007).

High Level Fusion or Late Fusion

Late fusion mainly seeks to merge the monomedia relevance scores or ranks by means of aggregation functions. It is frequently used as it is better to combine the respective decisions rather than attempting to bridge the semantic gap. High level fusion is further classified into similarity score-based fusion and rank-based fusion.

Similarity Score Based Fusion

In this method the similarity score for images and the similarity score based on text are calculated separately and then combined together using various approaches. Lee (1997, 1995) proposed a technique called MinMax for normalizing the scores which is widely in use.

$$S_{final} = x = \frac{S - S_{min}}{S_{max} - S_{min}}$$

where S_{max} and S_{min} are the highest and lowest scores.

Transmedia Fusion/ Re-Ranking

In transmedia fusion or re-ranking, the main idea is to use one of the modalities (for example text) and then use the other modality (image) (jeon et al., 2003; Maillot et al., 2006; Ah-Pine et al., 2009).

Image reranking can be obtained in two ways. The first way is to find the objects according to text similarity S_t and then reorder them according to the visual similarity S_v. Thus, this method of re-ranking constrains the visual system to search among the set of objects that was returned by the text search instead of the entire collection and can be represented using the following equation:

$$S_{Rerank}(q;d) = I_{\{d \in KNNt(q)\}} S_v(q,d)$$

where KNNt(q) denotes the set of the K most similar objects to q according to the textual similarities S_t and, $I_{\{B\}} = 1$ if proposition B is true and $I_{\{B\}} = 0$ otherwise. Some of the examples of this type of fusion strategy can be seen in (Florea et al., 2006; Fakeri-Tabrizi et al., 2008; Simpson et al., 2009; Zhou et al., 2008, Benavent et al., 2010). In fact, by enforcing the visual system to search among the set of retrieved objects by the text expert, we somehow impose that images visually similar to the query images share a common semantic (given by the textual query). And hence an approach for combining re-ranking and late fusion has proven to work better than the late fusion or re-ranking alone (Clinchant et al., 2011).

Another way of reordering is to use image retrieval first and then reorder the results of visual retrieval by using text retrieval. Very few people have investigated this approach of re-ranking (Villena-Rom´an et al., 2005; Clinchant et al., 2007; Ah-Pine et al., 2009).

Fusion in Radiology Diagnostic Support Systems

Various attempts have been made in order to solve the problem of retrieving past similar cases in radiology based on image similarity and text associated with the radiology images such as radiology report, image annotations, clinical parameters and patient history. Different fusion approaches have been used.

Depeursinge et al. (2010) observed that the late fusion works better than the early fusion as well as the only visual approach for lung tissue classification. An example of low level fusion is described in Napel et al. (2010). The approach is designed for CT images of liver lesions. Similarity was calculated as the inverse of weighted sum of differences between corresponding feature vectors. Image features such as boundary sharpness, histogram and Gabor features and the semantic features generated from the annotations by radiologists using controlled vocabulary RadLex were used. The weights were learned using modified version of a machine learning method known as adaptive boosting (AdaBoost). The results show that combining semantic information features improve the precision and recall than the visual based features. However, the study used very small dataset (30 images) because the manual annotation is a time consuming process.

High level fusion or late fusion was attempted by Depeursinge et al. (2011) for 3D case based retrieval of interstitial lung disease. In this system, the similarity distance is obtained by weighted linear combination of distances calculated separately for volumes of the five different classes of lung tissue and 41 clinical parameters such as age, gender, smoking history, physical findings, medical history, and laboratory results. The limitations of the system are that the user interface is a bit complicated and the text query can only be chosen from the predefined alternatives.

The problem with radiology reports text is that different radiologists use different terms to express the same clinical feature/condition. Ontologies such as SNOMED-CT (Stearns et al., 2001), Foundational Model of Anatomy (FMA) (Rosse et al., 2003) and Radiology Lexicon (RadLex) (Langlotz, 2006) can be used to solve this problem. UMLS metathesaurus contains around 100 source vocabularies, some in multiple languages. Racoceanu et al. (2006) tried to map the image features and report text features into UMLS concepts. The final index for the case is determined by using the late fusion (weighted vectorial norm fusion) of the indexes according to visual UML concept and the text UML concept. The results show that this type of late semantic combination has increased the Mean Average Precision to 24% as compared to 16% for text only and 10% for image only. Liver lesions image retrieval using semantic similarities in an ontological fashion is investigated in Kurtz et al. (2014). On the similar lines we intend to map the report text into UMLS concept for increasing retrieval accuracy.

A different idea is using text query to guide the CBIR system (Wei et al., 2011). User can give an image query lesion and enter text to describe the lesion (mass, calcification). This text is then used to decide which features to extract from the image (For example shape, sharpness, margin, density for mass and spotsize, spot shape, brightness, contrast for calcification). SVM is used to classify the mammograms into relevant and irrelevant sets.

Another scenario for hybrid, textual and visual queries is proposed in the CBIR2 system (Antani et al., 2002). This system allows automatic segmentation of vertebrae from the spine x-ray images where similarity is based on shape features and the text retrieval using MySQL database for the associated survey data such as age, sex, back pain etc.

A system for using text to search in the metadata such as patient name, gender, age, modality and study date associated with a DICOM image is presented in (El-Kwae et al., 2000). Use of modality information (metadata) from the DICOM file for deciding the feature extraction algorithm is demonstrated in Dicoogle (Valente et al., 2013). It uses two indexes, one to index the metadata in DICOM file and the other to store the image features.

To summarize, fusion of image and text has shown to improve the classification/retrieval performance in multimedia applications. Few radiological systems have tried fusion of the image and associated text. It is possible to utilize correlation between multiple modalities at an early stage using low level fusion. However, it suffers from the curse of dimensionality problem. High level fusion approaches have performed better than text based search. High level fusion is comparatively easier than trying to bridge the semantic gap at feature level. The strength of image re-ranking is to realign the visual system to search in a relevant subset with respect to the semantic viewpoint, while the strength of late fusion relies on a well performing text expert. The cross media similarities attempt to bridge the semantic gap between visual and textual information. Semantic filtering approach (Clinchant et al., 2011) has outperformed other high level fusion and image re-ranking approaches. Moreover, graph based methods have proven to be the state-of-the-art techniques for multimedia retrieval tasks (Zha et al., 2012, Csurka et al., 2014). Graph based techniques take into account the cross media relevance scores thereby reducing the semantic gap and increasing the retrieval performance. Therefore, we intend to use the graph based transmedia pseudo-relevance technique for fusion.

PROPOSED FRAMEWORK

This section describes the proposed methodology in three stages. Stage 1 represents retrieval of radiology images based on *Visual Character N-gram* features; stage 2 details retrieval of associated radiology reports based on UMLS concepts; and stage 3 reveals the fusion approach used for effective case retrieval.

Stage 1: Retrieval by Image Similarity

Mammographic Image Database

The database consists of the mammographic images. The regions of interests are marked and annotated by one of the experienced radiologist at LakeImaging, a Ballarat based imaging facility. The annotations are saved as DICOM presentation state object. The DICOM images are exported into portable grey-map format and stored in our database. The images consist of the following types of cases: Circumscribed lesions, Speculation, Calcification, and Normal.

Image Pre-Processing

In order to calculate the visual N-gram features the mammographic images need to go pre-processing. The pre-processing consists of downscaling, region of interest (ROI) extraction and grey scale reduction as explained below.

Figure 3. Retrieval by image similarity

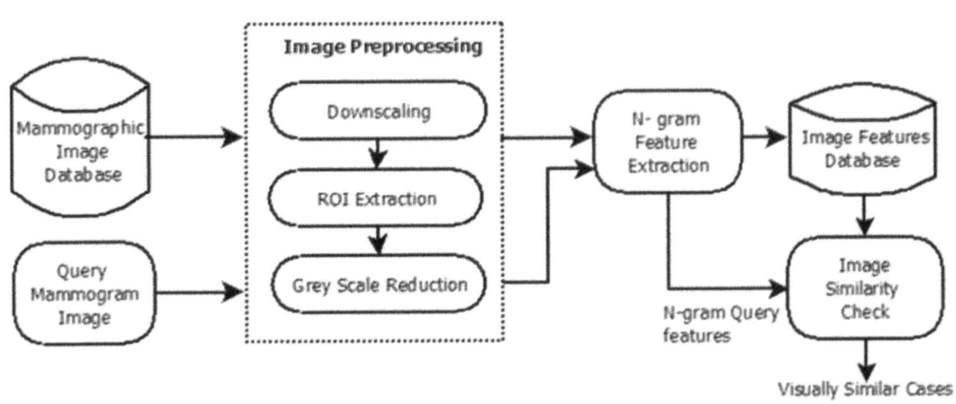

Downscaling

The mammographic images are not of same resolution. In order to have the same resolution of all the images, we decided to scale the images to the lowest resolution image available in the dataset. This downscaling of images is carried out by using Bi-cubic interpolation technique.

Interpolation means using known data to estimate values at unknown points. Grey scale image interpolation works in two directions. It uses the intensities of the surrounding pixels and tries to estimate a best value for a pixel's intensity. There are different rescaling algorithms such as nearest neighbour, bi-linear interpolation, bi-cubic interpolation, spline and sync. Bi-cubic considers the closest 4x4 neighbourhood of known pixels (16 pixels) to estimate the value of unknown pixel. Depending on the distance of the known pixel from the unknown pixel, these intensity values are given different weighting in the calculation. Bi-cubic interpolation produces noticeably sharper images than nearest neighbour and bilinear interpolation technique, and is the ideal combination of processing time and output quality. Also, a recent study shows that detection of masses and clustered microcalcifications on digital mammograms was unaffected by bi-cubic interpolation image reduction (Takane et al., 2013). Therefore, we choose Bi-cubic interpolation technique for downscaling the images.

Region Of Interest (ROI) Extraction

The abnormalities are marked as circles by the experienced radiologist and they are available as DICOM presentation state objects. After downscaling the images, equal sized square regions surrounding the abnormalities are cropped using MATLAB software. These images are called Regions of Interests (ROIs) and are saved in the database. For normal mammograms the same size regions of interest are extracted from the centre of the image.

Grey Scale Reduction

In ROI images each pixel is represented with a grey level between 0 and 255. To reduce computational complexity, the images are reduced to G number of grey level bins. To reduce the images to G number of grey level bins, the ith bin is composed of grey levels illustrated by following equation:

$$Bin_i = (i-1) * binsize \text{ to } (i * binsize) - 1$$

where

$$binsize = \frac{\text{highest grey level - lowest grey level}}{\text{number of bins}}$$

N-Gram Image Representation

The idea of visual character N-grams is inspired from the character N-gram model for text retrieval. Figure 5 describes the process of Visual Character N-gram representation of ROIs. It is achieved in two steps. First step is the creation of the Visual Character N-gram codebooks. All the images are considered

Figure 4. Grey scale reduction using 8 bins

30	55	62	131	140	102	145
28	48	25	75	78	83	58
25	180	200	205	104	108	88
63	196	220	210	99	74	69

Original Image

1	2	2	5	5	4	5
1	2	1	3	3	3	2
1	6	7	7	4	4	3
3	7	8	8	4	3	3

Grey Scale reduced image with 8 bins

Figure 5. Image Representation using visual character N-grams

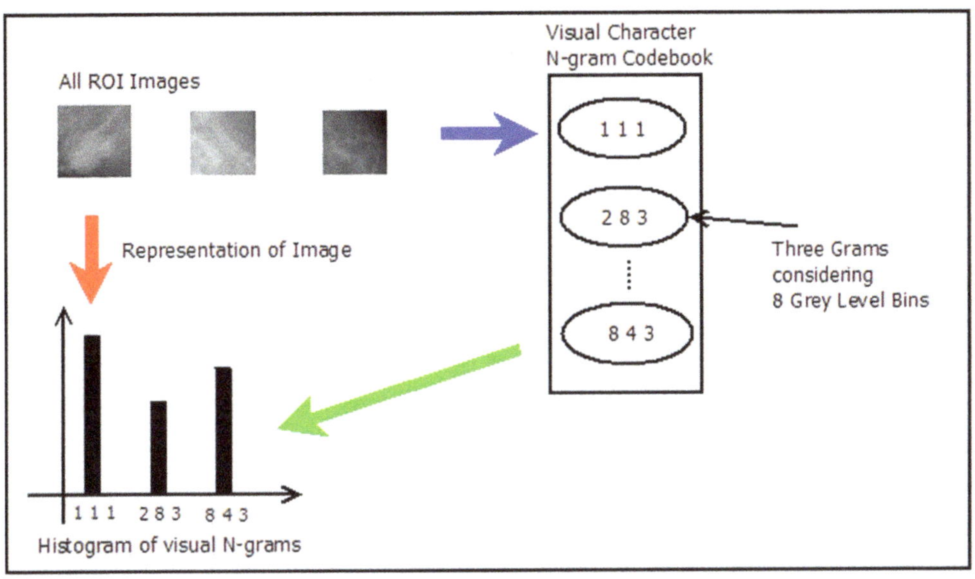

during this step. The Grey scale reduction of ROIs is achieved using 8 grey level bins as explained in the aforementioned section. Each pixel value is considered a visual character. The number of possible phrases is dependent on the grey level bins used to represent the image and can be calculated with the following equation.

$$\text{Num of possible phrases in n gram} = (\text{Num of grey level bins})^n$$

Thus, if we want to use all the possible N-grams then the dimensions of the feature vector get bigger and bigger (for example three grams equal $8^3 = 512$). Moreover, as all the possible N-grams are not necessarily present in the given corpus many of these counts would be zero. This creates a sparse vector problem. In order to solve the sparse vector problem, we would consider the N-grams present in the given corpus by generating the codebook.

As opposed to text document, an image can be read in several different directions (for example, horizontal, vertical or at an angle of θ degrees). For preliminary experiments we strictly followed the text analogy and hence we only considered reading the image in horizontal direction from left to right. For detailed analysis we will consider the N-grams in horizontal (left to right), vertical (top to bottom) and at an angle of 45 degrees (diagonal) directions. Although, N-grams having same order but different orientations convey totally different meanings in case of text, for an image they may correspond to the same pattern. Figure 6 shows three grams of the given image in horizontal and vertical directions. Consider if the image is rotated by 90 degrees then the pattern 4-3-2 explains the distribution of the same pixels which generated the 2-3-4 pattern. Thus we consider these both patterns the same N-gram.

A sliding window of size N characters is used to extract the N-gram codebook. Figure 7 shows the sliding window for calculating three gram features of a ROI in horizontal direction. We consider two, three and four grams for our experiments. Firstly, with the longer sequences the computational complexity increases rapidly and secondly using longer sequences produce large vocabularies and therefore also create sparse feature vector as longer sequences are hard to find. Thus the two gram, three gram and four gram codebooks are generated separately. In the second step using the visual character N-gram codebook, histogram of occurrence of N-grams is calculated for every ROI. The N-gram counts are normalized

Figure 6. Effect of rotation of image on visual character N-grams

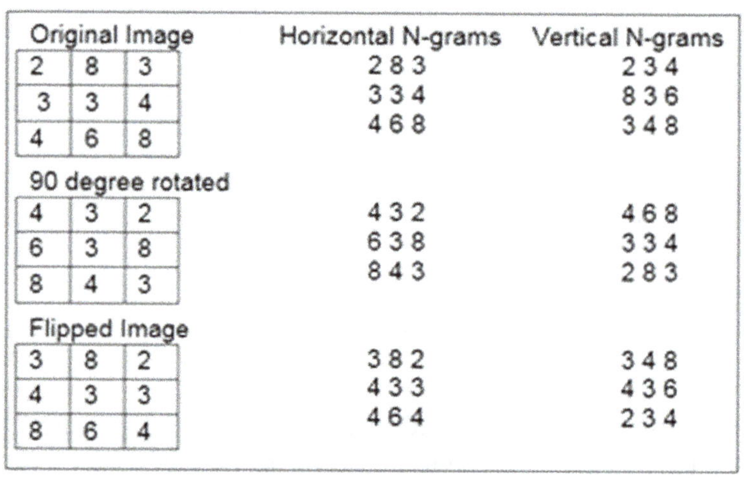

Figure 7. Sliding window for calculating three gram features

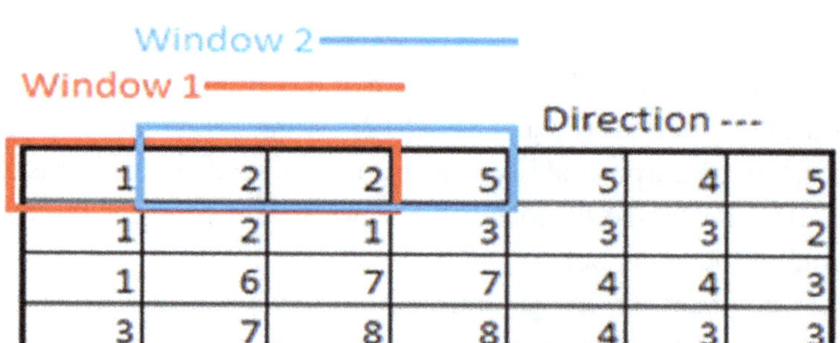

using Term Frequency/Total number of N-gram counts in an image so that they fall in the range of zero to one. These N-gram features are stored in the image features database.

Image Similarity Check

Query mammographic image undergoes the same pre-processing steps (downscaling, ROI extraction, Grey scale reduction). The N-gram features are then calculated for the query ROI. The query image is represented using the N-gram feature vector. The query feature vector is then compared with the feature vectors in the features database for similarity. Image similarity measures are distances between the feature vectors of query image and images in the database. Smaller the distance more similar is the image with the query image. Various distance measures have been used for CBIR such as Euclidean distance, Cityblock distance, Manhattan distance, Cosine similarity measure, Pearsons Correlation Coefficient, Earth Movers distance and Chi-Square distance. The Euclidean distance is simple and most commonly used distance measure for CBIR (Muller et al., 2004). Also according to recent study about similarity measures for breast masses, Euclidean distance has performed quite well (Cho et al., 2011). Therefore, visual similarity score would be calculated using Euclidean distance (Jain et al. 1996). Thus, the first stage of the experiment will retrieve the most similar images by content.

Stage 2: Retrieval by Text Similarity

Figure 8 shows a block diagram of case retrieval by report text similarity. Concept based approach has been adopted as explained below.

Figure 8. Retrieval by text similarity

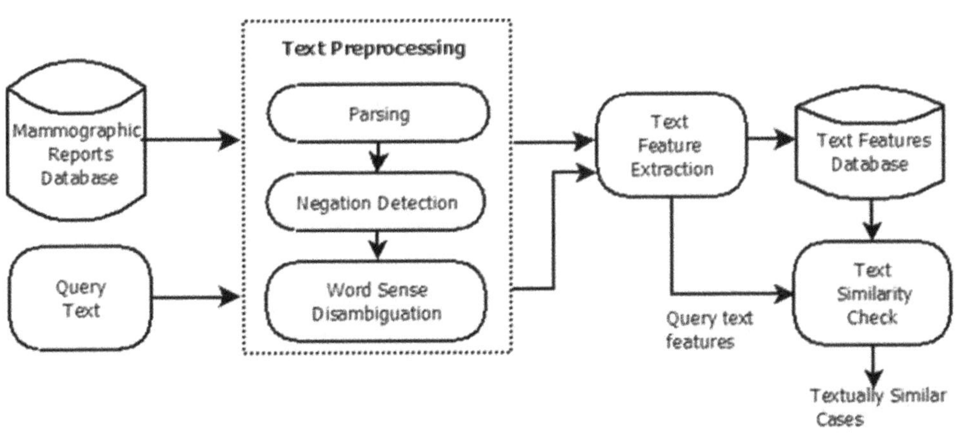

Mammogram Reports Database

The radiology reports (English language) associated with the mammographic images (Image database) are stored in the mammographic reports database. For every image we have an associated mammogram report.

Text Pre-Processing

In order to extract text features, the radiology reports undergo pre-processing steps. The pre-processing includes parsing of reports, negation detection, word sense disambiguation as explained below.

Parsing of Reports

Stop words and other punctuation characters are removed as the first step of parsing the reports. Then the reports are parsed into different sections such as modality, findings, diagnosis, recommendations. Tokenizer separates the text into different tokens and tags them as nouns, pro-nouns, verbs, adjectives, prepositions etc. The phrases are formed by combination of adjacent words that make sense.

Negation Detection

Negation detection is very important in radiology reports as they often contain a multitude of negative and excluded findings. The radiologists usually write phrases such as "no sign of cancer", "no evidence of". Moreover, negations can also represent positive expressions as in "no significant changes". Hence, for our project negation detection is carried out using Wendy Chapman's NegEx algorithm (Chapman et al., 2001).

Word Sense Disambiguation (WSD)

Lexical ambiguity is a fundamental characteristic of a language. Words can have more than one distinct meaning. Word Sense Disambiguation is determining the meaning of every word in the context. This is also a very important step in retrieval of radiology reports. The word sense disambiguation is achieved by using the Journal Descriptor Indexing (JDI) algorithm (Humphrey et al. 2006).

Text Feature Extraction

The text phrases are mapped to the UMLS concepts. The UMLS is developed by U.S. National Library of Medicine (NLM) and it includes the Metathesaurus, the Specialist Lexicon and Semantic Network. The Metathesaurus is organized by concept, and each concept has specific attributes defining its meaning and is linked to the corresponding concept names in the various source vocabularies (for example SNOMED CT, MeSH). Each concept in the Metathesaurus is assigned one or more categories, which are linked with one another through *semantic relationships.* The Semantic Network is a catalog of these semantic types and relationships. The Specialist Lexicon contains information about common English vocabulary, biomedical terms, terms found in the UMLS Metathesaurus.

While retrieving text we only consider two scenarios:

- Radiologist is interested in searching for a similar past case(s) based on specific clinical finding.
- Radiologist is interested in searching for a similar past case(s) based on specific diagnosis.

Therefore, only pathology UML concepts such as [Acquired Abnormality, Disease or Syndrome] are extracted. The text features of the report consist of a UML pathology concept and their frequencies. These text features are stored in the text features database. These text features will be extracted using readily available software called METAMAP.

METAMAP is software developed by the NLM. It maps biomedical text to concepts from UMLS. It supports parsing, Negation Detection based on NegEx algorithm (Chapman et al., 2001) and Word Sense Disambiguation based on JDI (Humphrey et al., 2006). Following is an example of how METAMAP software maps a phrase into a concept.

- **Phrase:** “lung cancer.”
- Meta Candidates (8):
- 1000 Lung Cancer (Malignant neoplasm of lung) [Neoplastic Process]
- 1000 Lung Cancer (Carcinoma of lung) [Neoplastic Process]
- 861 Cancer (Malignant Neoplasms) [Neoplastic Process]
- 861 Lung [Body Part, Organ, or Organ Component]
- 861 Cancer (Cancer Genus) [Invertebrate]
- 861 Lung (Entire lung) [Body Part, Organ, or Organ Component]
- 861 Cancer (Specialty Type - cancer) [Biomedical Occupation or Discipline]
- 768 Pneumonia [Disease or Syndrome]
- Meta Mapping (1000):
- 1000 Lung Cancer (Carcinoma of lung) [Neoplastic Process]
- Meta Mapping (1000):
- 1000 Lung Cancer (Malignant neoplasm of lung) [Neoplastic Process]

Text Similarity Check

The text query undergoes the same text pre-processing steps including parsing, negation detection and word sense disambiguation. Then the pathology UML concepts and the corresponding frequencies are obtained using Metamap software. The query text features are then compared with the corresponding text features of report in the database to calculate textual similarity. Again a simple Euclidean distance measure is employed for similarity calculation.

Stage 3: Fusion of CBIR and Text for Similar Case Retrieval

As depicted in the literature review section, the graph based techniques have been working better than low level and high level fusion approaches for multimedia datasets. Also, it is difficult to achieve low level fusion due to the curse of dimensionality problem. We therefore focus on graph based transmedia fusion technique for mammographic case retrieval. Our technique uses graphs to calculate the cross-media similarities inspired by the work of Csurka et al. (2014).

First, let us consider there is n number of cases in the database. We calculate the visual similarity matrix S_v between pairs of images (size n × n) and the textual similarity matrix S_t between pairs of reports (size n × n). Then we calculate the textual similarity between query text and the reports in the database S_{tq} (size 1 × n) and the visual similarity between query image and the images in the database S_{vq} (size 1 × n).

Given a text query q_t, we find the most similar cases according to the textual similarity. We then consider the set of k nearest neighbours as pseudo-relevant cases. The visual parts of these pseudo-relevant cases can thus feedback the visual retrieval process. Taking this pseudo relevance feedback, cross media similarity S_{tv} can be calculated as dot product of two similarity matrices as follows:

$$S_{tv} = S_{tq} . S_v$$

Where the similarity scores in matrix S_{tq} are replaced by zero where these values are lower than the kth highest score. Thus the cross media similarity of Ith case C_i with respect to query case C_q using text query first can be calculated as

$$CMtv = \sum_1^k (S_t(q,i).S_v(i,k))$$

(refer to Figure 9)

Similarly, in the next step given a visual query q_v, we find the most similar cases according to visual similarity. Again, the set of k nearest neighbours are considered as pseudo-relevant cases. Now the text part of the pseudo relevant cases act as feedback for the text retrieval process. This propagation of visual

Figure 9. Cross media similarity calculation using text query first (k =3)

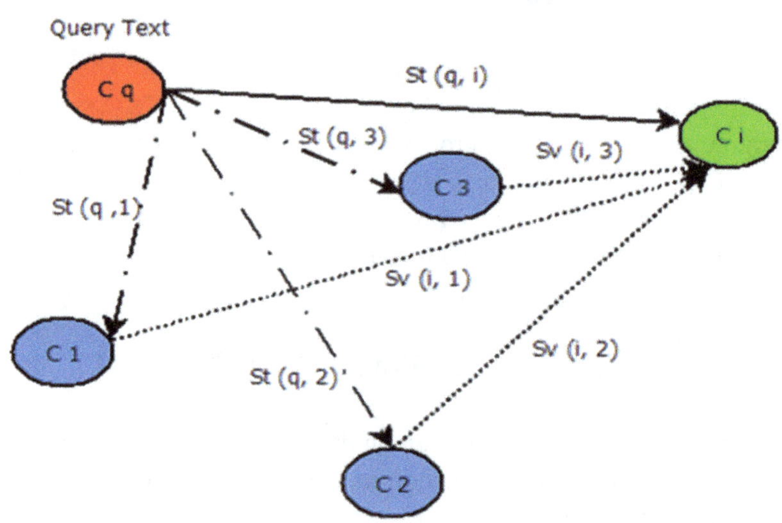

similarities to textual similarities can be achieved by calculating the cross-media similarity score S_{vt} as follows:

$$S_{vt} = S_{vq}.S_t$$

Where the similarity scores in matrix S_{vq} are replaced by zero if these are lower than k^{th} highest score. Thus the cross media similarity of Ith case C_i with respect to query case C_q using image query first can be calculated as:

$$CMvt = \sum_1^k (S_v(q,i).S_t(i,k))$$

(refer to Figure 10)

The final similarity score matrix for cases in the database against a query case can then be calculated by combining textual similarity matrix, visual similarity matrix and the cross-media similarity matrices as follows:

$$S_{case} = W_t S_{tq} + W_v S_{vq} + W_{tv} S_{tv} + W_{vt} S_{vt}$$

where the $W_t + W_v + W_{tv} + W_{vt} = 1$

The cases are then presented with the descending order of final similarity score. Thus the inter-media feedback mechanism is achieved by working at the similarities levels rather than trying to bridge the semantic gap at the feature level.

Figure 10. Cross media similarity calculation using Image query first (k=3)

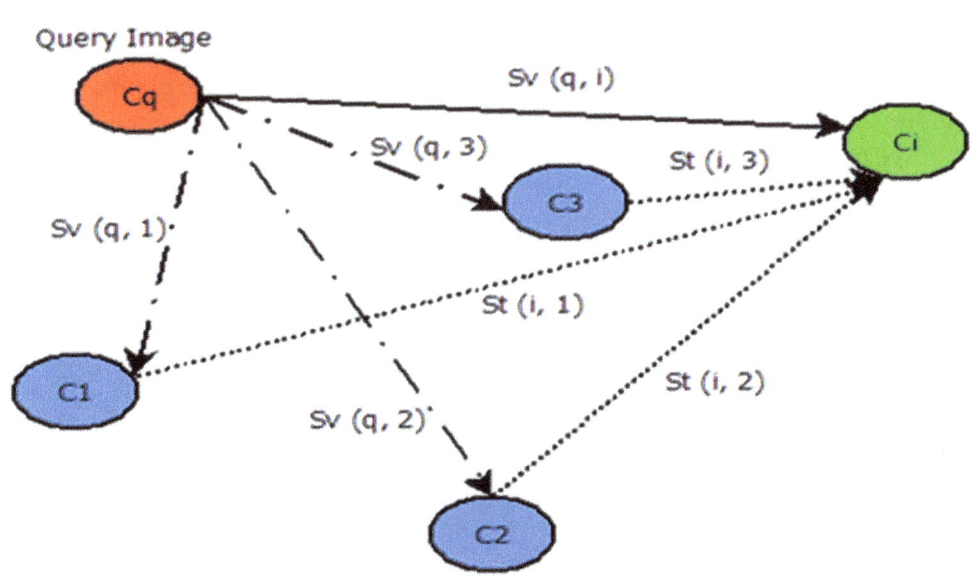

EXPERIMENTAL SET UPS AND EVALUATION TECHNIQUES

Dataset for Experiments

Lake Imaging provides a comprehensive radiology service, by means of referrals from Doctors and allied health professionals, using innovative infrastructure, systems and procedures to deliver industry leading patient care, clinical outcomes and business efficiencies. LakeImaging, Ballarat has agreed to provide us non-identifiable radiology images and their associated radiology reports for this project. The images would be annotated by an experienced radiologist and are provided as DICOM presentation state files. Use of pre-existing data from Lakeimaging is approved by the Ethics committee of Federation University.

Experiment 1

Hypothesis: Three gram features are at least as accurate as any other n-gram features for classification of mammograms.

For this experiment the dataset consist of 120 mammograms annotated by the radiologist into circumscribed lesion (20), Speculation (20), Calcification (20), and Normal (60).

All the images are downsized using bi-cubic interpolation technique. The regions of interests (ROI) are extracted from the images and reduced to 8 grey levels for ease of computation. The three gram features are then calculated for every region of interest. There would be $8^3 = 512$ three gram features for every ROI. The normalized three gram features are fed to the neural network for classification. The neural network is trained using 90 ROIs such that the training data contains ¾ th of the number of each category of images (for example for circumscribed ¾ of 20 = 15, for normal ¾ of 60 = 45). The remaining 30 ROI's are used for testing and the classification accuracy is calculated. In the next step 90 different ROI's are used for training and the remaining 30 are used for testing. This process is repeated five times and the average classification accuracy is noted.

The same process of five-fold cross validation is repeated for one gram, two gram, four gram and five gram features. The classification accuracy is noted each time. The error for each ROI is also recorded for 'T Test of significance' every time. The classification accuracy with three gram features is then compared with the classification accuracy using one gram, two gram, four gram and five gram features. Similarly the error with the three gram representation is compared with error while using one gram, two gram, four gram and five gram representation

Experiment 2

Hypothesis: A Neural network based classifier is more accurate than SVM for classification of mammograms using three gram features.

For this experiment the dataset consist of 120 mammograms annotated by the radiologist into circumscribed lesion (20), Speculation (20), Calcification (20), and Normal (60).

Three gram feature for all the 120 ROIs are calculated and stored in the database. Firstly, the back propagation neural network is used for classification of ROI's into four different categories. The three gram features are used as inputs of the neural network classifier. A supervised learning strategy with five-fold cross-validation technique is used to calculate the classification accuracy. The average classification accuracy is noted.

Secondly, the same three gram features are applied as inputs to SVM. Again, the five-fold cross validation technique is used to calculate the classification accuracy. The average classification accuracy is noted. The error of each ROI is noted in both cases. The classification accuracies are then compared. The errors are then compared using T test of significance.

Experiment 3

Hypothesis: Three gram based image classification is at least as accurate as classification based on co-occurrence matrix features.

Three gram features are calculated for all the 120 mammograms. These three gram features are then normalized and used as input to the neural network for classification into four categories (circumscribed lesion, speculation, calcification, normal). Five-fold cross-validation technique is used for reporting the average classification accuracy.

Co-occurrence matrix features based on adjacency distance of one in four different directions (0, 45, 90, 135 degrees) are used for classification of mammograms into four different categories using neural network. The average classification accuracy is again noted for this case.The average classification accuracies using three gram features and co-occurrence based features are then compared.

Experiment 4

Hypothesis: N-grams are computationally less expensive than co-occurrence based features.

Regions of interests of three different sizes are considered. The time required to calculate N-gram features is noted and plotted as a function of N. Similarly, for the same three sizes of ROIs time required to calculate the co-occurrence based features is noted and plotted against N. By analysing these two graphs (Linear, squared, exponential) computational complexity of the two feature extraction techniques will be compared.

Experiment 5

Hypothesis: Three-gram based image matching is accurate for matching circumscribed lesion, speculation lesion, calcification and normal mammographic images.

For this experiment the dataset consist of 120 mammograms annotated by the radiologist into Circumscribed lesion (20), Speculation (20), Calcification (20), and Normal (60).

All the images are downsized using bi-cubic interpolation technique. The regions of interests are extracted from the images and reduced to 8 grey levels for ease of computation. The three gram features are then calculated for every region of interest. There would be $8^3 = 512$ three gram features for every ROI. The normalized three gram features are used to classify the images into four different categories (circumscribed lesion, Speculation, calcification, normal) using trained ANN classifier. When the query ROI is given, the three-gram features of the query ROI are calculated and used to determine the class of the ROI. Euclidean distance is used for calculating the distance between the query ROI and the ROIs in the database. The images are ranked in the ascending order of the similarity distance. Precision and Recall are calculated for each query image and the F-score is used as a measure of accuracy.

Average precision is the area under the precision- recall curve. The mean average precision for set of queries is calculated as mean of averaged precision scores for each query.

Experiment 6

Hypothesis: Text retrieval using ontologies enhance the accuracy of image retrieval.

For this experiment, the dataset consist of the 120 mammograms of four different categories and the corresponding radiology reports.

Three-gram features are calculated from the ROIs of 120 images and stored in the database. Euclidean distance is used for determining similarity between the query image and images in the database. Precision, Recall and F-score are noted.

The reports are parsed to acquire the phrases. The negation detection and mapping with the UMLS (meta-thesaurus) concept is achieved using Metamap software developed by NLM. The concept and its frequency are used as the text features. These features are used to calculate the similarity between the query text and the reports in the dataset. The final similarity score is calculated by using graph based transmedia pseudo-relevance technique described in the introduction section.

Axis 1: Show me the lesion that looks similar but have different clinical features

With the help of Dr. Manish Mittal (Senior Radiologists) several queries consisting of an image and keywords are formed to test this scenario. Precision, Recall and F-score is noted down. The ROI's annotations for the clinical feature are used to verify which results are relevant to the query. The average precision, recall and F-score are then calculated for all the queries.

Axis 2: Show me the lesion that looks similar but have different diagnosis

Again several queries are formed to test this scenario. The queries consist of region of interest and keywords representing possible diagnosis. The annotations from the expert about the disease are used for verification of relevant results. Precision, Recall and F-score are noted down. The average precision, recall and F-score are then calculated.

For both the scenarios the precision, recall and the F-score is compared with the same obtained by using image only retrieval.

Experiment 7

Hypothesis: Graph based trans-media fusion performs better than high level fusion.

For this experiment, the dataset consist of the 120 mammograms of four different categories and the corresponding radiology reports. The image and report similarity is calculated in a similar way mentioned in experiment 5. The high level fusion approach is used to calculate final similarity and rank the cases.

The precision, recall and retrieval accuracy is noted for each query. In the second part the graph based transmedia pseudo-relevance feedback technique is used to calculate the final similarity. The precision, recall and retrieval accuracy is again noted for each query. The retrieval accuracies using two fusion techniques are then compared.

EVALUATION TECHNIQUES

Quantitative Evaluation Measures

For evaluating the performance of the classification stage of our CBIR we will use the precision, recall and the classification accuracy for each class. The confusion matrix for the circumscribed lesion is shown in Table 2. The average classification accuracy is then noted as overall classification accuracy.

In information retrieval, precision and recall are the most commonly used evaluation measures. Usually these are presented as precision versus recall curve/graph (Salton, 1971):-

$$\text{Precision}=\frac{\text{No. of relevant documents or images retrieved}}{\text{Total number of documents or images retrieved}}$$

$$\text{Recall}=\frac{\text{No. of relevant documents or images retrieved}}{\text{Total number of relevant documents or images in the collection}}$$

We will be using the precision recall curve to evaluate our text based, image based and combined retrieval system. The area under the curve will be used to calculate the average precision. Mean Average Precision (MAP) for query collection is the arithmetic average of average precisions for each query and it summarizes ranking from multiple queries.

Table 2. Confusion matrix and evaluation measures for circumscribed lesion class

		Actual Output		
		Circumscribed lesion	**Other**	
Predicted output	Circumscribed lesion	True positive	False positive	Precision $=\frac{\text{True positive}}{\text{True positive}+\text{False positive}}$
	Other	False negative	True negative	
		Recall or sensitivity $=\frac{\text{True positive}}{\text{True positive}+\text{False negative}}$		Accuracy $=\frac{\text{Precision}\times\text{Recall}}{\text{Precision}+\text{Recall}}$

Accuracy of our retrieval system would be measured using F-score value. The traditional F-measure or balanced F-score (F1 score) is the harmonic mean of precision and recall. It can be interpreted as a weighted average of the precision and recall. The F1 score reaches its best value at 1 and worst score at 0 and is calculated as:

$$F1 = 2 \times \frac{\text{precision} \times \text{recall}}{\text{precision} + \text{recall}}$$

Qualitative Evaluation Measures

We would be allowing online access to our system to a group of two less experienced and two experienced radiologists. We will get them to describe their feedback regarding the system. The following open questions would be used to guide and analyse the feedback. The merits and demerits of using our system would then be summarized and used for future research.

- How useful do you think the system is for diagnosis?
- Do you think the system will be useful in increasing your confidence level while diagnosing? How?
- Do you think the system will help increase the diagnostic accuracy?
- How do you think the system is helpful in saving some time and increasing your diagnostic throughput?
- How useful was the system in improving your radiology report?
- How user friendly is the system?
- How accurately do you think the system retrieved the desired images?
- Did the system created ambiguity in some cases or increased confusion in diagnosis? What are these?

CONCLUSION

This chapter has proposed a Content-based Image Retrieval approach to assist radiologist for the improvement in diagnosis. It is important to retrieve accurate information based on textual and image queries. Image and textual queries are expressed at different semantic levels, therefore it is a challenging task to correlate both representations in order to satisfy the information need of a user. The appropriate fusion of text and image content has been found to be more effective than using purely text or visual content separately. The proposed framework is divided in three stages, Stage 1 was represented for retrieval of radiology images based on Visual Character N-gram features; stage 2 has provided details the retrieval of associated radiology reports based on UMLS concepts; and stage 3 detailed the fusion approach used for effective case retrieval. In transmedia fusion or re-ranking is used one of the modalities either text or image and then use the other modality. Cross media similarity is calculated using image query and text query. The final similarity score matrix for cases in the database against a query case can then be calculated by combining textual similarity matrix, visual similarity matrix and the cross-media similarity matrices. Various experiments are proposed for checking the retrieval of the similar cases and system will be evaluated using quantitative and qualitative approaches.

REFERENCES

Ah-Pine, J., Bressan, M., Clinchant, S., Csurka, G., Hoppenot, Y., & Renders, J. (2009). Crossing Textual and Visual content in different application scenarios. *Multimedia Tools and Applications*, *42*(1), 31–56. doi:10.1007/s11042-008-0246-8

Aisen, M., Broderick, L., Winer-Muram, H., Brodley, C., Kak, A., Pavlopoulou, C., & Marchori, A. et al. (2003). Automated Storage and Retrieval of thin-section CT images to assist diagnosis:System description and Preliminary Assessment. *Radiology*, *228*(1), 265–270. doi:10.1148/radiol.2281020126 PMID:12832587

Akgül, C., Rubin, D., Napel, S., Beaulieu, C., Greenspan, H., & Acar, B. (2011). Content-based image retrieval in radiology: Current status and future directions. *Journal of Digital Imaging*, *24*(2), 208–222. doi:10.1007/s10278-010-9290-9 PMID:20376525

Antani, S., Lee, D., Long, L., & Thoma, G. (2004). Evaluation of shape similarity measurement methods for spine X-ray images. *Journal of Visual Communication and Image Representation*, *15*(3), 285–302. doi:10.1016/j.jvcir.2004.04.005

Aronson, A. (2006). Metamap: Mapping text to the UMLS metathesaurus. Bethesda, MD: NLM, NIH, DHHS.

Atrey, P., Hossain, M., El Saddik, A., & Kankanhalli, M. (2010). Multimodal fusion for multimedia analysis: A survey. *Multimedia Systems*, *16*(6), 345–379. doi:10.1007/s00530-010-0182-0

Avni, U., Greenspan, H., Konen, E., Sharon, M., & Goldberger, J. (2011). X-ray categorization and retrieval on the organ and pathology level, using patch- based visual words. *IEEE Transactions on Medical Imaging*, *30*(3), 733–746. doi:10.1109/TMI.2010.2095026 PMID:21118769

Bach, J., Fuller, C., Gupta, A., Hampapur, A., Horowitz, B., Humphrey, R., & Shu, C. (1996, March). Virage image search engine: An open framework for image management. In Electronic Imaging: Science & Technology (pp. 76-87). International Society for Optics and Photonics.

Berber, T., & Alpkoc¸ak, A. (2009). DEU at ImageCLEFmed 2009: Evaluating re–ranking and integrated retrieval model. Working Notes of CLEF 2009.

Benavent, J., Benavent, X., de Ves, E., Granados, R., & García-Serrano, A. (2010). Experiences at ImageCLEF 2010 using CBIR and TBIR Mixing Information Approaches. CLEF (Notebook Papers/LABs/Workshops).

Besancon, R., & Millet, C. (2005). Merging results from different media: Lic2m experiments at ImageCLEF 2005. *Cross Language Evaluation Forum 2005 Workshop.*

Caicedo, J., Cruz, A., & Gonzalez, F. (2009). Histopathology image classification using bag of features and kernel functions. In *Artificial Intelligence in Medicine* (pp. 126–135). Berlin: Springer. doi:10.1007/978-3-642-02976-9_17

Caritá, E., Seraphim, E., Honda, M., & Azevedo-Marques, P. (2008). Implementation and evaluation of a medical image management system with content-based retrieval support. *Radiologia Brasileira*, *41*(5), 331–336.

Carpineto, C., & Romano, G. (2012). A survey of automatic query expansion in information retrieval. *ACM Computing Surveys*, *44*(1), 1–23. doi:10.1145/2071389.2071390

Chandy, D., Johnson, J., & Selvan, S. (2013). Texture feature extraction using gray level statistical matrix for content-based mammogram retrieval. *Multimedia Tools and Applications*, 1–14.

Chapman, W., Bridewell, W., Hanbury, P., Cooper, G., & Buchanan, B. (2001). A simple algorithm for identifying negated findings and diseases in discharge summaries. *Journal of Biomedical Informatics*, *34*(5), 301–310. doi:10.1006/jbin.2001.1029 PMID:12123149

Cheng, P., Chien, B., Ke, H., & Yang, W. (2005). NCTU-DBLAB@ImageCLEFmed 2005: Automatic annotation task. Working Notes of CLEF 2005.

Chevallet, J., Lim, J., Radhouani, S., & France, C. (2005). *Using ontology dimensions and negative expansion to solve precise queries in clef medical task*. Vienna, Austria: CLEF Workhop, Working Notes Medical Image Track.

Cho, H., Hadjiiski, L., Sahiner, B., Chan, H., Helvie, M., Paramagul, C., & Nees, A. (2011). Similarity evaluation in a content-based image retrieval (CBIR) CADx system for characterization of breast masses on ultrasound images. *Medical Physics*, *38*(4), 1820–1831. doi:10.1118/1.3560877 PMID:21626916

Chu, S., & Cesnik, B. (2001). Knowledge representation and retrieval using conceptual graphs and free text document self-organisation techniques. *International Journal of Medical Informatics*, *62*(2-3), 121–133. doi:10.1016/S1386-5056(01)00156-3 PMID:11470615

Clinchant, S., Renders, J., & Csurka, G. (2007). XRCE's Participation to ImageCLEFphoto 2007. *Working Notes of the CLEFWorkshop*.

Clinchant, S., Ah-Pine, J., & Csurka, G. (2011, April). Semantic combination of textual and visual information in multimedia retrieval. In *Proceedings of the 1st ACM International Conference on Multimedia Retrieval* (p. 44). ACM. doi:10.1145/1991996.1992040

Cohn, A., Miller, P., Fisher, P., Mutalik, P., & Swett, H. (1990). Knowledge-based radiologic image retrieval using axes of clinical relevance. *Computers and Biomedical Research, an International Journal*, *23*(3), 199–221. doi:10.1016/0010-4809(90)90017-7 PMID:2350958

Csurka, G., Ah-Pine, J., & Clinchant, S. (2014). *Unsupervised Visual and Textual Information Fusion in Multimedia Retrieval-A Graph-based Point of View*. arXiv preprint arXiv:1401.6891

Dang, P., Kalra, M., Schultz, T., Graham, S., & Dreyer, K. (2009). Informatics in radiology: Render: An online searchable radiology study repository. *Radiographics*, *29*(5), 1233–1246. doi:10.1148/rg.295085036 PMID:19564253

Datta, R., Joshi, D., Li, J., & Wang, J. (2008). Image retrieval: Ideas, Influences, and trends of the new age. *ACM Computing Surveys*, *40*(2), 1–60. doi:10.1145/1348246.1348248

de Herrera, A., Kalpathy–Cramer, J., Demner-Fushman, D., Antani, S., & Müller, H. (2013). Overview of the ImageCLEF 2013 medical tasks. *Working Notes of CLEF*.

Demner-Fushman, D., Chapman, W., & McDonald, C. (2009). What can natural language processing do for clinical decision support? *Journal of Biomedical Informatics*, *42*(5), 760–772. doi:10.1016/j.jbi.2009.08.007 PMID:19683066

Deng, Y., & Manjunath, B. (2001). Unsupervised segmentation of color-texture regions in images and video. *IEEE Transactions on Pattern Analysis and Machine Intelligence*, *23*(8), 800–810. doi:10.1109/34.946985

Depeursinge, A., & Müller, H. (2010). Fusion techniques for combining textual and visual information retrieval. In *ImageCLEF* (pp. 95–114). Berlin: Springer. doi:10.1007/978-3-642-15181-1_6

Depeursinge, A., Racoceanu, D., Iavindrasana, J., Cohen, G., Platon, A., Poletti, P., & Müller, H. (2010). Fusing visual and clinical information for lung tissue classification in HRCT data. *Artificial Intelligence in Medicine*. doi:10.1016/j.artmed.2010.04.006

Depeursinge, A., Vargas, A., Gaillard, F., Platon, A., Geissbuhler, A., Poletti, P., & Müller, H. (2011). Case-based lung image categorization and retrieval for interstitial lung diseases: Clinical workflows. *International Journal of Computer Assisted Radiology and Surgery*, *7*(1), 97–110. doi:10.1007/s11548-011-0618-9 PMID:21629982

Deselaers, T., Weyand, T., Keysers, D., Macherey, W., & Ney, H. (2005). FIRE in ImageCLEF 2005: Combining content–based image retrieval with textual information retrieval. *Working Notes of the CLEF Workshop*.

Deselaers, T., Weyand, T., & Ney, H. (2006). Image retrieval and annotation using maximum entropy. Working Notes of CLEF 2006.

Deselaers, T., Gass, T., Weyand, T., & Ney, H. (2007). FIRE in ImageCLEF 2007. Working Notes of CLEF 2007.

Eakins, J. P. (2002). Towards intelligent image retrieval. *Pattern Recognition*, *35*(1), 3–14. doi:10.1016/S0031-3203(01)00038-3

El-Kwae, E., Xu, H., & Kabuka, M. (2000). Content-based retrieval in picture archiving and communication systems. *Journal of Digital Imaging*, *13*(2), 70–81. doi:10.1007/BF03168371 PMID:10843252

Endo, M., Aramaki, T., Asakura, K., Moriguchi, M., Akimaru, M., Osawa, A., & Yamaguchi, K. (2012). Content-based image- retrieval system in chest computed tomography for a solitary pulmonary nodule: Method and preliminary experiments. *International Journal of Computer Assisted Radiology and Surgery*, *7*(2), 331–338. doi:10.1007/s11548-011-0668-z PMID:22258753

Escalante, H., González, J., Hernández, C., López, A., Montes, M., Morales, E., & Villasenor, L. (2008, September). TIA-INAOE's Participation at ImageCLEF 2008. *Working Notes of the CLEF 2008 Workshop*.

Fakeri-Tabrizi, A., Amini, M., Tollari, S., & Gallinari, P. (2008). *UPMC/LIP6 at ImageCLEF's WikipediaMM: An image–annotation model for an image search–engine. Working Notes of CLEF.*

Ferecatu, M., & Sahbi, H. (2008, September). TELECOM ParisTech at ImageClefphoto 2008: Bi-modal text and image retrieval with diversity enhancement. Working Notes for the CLEF 2008 Workshop.

Fischer, B., Welter, P., Günther, R., & Deserno, T. (2012). Web-based bone age assessment by content-based image retrieval for case-based reasoning. *International Journal of Computer Assisted Radiology and Surgery*, *7*(3), 389–399. doi:10.1007/s11548-011-0627-8 PMID:21671096

Flickner, M., Sawhney, H., Niblack, W., Ashley, J., Huang, Q., Dom, B., & Yanker, P. (1995). Query by image and video content: The QBIC system. *Computer*, *28*(9), 23–32. doi:10.1109/2.410146

Florea, F., Rogozan, A., Cornea, V., Bensrhair, A., & Darmoni, S. (2006, September). MedIC/CISMeF at ImageCLEF 2006: Image annotation and retrieval tasks. *Working Notes of the 2006 CLEF Workshop.*

Friedman, C. (2005). Semantic text parsing for patient records. *Medical Informatics*, *8*, 423–448.

Friedman, C., & Elhadad, N. (2014). Natural language processing in health care and biomedicine. In Biomedical. Informatics: Computer Applications in Health Care and Biomedicine. Springer London. doi:10.1007/978-1-4471-4474-8_8

Gerstmair, A., Daumke, P., Simon, K., Langer, M., & Kotter, E. (2012). Intelligent image retrieval based on radiology reports. *European Radiology*, *22*(12), 2750–2758. doi:10.1007/s00330-012-2608-x PMID:22865274

Ghosh, P., Antani, S., Rodney, L., & Thoma, G. (2011). Review of medical Image retrieval systems and future. *Computer Based Medical Systems*, *24*, 1–6. doi:10.1109/CBMS.2011.5999142

Gobeill, J., Müller, H., & Ruch, P. (2006). *Query and document translation by automatic text categorization: A simple approach to establish a strong textual baseline for ImageCLEFmed 2006. ImageCLEF Working Notes.*

Haralick, R., Shanmugam, K., & Dinstein, I. (1973). Textural features for image classification. *IEEE Transactions on Systems, Man, and Cybernetics*, *3*(6), 610–621. doi:10.1109/TSMC.1973.4309314

Hermitage Museum. (2003). *QBIC colour and layout searches.* Retrieved from http://www.hermitagemuseum.org/fcgi-bin/db2www/qbicSearch.mac/qbic?selLang=English

Hersh, W., & Hickam, D. (1995). Information retrieval in medicine: The SAPHIRE experience. *JASIS*, *46*(10), 743–747. doi:10.1002/(SICI)1097-4571(199512)46:10<743::AID-ASI5>3.0.CO;2-C PMID:8591469

Ho, T., Hull, J., & Srihari, S. (1994). Decision combination in multiple classifier systems. *IEEE Transactions on Pattern Analysis and Machine Intelligence*, *16*(1), 66–75. doi:10.1109/34.273716

Horsch, K., Giger, M., Vyborny, C., Lan, L., Mendelson, E., & Hendrick, R. (2006). Classification of breast lesions with multimodality computer-aided diagnosis: Observer study results on an independent clinical data set 1. *Radiology*, *240*(2), 357–368. doi:10.1148/radiol.2401050208 PMID:16864666

Houston, A., Chen, H., Schatz, B., Hubbard, S., Sewell, R., & Ng, T. (2000). Exploring the use of concept spaces to improve medical information retrieval. *Decision Support Systems*, *30*(2), 171–186. doi:10.1016/S0167-9236(00)00097-X

Huang, H., Nielsen, J., Nelson, M., & Liu, L. (2005). Image-matching as a medical diagnostic support tool (DST) for brain diseases in children. *Computerized Medical Imaging and Graphics*, *29*(2), 195–202. doi:10.1016/j.compmedimag.2004.09.008 PMID:15755537

Humphrey, S., Rogers, W., Kilicoglu, H., Demner-Fushman, D., & Rindflesch, T. (2006). Word sense disambiguation by selecting the best semantic type based on Journal Descriptor Indexing: Preliminary experiment. *Journal of the American Society for Information Science and Technology*, *57*(1), 96–113. doi:10.1002/asi.20257 PMID:19890434

Hussain, M., Khan, S., Muhammad, G., Berbar, M., & Bebis, G. (2012, July). Mass detection in digital mammograms using gabor filter bank. *IET Conference on Image Processing (IPR 2012)*, 1-5. doi:10.1049/cp.2012.0465

Hwang, K., Lee, H., & Choi, D. (2012). Medical image retrieval: Past and present. *Healthcare Informatics Research*, *18*(1), 3–9. doi:10.4258/hir.2012.18.1.3 PMID:22509468

Inkpen, D., Stogaitis, M., DeGuire, F., & Alzghool, M. (2009). Clustering for photo retrieval at Image CLEF 2008. In *Evaluating Systems for Multilingual and Multimodal Information Access* (pp. 685–690). Berlin: Springer. doi:10.1007/978-3-642-04447-2_86

Jain, A., & Vailaya, A. (1996). Image retrieval using color and shape. *Pattern Recognition*, *29*(8), 1233–1244. doi:10.1016/0031-3203(95)00160-3

Jeon, J., Lavrenko, V., & Manmatha, R. (2003, July). Automatic image annotation and retrieval using cross-media relevance models. In *Proceedings of the 26th annual international ACM SIGIR conference on Research and development in informaion retrieval* (pp. 119-126). ACM. doi:10.1145/860435.860459

Jégou, H., Douze, M., & Schmid, C. (2010). Improving bag-of-features for large scale image search. *International Journal of Computer Vision*, *87*(3), 316–336. doi:10.1007/s11263-009-0285-2

Jones, G., Groves, D., Khasin, A., Lam-Adesina, A., Mellebeek, B., & Way, A. (2005). Dublin City University at CLEF 2004: Experiments with the ImageCLEF St. Andrew's Collection. In *Multilingual Information Access for Text, Speech and Images* (pp. 653–663). Berlin: Springer. doi:10.1007/11519645_64

Kanaris, I., Kanaris, K., Houvardas, I., & Stamatatos, E. (2007). Words versus character n-grams for anti-spam filtering. *International Journal of Artificial Intelligence Tools*, *16*(06), 1047–1067. doi:10.1142/S0218213007003692

Kelly, P., Cannon, T., & Hush, D. (1995). Query by image example: the CANDID approach. *SPIE 2420 Storage and Retrieval for Image and Video Databases III*, 238-248. doi:.10.1117/12.205289

Keysers, D., Dahmen, J., Ney, H., Wein, B. B., & Lehmann, T. M. (2003). Statistical framework for model-based image retrieval in medical applications. *Journal of Electronic Imaging*, *12*(1), 59–68. doi:10.1117/1.1525790

Kludas, J., Bruno, E., & Marchand-Maillet, S. (2008). Information fusion in multimedia information retrieval. In *Adaptive Multimedial Retrieval: Retrieval, User, and Semantics* (pp. 147–159). Berlin: Springer. doi:10.1007/978-3-540-79860-6_12

Kulkarni, P., Stranieri, A., Kulkarni, S., Ugon, J., & Mittal, M. (2014a, February). Hybrid technique based on n-gram and neural networks for classification of mammographic images. *Second International Conference on Signal, Image Processing and Pattern Recognition*, 297–306. doi:10.5121/csit.2014.4225

Kulkarni, P., Stranieri, A., Kulkarni, S., Ugon, J., & Mittal, M. (2014b, April). Visual character n-grams for classification and retrieval of radiological images. *International Journal of Multimedia and its Applications*, *6*(2), 35-49

Kulkarni, S., & Verma, B. (2003, September). Fuzzy logic based texture queries for CBIR. *Proceedings of Fifth International Conference on Computational Intelligence and Multimedia Applications*, 223-228. doi:10.1109/ICCIMA.2003.1238129

Kurtz, C., Beaulieu, C., Napel, S., & Rubin, D. (2014). A hierarchical knowledge-based approach for retrieving similar medical images described with semantic annotations. *Journal of Biomedical Informatics*, *49*, 227–244. doi:10.1016/j.jbi.2014.02.018 PMID:24632078

Langlotz, C. P. (2006). RadLex: A new method for indexing online educational materials1. *Radiographics*, *26*(6), 1595–1597. doi:10.1148/rg.266065168 PMID:17102038

Lavrenko, V., Manmatha, R., & Jeon, J. (2003). A model for learning the semantics of pictures. Advances in Neural Information Processing Systems.

Lee, J. (1995, July). Combining multiple evidence from different properties of weighting schemes. In *Proceedings of the 18th annual international ACM SIGIR conference on Research and development in information retrieval* (pp. 180-188). ACM. doi:10.1145/215206.215358

Lee, J. H. (1997, July). Analyses of multiple evidence combination. *ACM SIGIR Forum, 31*, 267-276. doi:10.1145/258525.258587

Li, Q., Li, F., Shiraishi, J., Katsuragawa, S., Sone, S., & Doi, K. (2003). Investigation of new psychophysical measures for evaluation of similar images on thoracic computed tomography for distinction between benign and malignant nodules. *Medical Physics*, *30*(10), 2584–2593. doi:10.1118/1.1605351 PMID:14596294

Li, J., & Wang, J. Z. (2006). *ALIPR: Automatic photo tagging and visual image search.* Retrieved from http://www.alipr. com

Li, Q., & Wu, Y. (2006). Identifying important concepts from medical documents. *Journal of Biomedical Informatics*, *39*(6), 668–679. doi:10.1016/j.jbi.2006.02.001 PMID:16545986

Lim, J. H., & Chevallet, J. P. (2005). Vismed: a visual vocabulary approach for medical image indexing and retrieval. In Information Retrieval Technology (pp. 84-96). Springer Berlin Heidelberg. doi:10.1007/11562382_7

Liu, C. T., Tai, P. L., Chen, A. Y. J., Peng, C. H., Lee, T., & Wang, J. S. (2001, August). A content-based ct lung image retrieval system for assisting differential diagnosis images collection. *2001 IEEE International Conference on Multimedia and Expo (ICME'01).*

Liu, Y., Zhang, D., Lu, G., & Ma, W. Y. (2007). A survey of content-based image retrieval with high-level semantics. *Pattern Recognition*, *40*(1), 262–282. doi:10.1016/j.patcog.2006.04.045

Long, F., Zhang, H., & Feng, D. D. (2003). Fundamentals of content-based image retrieval. In *Multimedia Information Retrieval and Management* (pp. 1–26). Berlin: Springer. doi:10.1007/978-3-662-05300-3_1

Ma, W., Deng, Y., & Manjunath, B. (1997, June). Tools for texture-and color-based search of images. *Human Vision and Electronic Imaging II, SPIE*, *3016*, 496–507.

Mao, W., & Chu, W. (2007). The phrase-based vector space model for automatic retrieval of free-text medical documents. *Data & Knowledge Engineering*, *61*, 76–92.

Maillot, N., Chevallet, J., Valea, V., & Lim, J. (2006). *IPAL inter-media pseudo-relevance feedback approach to imageclef 2006 photo retrieval. CLEF Working Notes.*

Martínez-Fernández, J., Serrano, A., Villena, J., Sáenz, V., Tortosa, S., Castagnone, M., & Alonso, J. (2004, September). MIRACLE at ImageCLEF 2004. *Working Notes for the CLEF 2004 Workshop,* 545-553.

Magalh˜aes, J., Overell, S., & Rüger, S. (2007). Exploring image, text and geographic evidences. *ImageCLEF 2007.*

Millar, E., Shen, D., Liu, J., & Nicholas, C. (2006). Performance and scalability of a large-scale n-gram based information retrieval system. *Journal of Digital Information*, *1*(5), 1–25.

Mori, Y., Takahashi, H., & Oka, R. (1999, October). Image-to-word transformation based on dividing and vector quantizing images with words. *First International Workshop on Multimedia Intelligent Storage and Retrieval Management.*

Montani, S., & Bellazzi, R. (2002). Supporting decisions in medical applications: The knowledge management perspective. *International Journal of Medical Informatics*, *68*(1), 79–90. doi:10.1016/S1386-5056(02)00067-9 PMID:12467793

Moulin, C., Barat, C., Géry, M., Ducottet, C., & Largeron, C. (2009). UJM at ImageCLEFwiki 2008. In *Evaluating Systems for Multilingual and Multimodal Information Access* (pp. 779–786). Berlin: Springer. doi:10.1007/978-3-642-04447-2_101

Müller, H. (2013). Medical (visual) information retrieval. In *Information Retrieval Meets Information Visualization* (pp. 155–166). Berlin: Springer. doi:10.1007/978-3-642-36415-0_10

Müller, H., Clough, P., Deselaers, T., & Caputo, B. (Eds.). (2010). *ImageCLEF: Experimental Evaluation in Visual Information Retrieval.* Springer. doi:10.1007/978-3-642-15181-1

Müller, H., Michoux, N., Bandon, D., & Geissbuhler, A. (2004). A review of content-based image retrieval systems in medical applications—clinical benefits and future directions. *International Journal of Medical Informatics*, *73*(1), 1–23. doi:10.1016/j.ijmedinf.2003.11.024 PMID:15036075

Müller, H., Rosset, A., Vallée, J., & Geissbuhler, A. (2002). Integrating content-based visual access methods into a medical case database. *Studies in Health Technology and Informatics*, *95*, 480–485. PMID:14664033

Muramatsu, C., Schmidt, R., Shiraishi, J., Li, Q., & Doi, K. (2010). Presentation of similar images as a reference for distinction between benign and malignant masses on mammograms: Analysis of initial observer study. *Journal of Digital Imaging*, *23*(5), 592–602. doi:10.1007/s10278-009-9263-z PMID:20054606

Muramatsu, C., Suzuki, K., Schmidt, R., Shiraishi, J., Newstead, G., & Doi, K. (2005). Investigation of psychophysical measure for evaluation of similar images for mammographic masses: Preliminary results. *Medical Physics*, *32*(7), 2295–2304. doi:10.1118/1.1944913 PMID:16121585

Nadkarni, P., Ohno-Machado, L., & Chapman, W. (2011). Natural language processing: An introduction. *Journal of the American Medical Informatics Association*, *18*(5), 544–551. doi:10.1136/amiajnl-2011-000464 PMID:21846786

Nakayama, R., Abe, H., Shiraishi, J., & Doi, K. (2009). Potential usefulness of similar images in the differential diagnosis of clustered Microcalcifications on Mammograms. *Radiology*, *253*(3), 625–631. doi:10.1148/radiol.2533090373 PMID:19789245

Napel, S., Beaulieu, C., Rodriguez, C., Cui, J., Xu, J., Gupta, A., & Rubin, D. (2010). Automated retrieval of CT images of liver lesions on the basis of image similarity: Method and preliminary results. *Radiology*, *256*(1), 243–252. doi:10.1148/radiol.10091694 PMID:20505065

Nassif, H., Woods, R., Burnside, E., Ayvaci, M., Shavlik, J., & Page, D. (2009, December). Information extraction for clinical data mining: A mammography case study. *IEEE International Conference on Data Mining Workshops*, 37-42. doi:10.1109/ICDMW.2009.63

National Library of Medicine NLM. (2014). Retrieved from http://www.nlm.nih.gov/

Niblack, C., Barber, R., Equitz, W., Flickner, M., Glasman, E., Petkovic, D., & Taubin, G. (1993, April). QBIC project: Querying images by content, using color, texture, and shape. *IS&T/SPIE's Symposium on Electronic Imaging: Science and Technology*, 173-187.

Nister, D., & Stewenius, H. (2006). Scalable recognition with a vocabulary tree. *IEEE Computer Society Conference on Computer Vision and Pattern Recognition*, *2*, 2161-2168.

Pentland, A., Picard, R., & Sclaroff, S. (1996). Photobook: Content-based manipulation of image databases. *International Journal of Computer Vision*, *18*(3), 233–254.

Pedrosa, G., & Traina, A. (2013, August). From Bag-of-Visual-Words to Bag-of-Visual-Phrases Using n-Grams. *SIBGRAPI-Conference on Graphics, Patterns and Images,* 304-311. doi:10.1109/SIBGRAPI.2013.49

Pham, D., Xu, C., & Prince, J. (2000). Current methods in medical image segmentation 1. *Annual Review of Biomedical Engineering Arequipa, Peru, 2*(1), 315-337.

Philbin, J., Chum, O., Isard, M., Sivic, J., & Zisserman, A. (2007, June). Object retrieval with large vocabularies and fast spatial matching. *Proceedings of IEEE Conference on Computer Vision and Pattern Recognition*, 1-8. doi:10.1109/CVPR.2007.383172

Piraino, D. (2013). *Evaluation of Free text search of radiology reports for clinical decision support during radiology reporting using open source software.* Society for Imaging Informatics In Medicine Annual Meeting, Grapevine, TX.

Pires, R., Jelinek, H., Wainer, J., Goldenstein, S., Valle, E., & Rocha, A. (2013). Assessing the Need for Referral in Automatic Diabetic Retinopathy Detection. *IEEE Transactions on Bio-Medical Engineering, 60*(12), 3391–3398. doi:10.1109/TBME.2013.2278845 PMID:23963192

Porter, M. (1980). An algorithm for suffix stripping. *Program: Electronic Library and Information Systems, 14*(3), 130-137.

Quellec, G., Lamard, M., Cazuguel, G., Cochener, B., & Roux, C. (2010). Wavelet optimization for content-based image retrieval in medical databases. *Medical Image Analysis, 14*(2), 227–241. doi:10.1016/j.media.2009.11.004 PMID:20007020

Racoceanu, D., Lacoste, C., Teodorescu, R., & Vuillemenot, N. (2006). A semantic fusion approach between medical images and reports using UMLS. In *Information Retrieval Technology* (pp. 460–475). Berlin: Springer. doi:10.1007/11880592_35

Rasiwasia, N., Costa Pereira, J., Coviello, E., Doyle, G., Lanckriet, G., Levy, R., & Vasconcelos, N. (2010, October). A new approach to cross-modal multimedia retrieval. *Proceedings of the international conference on Multimedia*, 251-260. doi:10.1145/1873951.1873987

Ramaswamy, M., Patterson, D., Yin, L., & Goodacre, B. W. (1996). MoSearch: A radiologist-friendly tool for finding-based diagnostic report and image retrieval. *Radiographics, 16*(4), 923–933. doi:10.1148/radiographics.16.4.8835980 PMID:8835980

Rahman, M., Antani, S., & Thoma, G. (2011, June). Biomedical CBIR using "bag of keypoints" in a modified inverted index. *IEEE 24th International Symposium on Computer-Based Medical Systems (CBMS),* 1-6.

Ren, J. (2012). ANN vs. SVM: Which one performs better in classification of MCCs in mammogram imaging. *Knowledge-Based Systems, 26*, 144–153. doi:10.1016/j.knosys.2011.07.016

Robertson, S. E., & Jones, K. S. (1997). *Simple, proven approaches to text retrieval.* UK Computer Laboratory, University of Cambridge.

Rogers, E., & Arkin, R. C. (1991, October). Visual interaction: A link between perception and problem solving. *Proceedings of IEEE International Conference on Systems, Man, and Cybernetics, Decision Aiding for Complex Systems*, 1265-1270. doi:10.1109/ICSMC.1991.169861

Rosse, C., & Mejino, J. Jr. (2003). A reference ontology for biomedical informatics: The Foundational Model of Anatomy. *Journal of Biomedical Informatics, 36*(6), 478–500. doi:10.1016/j.jbi.2003.11.007 PMID:14759820

Rubin, G. (2000). Data explosion: The challenge of multidetector-row CT. *European Journal of Radiology, 36*(2), 74–80. doi:10.1016/S0720-048X(00)00270-9 PMID:11116170

Salton, G. (1971). *The SMART retrieval system—experiments in automatic document processing.* Academic Press.

Srinivasan, S., Rindflesch, T., Hole, W., Aronson, A., & Mork, J. (2002). Finding UMLS Metathesaurus concepts in MEDLINE. *Proceedings of AMIA Symposium*, 727–31.

Shyu, C., Brodley, C., Kak, A., Kosaka, A., Aisen, A., & Broderick, L. (1999). ASSERT, A physician-in-the-loop content-based image retrieval system for HRCT image databases. *Computer Vision and Image Understanding*, *75*(1), 111–132. doi:10.1006/cviu.1999.0768

Shaw, J., & Fox, E. (1995). Combination of multiple searches. *NIST Special Publication SP*, 105-105.

Sickles, E., Miglioretti, D., Ballard-Barbash, R., Geller, B., Leung, J., Rosenberg, R., & Yankaskas, B. et al. (2005). Performance benchmarks for diagnostic mammography. *Radiology*, *235*(3), 775–790. doi:10.1148/radiol.2353040738 PMID:15914475

Siegle, R., Baram, E., Reuter, S., Clarke, E., Lancaster, J., & McMahan, C. (1998). Rates of disagreement in imaging interpretation in a group of community hospitals. *Academic Radiology*, *5*(3), 148–154. doi:10.1016/S1076-6332(98)80277-8 PMID:9522880

Simpson, M., Rahman, M., Demner-Fushman, D., Antani, S., & Thoma, G. (2009, September). Text-and content-based approaches to image retrieval for the ImageCLEF 2009 medical retrieval track. *CLEF2009 Working Notes. CLEF 2009 Workshop,* (30).

Sivic, J., & Zisserman, A. (2003, October). Video Google: A text retrieval approach to object matching in videos. *Proceedings of Ninth IEEE International Conference on Computer Vision*, 1470-1477. doi:10.1109/ICCV.2003.1238663

Sklansky, J., Tao, E., Bazargan, M., Ornes, C., Murchison, R., & Teklehaimanot, S. (2000). Computer-aided, case-based diagnosis of mammographic regions of interest containing microcalcifications. *Academic Radiology*, *7*(6), 395–405. doi:10.1016/S1076-6332(00)80379-7 PMID:10845398

Smeulders, A., Worring, M., Santini, S., Gupta, A., & Jain, R. (2000). Content-based image retrieval at the end of the early years. *IEEE Transactions on Pattern Analysis and Machine Intelligence*, *22*(12), 1349–1380. doi:10.1109/34.895972

Snoek, C., Worring, M., & Smeulders, A. (2005, November). Early versus late fusion in semantic video analysis. *Proceedings of the 13th annual ACM international conference on Multimedia*, 399-402. doi:10.1145/1101149.1101236

Soffa, D., Lewis, R., Sunshine, J., & Bhargavan, M. (2004). Disagreement in interpretation: A method for the development of benchmarks for quality assurance in imaging. *Journal of the American College of Radiology*, *1*(3), 212–217. doi:10.1016/j.jacr.2003.12.017 PMID:17411562

Stearns, M., Price, C., Spackman, K., & Wang, A. (2001). SNOMED clinical terms: Overview of the development process and project status. *Proceedings of the* American Medical Informatics Association *(AMIA) Symposium*, 662.

Suckling, J., Parker, J., Dance, D., Astley, S., Hutt, I., Boggis, C., & Savage, J. (1994). The mammographic image analysis society digital mammogram database. In *Proceedings of Second International Workshop on Digital Mammography*. Excerta Medica.

Swett, H., Fisher, P., Cohn, A., Miller, P., & Mutalik, P. (1989). Expert system-controlled image display. *Radiology*, *172*(2), 487–493. doi:10.1148/radiology.172.2.2664871 PMID:2664871

Takane, Y., Kawasumi, Y., Horie, T., & Ishibashi, T. (2013, March). Does image reduction affect the diagnostic accuracy of digital mammograms? In *SPIE Medical Imaging* (p. 867319–867319). International Society for Optics and Photonics. doi:10.1117/12.2008169

Tirilly, P., Claveau, V., & Gros, P. (2008, July). Language modeling for bag-of-visual words image categorization. In *Proceedings of the 2008 international conference on Content-based image and video retrieval* (pp. 249-258). ACM doi:10.1145/1386352.1386388

Teng, S., & Lu, G. (2007). Image indexing and retrieval based on vector quantization. *Pattern Recognition*, *40*(11), 3299–3316. doi:10.1016/j.patcog.2007.01.029

Tommasi, T., Orabona, F., & Caputo, B. (2008). CLEF2008 image annotation task: An SVM confidence-based approach. Working Notes of the 2008 CLEF Workshop.

Traina, A., Castanon, C., & Traina, C. Jr. (2003, June). Multiwavemed: A system for medical image retrieval through wavelets transformations. *Proceedings of 16th IEEE Symposium on Computer-Based Medical Systems*, 150-155. doi:10.1109/CBMS.2003.1212781

Unified Medical Language System. (2014). Retrieved from http://www.nlm.nih.gov/research/umls/

Valente, F., Costa, C., & Silva, A. (2013). Dicoogle, a PACS featuring profiled content based image retrieval. *PLoS ONE*, *8*(5), e61888. doi:10.1371/journal.pone.0061888 PMID:23671578

Van Erp, M., & Schomaker, L. (2000). Variants of the borda count method for combining ranked classifier hypotheses. *Seventh International Workshop on Frontiers in Handwriting Recognition.*

van Zaanen, & de Croon. (2005). Multi-modal information retrieval using FINT. In *Multilingual Information Access for Text, Speech and Images* (pp. 728-739). Berlin: Springer.

Villena Román, J., González Cristóbal, J., Goñi Menoyo, J., Martínez Fernández, J., & Fernández, J. (2005). MIRACLE's combination of visual and textual queries for medical images retrieval. *Working Notes for the CLEF 2005 Workshop.*

Villena-Román, J., Lana-Serrano, S., & González-Cristóbal, J. (2008). MIRACLE at ImageCLEFmed 2007: Merging textual and visual strategies to improve medical image retrieval. In *Advances in Multilingual and Multimodal Information Retrieval* (pp. 593–596). Berlin: Springer. doi:10.1007/978-3-540-85760-0_74

Vinokourov, A., Hardoon, D., & Shawe-Taylor, J. (2003). Learning the semantics of multimedia content with application to web image retrieval and classification. *Fourth International Symposium on Independent Component Analysis and Blind Source Separation.*

Wang, J., Li, Y., Zhang, Y., Xie, H., & Wang, C. (2011, August). Bag-of-features based classification of breast parenchymal tissue in the mammogram via jointly selecting and weighting visual words. *Sixth IEEE International Conference on Image and Graphics (ICIG)*, 622-627. doi:10.1109/ICIG.2011.192

Wee, C., & Paramesran, R. (2007). On the computational aspects of Zernike moments. *Image and Vision Computing*, *25*(6), 967–980. doi:10.1016/j.imavis.2006.07.010

Wei, C., Li, C., & Wilson, R. (2005, April). A general framework for content-based medical image retrieval with its application to mammograms. In *Medical Imaging* (pp. 134–143). International Society for Optics and Photonics. doi:10.1117/12.594929

Wei, C., Li, Y., & Huang, P. (2011). Mammogram retrieval through machine learning within BI-RADS standards. *Journal of Biomedical Informatics*, *44*(4), 607–614. doi:10.1016/j.jbi.2011.01.012 PMID:21277387

Wei, C., Chen, S., & Liu, X. (2012). Mammogram retrieval on similar mass lesions. *Computer Methods and Programs in Biomedicine*, *106*(3), 234–248. doi:10.1016/j.cmpb.2010.09.002 PMID:20933295

Welter, P., Deserno, T. M., Fischer, B., Günther, R. W., & Spreckelsen, C. (2011). Towards case-based medical learning in radiological decision making using content-based image retrieval. *BMC Medical Informatics and Decision Making*, *11*(1), 68. doi:10.1186/1472-6947-11-68 PMID:22032775

Weyand, T., & Deselaers, T. (2005, October). *Combining Content-based Image Retrieval with Textual Information Retrieval.* RWTH Aachen.

Wilhelm, T., Kürsten, J., Eibl, M., & der Nationen, S. (2007). *Experiments for the ImageCLEF 2007 photographic retrieval task. Working Notes for the CLEF.*

Wu, H., Sun, T., Wang, J., Li, X., Wang, W., Huo, D., & Guo, X. (2013). Combination of radiological and gray level co-occurrence matrix textural features used to distinguish solitary pulmonary nodules by computed tomography. *Journal of Digital Imaging*, *26*(4), 797–802. doi:10.1007/s10278-012-9547-6 PMID:23325122

Xue, Z., Antani, S., Long, L., & Thoma, G. (2009, August). A system for searching uterine cervix images by visual attributes. *22nd IEEE International Symposium on Computer-Based Medical Systems (CBMS 2009)*, 1-5. doi:10.1109/CBMS.2009.5255319

Zha, Z., Wang, M., Shen, J., & Chua, T. (2012). Text Mining in Multimedia. In *Mining Text Data* (pp. 361–384). Springer. doi:10.1007/978-1-4614-3223-4_11

Zheng, Q., Wang, W., & Gao, W. (2006, October). Effective and efficient object-based image retrieval using visual phrases. *Proceedings of the 14th annual ACM international conference on Multimedia*, 77-80. doi:10.1145/1180639.1180664

Zhou, X., Gobeill, J., & Müller, H. (2008). *MedGIFT at ImageCLEF 2008. Working Notes of CLEF.*

Zhou, X., Stern, R., & Müller, H. (2012). Case-based fracture image retrieval. *International Journal of Computer Assisted Radiology and Surgery*, *7*(3), 401–411. doi:10.1007/s11548-011-0643-8 PMID:21800188

Chapter 7
Image Registration in Ultrasound-Assisted Brain Surgery:
Its Prospects, Challenges, and Techniques

Haradhan Chel
Central Institute of Technology Kokrajhar, India

Prabin Kumar Bora
Indian Institute of Technology Guwahati, India

ABSTRACT

Image registration is an essential step in the image guided brain surgery. A preoperative magnetic resonance (MR) image guides the neurosurgeon about the size and the location of the tumor inside the brain of the diseased person. Due to several reasons, brain shift occurs during the surgery, results in the shift of the actual position of the tumor. Intra-operative MR imaging is expensive and may not be financially viable for many hospitals. An effective intraoperative US can be used in replacement of MR. For performing registration of US and MR images, the most of the state-of-the-art methods use a suitable similarity or dissimilarity measure, a spline based deformation model, a smoothing technique and an effective fast optimization method. This chapter starts with a discussion on various types of brain tumors and their clinical significance. It also covers on various similarity measures, optimizations and the available database of US and MR brain images.

INTRODUCTION

Brain lesion is a broad term which includes *Brain Tumor*, *Cerebral Infarction*, *Multiple Sclerosis*, *Abscess* etc (Moore,K., Kim, Lyndon, 2009), (Radha, M.L, 2004) . The surgical treatment of a brain lesion is a complex task to a neurosurgeon. Such treatments differ depending on the types, the nature of growth, the criticality of location, shapes, sizes and the malignancy. When a brain tumor patient approaches for a

DOI: 10.4018/978-1-5225-2829-6.ch007

treatment from a neurologists, generally the patient is first advised for a imaging test with either a *computer Tomography (CT)* or a *magneto Resonance* (MR) imaging. If a surgery is advised based on those MR or CT images, neurosurgeon plans it accordingly based on those images. In spite of the availability of these high resolution preoperative MR or CT images, it is almost impossible to perform the surgery without the help of an intraoperative image assistance. The main reason is the brain shift during the craniotomy, and the leakage of *cerebro spinal fluid* (CSF) during surgery. In the field of brain surgery, preoperative and intraoperative imaging have equal importance. Both of these imaging modalities are the necessary assisting elements to a neuro-surgeon. For assisting the doctors with both preoperative and intraoperative imaging for surgery planning and execution, various types of neuro-navigational systems are used. Among all the brain imaging modalities, MR is the most popular modality for its better resolution and visibility of different tissue structures. In the field of clinical investigation of a brain lesion, the shape, the size and the location of the lesion become accurately available from the images. Ultrasound(US) is also suitable modality which can effectively be used for neurosurgical assistance. Experts trained in US imaging can differentiate between normal and abnormal tissues by looking into the echogenicity of different tissue structures. In spite of several advantages of ultrasound, MR imaging is preferred over US imaging as an intraoperative modality in neurosurgical assistance. The main reason is that most of the neuro surgeons are trained in either *axial computed tomography* slices or *magnetic resonance imaging* slices only. The limitations of MR images are the higher cost of and the larger time required to scan a volume. Building an infrastructure with intraoperative MR imaging involves a huge investment and the maintenance of such a system requires skilled engineers. This sometime creates financial limitation in many hospitals. For these reasons, such infrastructure is available in a very few locations or big cities in many underdeveloped countries like India. Before the year 2000, the medical community was of the opinion that ultrasound (US) is not a suitable modality for investigating the brain diseases. There are two main reasons behind that. Firstly US imagery has a poor resolution and certain textures of *low grade gliomas* are not separable from the speckle noises present in the US image. Another reason is that US cannot pass through the cranial bones. US image of brain can only be taken after the craniotomy. By the advancement of the US image acquisition sensors and signal processing techniques, the resolution of the US images have been improved a lot. However, no such technology is reported till now which can generate a better US brain image without craniotomy. In various studies it has shown that the intraoperative ultrasound can replace the intraoperative MR and it directly reduces the infrastructural cost which is easily implementable in all suburban areas. At the present situation, high level professional surgeons who are working in suburban areas face infrastructural issues in using intraoperative MR imaging. This can be minimized by using low cost US modality. For linking the missing space between using the US and MR images, continuous efforts from 1993 (Trobaugh, J.W, 1993) are carried out by this medical community. For using US as an intraoperative modality, this community has developed the state-of-the-art techniques. Beltagy *et.al, (*2010) proposed a method for registration between pre, during, and post-resection ultrasound images, as well as MR images. With the help of retrospective cohort study of intraoperative US on 25 patients they showed that the intraoperative US was useful in identifying tumor boundaries and minimizing residual tumor. Renovanz *et.al* (2014), Anokhin, *et.al,* (2015), Coburger *et. al. (*2015), and Moiyadi and Shetty (2016) performed a retrospective analysis of the g*ross total resection (GTR)* of patients who underwent ultrasound guided neurosurgery and concluded that ultrasound could be effective in achieving GTR, especially for low-grade glioma. Various literature are available in this field which can categorically be classified from two different views i) clinical point of view: (Moore,K.,Kim, L.,2009), (Radha, M.L, 2004), (Trobaugh *et.al*,2004), (Kaivukangas *et.al* 1993), (Maarouf *et.al.*, 1996), (Gronningsaeter *et.al.*, 1996), (Mercier *et.al.* 2011), (Unsgaard *.et.al.*, 2002), (Unsgaard *.et.al.*, 2005), (Unsgaard. *et.al*, 2002) and, ii) image processing point of view: (Forsberg, D., 2013), (Brown, L. G.,2002),(Maintz, J. B. A. and Viergever M.A., 1998), (Zitova, B., Flusser, J. 2003), (Sotiras *et.al.*, 2013), (Fatma *et.al.*, 2016), (Roche *et.al.*, 1999),(Roche *et.al.*, 2001), (Pennec *et.al.*, 2005),

This chapter focuses the techniques related with the image processing point of view.

The rest of this chapter is organized as follows. Section-2 describes the different types of brain tumors and their clinical significance. The image registration problem is presented in section-3 along with the issues related with registering brain images. A common setup for image guided neurosurgery is described in section-4. Section-5 outlines the challenges in US and MR image registration. State-of-the-art literature on preoperative US and preoperative /post-operation MR image registration is reviewed in section -6. Finally conclusion is drawn in section-7.

BRAIN LESIONS AND THEIR CLINICAL SIGNIFICANCE

Any kind of abnormal tissues are known as lesion. Various types of lesions are found in the brain which may be traumatic, benign (non-malignant tumors), malignant, genetic, plaques and brain ischemia etc (Moore,K, Kim, Lyndon, 2009). A Brain Tumor *(intracranial neoplasm)* is an assembly of abnormal tissues in the cranial cavity. It can grossly be grouped into two types *a) primary brain tumor* and *b) secondary brain tumors.* Primary tumors are benign (not fatal) in nature. Secondary tumors are generally malignant. A primary brain tumor can appear with a *cystic component* (a hollow space in brain filled with fluid). Secondary tumors mostly contain a *metastasis* (abnormal spread of tumor from primary region to secondary region). Sometime it contains a cystic element also. The nature of the malignancy of a tumor can easily be detected looking either a US or an MR image. There are various types of brain tumors as follows (Moore,K, Kim, Lyndon,2009), (M.L.Radha, 2004).

1. **Glioma:** A brain tumor formed in the *glial* cells in brain is known as *Glioma.* The glial cells surround neurons and provide insulation between them. Depending on the degree of abnormality in the cell structure, gliomas are classified into four grades i.e. Grade-I to IV. Grades-I and II are known to be benign. *Grade III* gliomas are malignant and they have abnormal and irregular shapes. The most fatal is the *Grade-IV* glioma which is also known as *Glioblastoma.* The main feature of a *Glioblastoma* is the existence of the necrosis (dead cells). Figure (1.a) and Figure(1.b) show grade-IV gliomas which are taken from BITE (Mercier et.al., 2012) data base.
2. **Astrocytoma:** Normally 20-40 percent of glial cells in the human brain and the spinal cord are of a star shapes. These cells are known as *astrocytes* and the group of such cells are known as *astroglia.* When a glioma is formed over such astrocytes or astroglia, they are known as *astrocytoma.* They have also similar classifications like gliomas. where grade-III and -IV are known as *anaplastic (cancerous) astrocytoma.* A grade-II astrocytoma of a patient is shown in Figure (1.c) and Figure (1.d) where Figure (1.c) is a T1 weighted MR image and Figure (1.d) is an US image of the same patient.

Figure 1. a. MR image of Grade-IV glioblastoma with necrosis, b. US image of Grade-IV glioblastoma with necrosis, (Image of patient-3, BITE Database, Mercier, et.al.,2012) c. MR image of Grade-II astrocytoma. Figure 1.d. US image of Grade-II astrocytoma, d. US image of Grade-II astrocytoma. (Image of Patient-2, BITE database,Mercier, et.al.,2012)

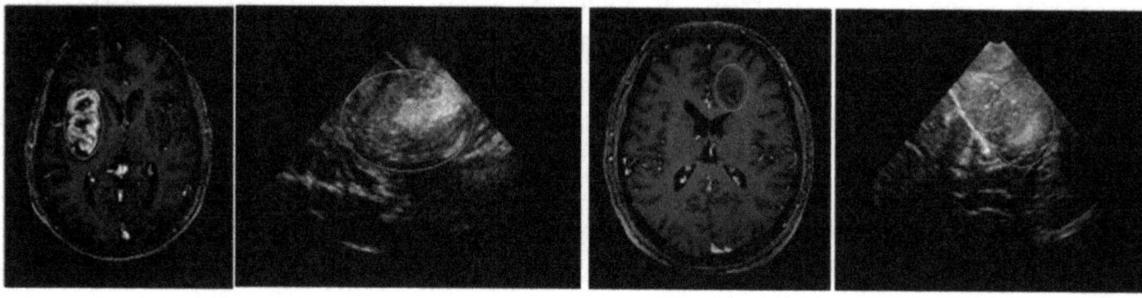

3. **Meningeoma:** Meningioma is a type of tumors which appears over the arachnoid villi, three layers of meninges. and the thick membrane, covers the layers of meninges known as *dura.* In 90 percent of the cases a meningioma is benign in nature and no surgery is required for this types of tumor. Frequent supervision is required using CT and MR imaging over time for watching the growth of the tumor.

IMAGE REGISTRATION FOR BRAIN SURGERY

Image registration (Forsberg, D., 2013), (Brown, L. G.,2002), (Maintz, J. B. A. and Viergever M.A., 1998), (Zitova, B., Flusser, J. 2003) is a technique of overlaying one or multiple input images with a reference image. The images are taken from different viewpoints or at different times. The images which undergo for image registration should have good structural similarity among themselves. Mathematically image registration is a method of estimating the spatial transformation $\left(T\right)$ which deforms the input image $\left(I_T\right)$ for making it similar to the reference image $\left(I_R\right)$. Suppose $\Omega \subset \mathbb{R}^d$ is the domain of a US image. Mathematically, image registration consists of two operations: i) spatial transformation $T = I_d + \boldsymbol{u}$, where I_d is the identity-transform and **u:** $\Omega \rightarrow \mathbb{R}^d$, a displacement operation and ii) a template mapping operation over I_T such that the composite operation $I_T \circ \left(I_d + \boldsymbol{u}\right)$ gives an image as similar as possible to the reference image I_R.

The displacement **u** that is of interest in image registration can be reformulated as,

$$\min_{u} J\left(\boldsymbol{u}\right) = D\left(I_R, I_T\ ; \boldsymbol{u}\right) + \alpha R\left(\boldsymbol{u}\right) \tag{1}$$

where J is the augmented cost function to be minimized. $D\left(I_R, I_T; u\right)$ is a distance measure, measuring the dissimilarity between I_R and $\left(I_T \circ \left(I_d + \boldsymbol{u}\right)\right)$. R measures the irregularity of T and α is the regularization parameter.

Image registration is essential in the field of brain surgery for the following reasons.

- During a surgical procedure, the ultrasound probe moves at various directions resulting in changes the view direction of the lesion. Hence an image registration method is required for automatically aligning the image into a suitable plane.
- Brain tissues are very soft and they change shapes due to minor pressure imparted during surgery.
- The process of removal of brain tumor is a *stereotactic surgery* procedure. During the surgery, with the help of a neuro navigation system and MR scanned images, a small hole is made for opening the cranial cavity (craniotomy) at a suitable location. If the ultrasound probe is to be fit into the same hole, the diameter of the hole is needed to be enlarged. The enlarged craniotomy is shown in Figure (2.a). For avoiding large opening, another small hole is made often in a suitable location wherefrom the lesion can be visualized better. This is known as *mini-craniotomy*. A mini craniotomy is shown in the Figure (2.b). It is a common phenomenon that brain shift occurs during craniotomy. It may mislead the neurosurgeon for finding the edges of the tumor. In such a scenario, a suitable registration method is required.
- During surgery, the *cerebro spinal fulid* (CSF) may get leaked and as a result the volume of the tissues surrounding to the *ventricles*, *arachnoid space* and *subaracnoid space* may get shrinked. In such a scenario, the original volume of the subject may get changed. Hence a suitable method for deformable registration between intraoperative US image and pre-operation US/MR images is required.

SETUP FOR IMAGE GUIDED NEUROSURGERY

IGNS system, there are three fixed reflectors and one moving reflector in the camera tracking system. The operating range of the system is around 70 cm. However, since the highest accuracy is achievable close to the transmitter, the transmitter is placed 15 – 20 cm away from the head of the examined subject. Image registration is an essential step in image guided neurosurgery (IGNS). A modern IGNS system is highly sophisticated. A typical surgical setup is shown in Figure (3) (Pherson, C. Mc, video lecture).

Figure 2 a. Enlarged craniotomy, b. Mini craniotomy with US probe

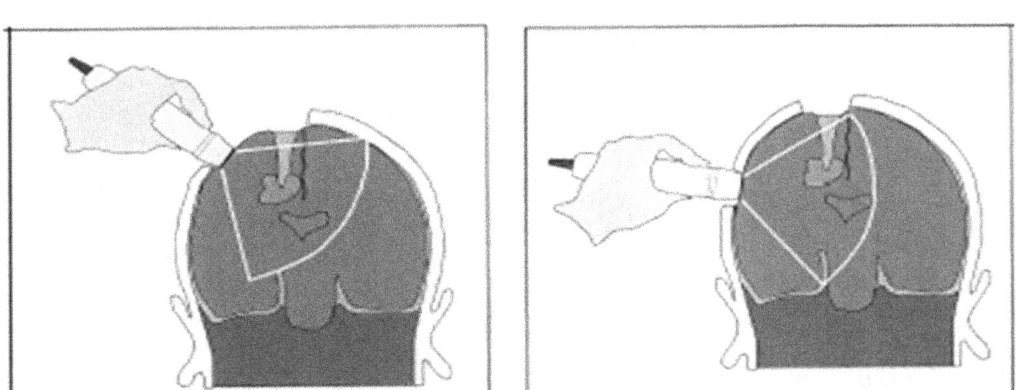

During the pre-surgery procedure, MRI scans are transferred to a neuro-navigation system. The first step is to scan the patient with the reference modality (MRI). The neuro-navigation unit is provided with the slice thickness and the spacing information. Based on these the IGNS system generates a homogeneous 3D volume showing the three orthogonal planes on which the surgical planning is done. The patient is positioned on the surgical table. A transmitter emitting infrared (IR) wave is rigidly attached to the surgical table by means of a fixed support. The position of the transmitter is treated as the origin of the world coordinate system. The patient head is kept stationary with a proper fixation support, while the actual position and orientation of the US probe and/or the pointer, moves freely in the generated three-dimensional (3D) space.

RESEARCH CHALLENGES IN THE BRAIN US AND MR IMAGE REGISTRATION

One of the major challenges in the research of US and MR brain image registration is the collection of data. The MR data can be obtained before surgery but the pre or post resection US images can be obtained during surgery only. Capturing such images it requires trained professionals. For such difficult data collection criteria, the researcher needs to collaborate with a super-spatiality hospital. A group of researchers under the supervision of Prof. Louis Collins of Montreal Neurological Institute has developed the BITE database for brain image registration. The purpose of the database was to provide the researchers with some ready images for performing various types of US and MR brain image registrations. The group reported BITE data base for MR-US brain image registration in 2012 (Mercier et.al., 2012) . The data base is completely an open source and can freely be downloaded from www.bic.mni.mcgill.ca/~laurence/data/. It contains both MR and US images of 14 different patients containing brain tumor of different types.

Figure 3. A typical IGNS system

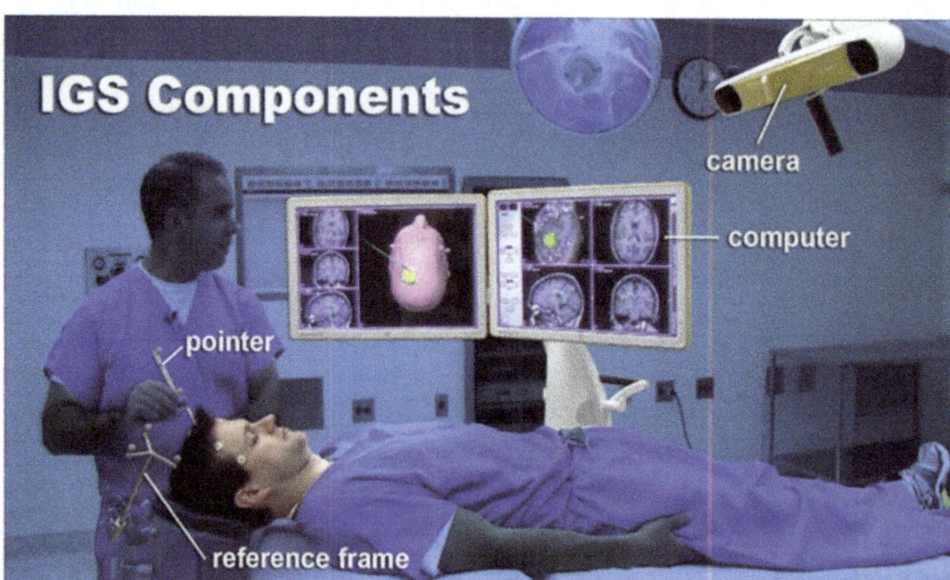

The data base is divided into three groups: Group-1 to 3. Group-1 contains both pre and post resection ultrasound data of 14 different patients. Both *pre* and *post* subfolders contain 3-4 different sweeps for each patients. The data folder of each patients contains a tag file indicating a few pair of 3D coordinates. A pair of coordinate represents one homologous point in two different images. One example of the tag file is as follows.

MNI Tag Point File
Volumes = 2;
%Volume: 4a.3dus.mnc
%Volume: 4u.3dus.mnc
Points =
43.6279754638672 214.060317993164 -96.5143280029297 41.5365791320801 216.671798706055 -100.06534576416 “”

The above text means that a point or an object has a homologous point coordinate (43.627,214.060, -96.514) in one image and the same homologous point or object has a coordinate (41.536,216.617,-100.065) in the other image. Those data are required to check the accuracy and efficiency of the registration algorithm.

Group-2 contains both the MRI and the 2D US stacks of 14 patients. For performing 3D registration, one 3D MR image is given in each folder. The dataset is useful for multimodal (US-MR) 2D and 3D registrations. The images are captured in the *Talairach space* (MIPAV, 2005). This space is a type of coordinate system which is used to represent a point inside the brain volume uniquely. The origin in this coordinate system is taken at the intersection of two lines. The first line joins the *anterior commissure* (AC) and *posterior commissure* (PC) as shown in the Figure (4.a). The second line is the vertical line through the posterior edge of the AC. In the Talairach system, AC and PC are the structures from which the system of reference is developed. The inter-hemispheric sagittal line passing through the origin as shown in Figure (4.b) is taken as the Z axis.

Group-3 contains both pre and post resection MR images. This dataset can be used for preoperative and post resection MRI image registration of 14 different patients. For performing 3D-MR registration, 3D volumes for pre and post resection are also included for each patient.

Figure 4. a Talairach horizontal and vertical reference line joining AC-PC, b. Talairach Space

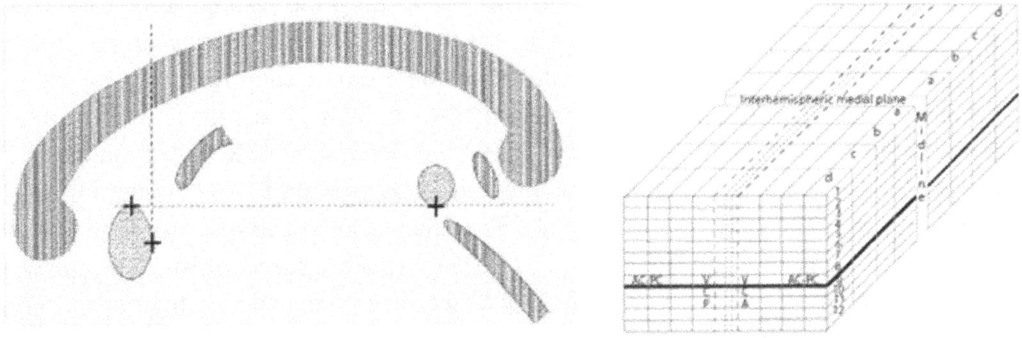

Apart from the limitation of data collection, there are some other challenges with US images. The usage of US as an intraoperative imaging modality during brain surgery was introduced in 1980s (KOIVUKANGAS J.; KELLY P.J., 1986) The major limitation, however, was the poor resolution of the US images and untrained professionals for diagnosing the brain US images. The delineation of a tumor boundary in US images is not a very easy task. The reason is the degradation of the image by speckle noise, produced due to acoustic multipath reflection from the layers of tissues (Lionello *et.al.,*2014) . Various adaptive filtering techniques (Michailovich,O. V., Tannenbaum. A., 2006), (Michailovich, O., Adam, D. (2003)) for speckle reduction increases the quality of images but the edge information does not get improved much. Secondly the image statistics of MR and US images are completely different and hence choosing a proper similarity or dissimilarity metric is really challenging. It is also required that, the registration procedure should be fast enough to fit in a real time system. For working in a real time operation, the minimum frame rate should be at least 30 frames/second which implies that to register one frame the maximum time available is 33 msec. Image registration is a combination of many steps viz. filtering, feature extraction, optimization etc. Completing all these steps within such a small time period is really challenging. In case of nonrigid registration, the local deformation model uses the *cubic Bspline* or the *thin plate spline* (Schwarz L. A., 2007), (Xie, Z. and Farin, G.E. (2004)" method. For modeling the local deformations, the number of control points should be higher and the estimation of the positions for these entities is computationally expensive. After the removal of the tumor tissues, the vacated region is filled with saline water and other blood clotting agents. This sometime creates a borderline artifact which has very similar appearance of malignant tumor tissues (Unsgaard *et.al.,* 2002). For overcoming these challenges various innovative methods have been described and they are outlined in the next section.

STATE-OF-THE-ART OF BRAIN IMAGE REGISTRATION

From the clinical point of view three types of image registrations are required: a) registration between preoperative and post-operation US images b) registration between intraoperative US image and preoperative MR images and c) registration between preoperative US image and preoperative MR images. We primarily focus over the first two requirements.

Preoperative and Post-Operation US Brain Image Registration

The detection of the residual tumor has a serious concern during brain tumor surgery. It has already been discussed that due to leakage of the CSF and brain shift, the exact boundary of a tumor gets shifted. In such a scenario, an intraoperative US image is effective in finding the residual tumor by seeking the echogenicity at the boundary of the resection cavity. As the image statistics between preoperative and post-operation US images are not much different, the residual tumor can effectively be identified by comparing the two images after performing registration between them. The image registration problems can be classified (Sotiras et.al., 2013), (Fatma *et.al.,* 2016) in various ways. Registration may be feature based (Sotiras et.al., 2013) (Bay *et.al.,*2008), (Morel et.al.,2009), (Juan, L. and Gwun, O. 2009) or intensity based (Carter *et.al.*2008), (Kim *et.al.,* 2004). They may also be classified as rigid (Roche *et.al.,* 2001), (Pennec *et.al.,* 2005) or nonrigid (Sotiras et.al., 2013). In feature based registration, corresponding points are found in different US images with the help of different feature matching methods (Sotiras et.al., 2013) In the case of intensity based methods, the intensity of pixels are used directly. The generalized approach is shown in Figure (5). The block diagram shows that a deformation model is estimated based on the optimization of a similarity or dissimilarity metric. Some of the popular metrics are *normalized correlation coefficient(NCC)* (Rivaz, H., Collins, D.L. 2015), *mutual information(MI),* (Pluim *et.al,* 2003), (Paul,V. *et.al,*1997), (Maes, F 1997), *local phase differences* (Nigris *et.al*, 2012) *and structural similarity index (SSIM),* (Sung-Hyuk, 2007), (Bovik *et.al.*,2004) *etc.* Among different optimization methods, *gradient descent optimization, stochastic gradient descent optimization* (Rivaz, H., Collins, D.L. 2015), (Penney,G.P. *et.al.*, 2004), *Powel optimization* (Roche *et.al.,* 2001), (Penney *et.al.*, 2004) and *particle swarm optimization* (Chel *et.al.*, 2015)are popular due to their faster convergence rates. The misalignment between a preoperative and an intraoperative US images occurs mainly due to two reasons: i) the capturing of frames by the US probes from different locations over the entire opened area of the craniotomy and ii) the combinational effect of brain shift and the leakage of the CSF. The misalignment due to the capturing of image frame over enlarged craniotomy is global in nature and it can grossly be matched by a rigid registration method. But the deformation in the images due to the brain shift and the leakage of the CSF is local and nonrigid. Mercier *et.al* (2013) proposed a cross-correlation based technique which uses nonrigid registration based *ANIMAL (Automatic Nonlinear Image Matching and Anatomical Labeling)* (Collins D.L, Evans, A.C., 1997) technique. The major limitation of their work is the requirement of manual segmentation which may not practically be feasible during surgery. Rivaz and Collins,2015 proposed a *cubic Bspline* based tool named as RESOUND (Non-Rigid-Registration of Ultrasound Volume) for nonrigid 3D registration between preoperative and post-operation US images.

The functional steps are shown in the block diagram in Figure (5). Here the negative of the square of the NCC $\left(-NCC^2\right)$ is minimized for obtaining the optimum matching. The cost function $\left(C\right)$ in

Figure 5. A generalized approach to US image registration
(Rivaz,H., Collins D.L. 2014)

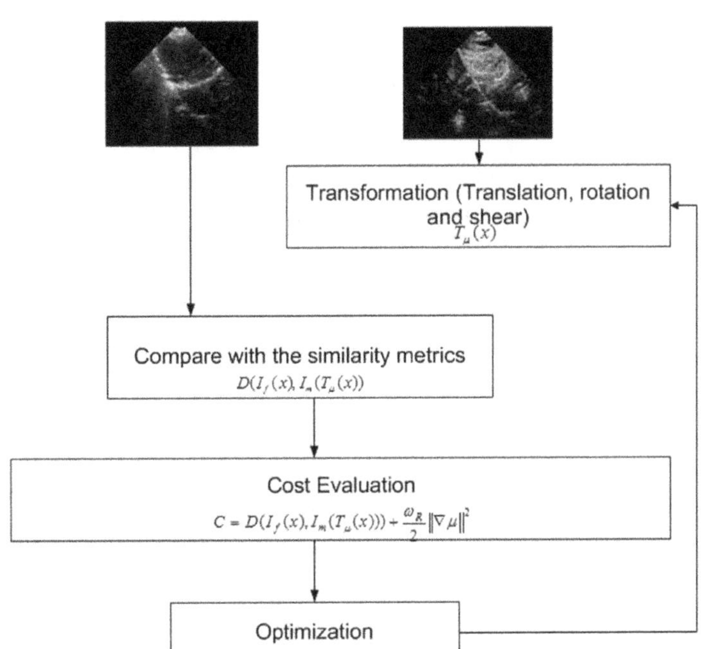

Figure (5) contains two different functions: the dissimilarity metric $D(I_f(x), I_m(T_\mu(x))$ and a regularization term $\frac{\omega_R}{2}\nabla\mu^2$ respectively. Here μ represents the transformation model for control points and the $\nabla\mu$ represents the difference between the B-spline nodes and their translations. But in practical cases, it is not always true that the forward transformation matrix (G) backward transformation matrix (H) are inverse consistent (Christensen, G. E. and Johnson, H. J. 2001). This was reported by Christensen and Johnson (Christensen, G. E. and Johnson, H. J. 2001).

For two different images $A\, and\, B$,

$$if\, A = (B^\circ G), then$$

$$B = (A^\circ H) \approx (A^\circ G^{-1}) \qquad (2)$$

This places a bias on the registration outcome and may additionally introduce an *inverse consistency error* (ICE) which can be written as,

Figure 6. (a)-(b) Pre- and post-resection ultrasound images. The misalignment in the superimposed images in (c) and (d) is mainly caused by the brain shift. Structures (1) and (2) are respectively the septum and ventricles. The tumor and the resection cavity are not present in these ultrasound slices *(Rivaz,H., Collins D.L. 2014).*

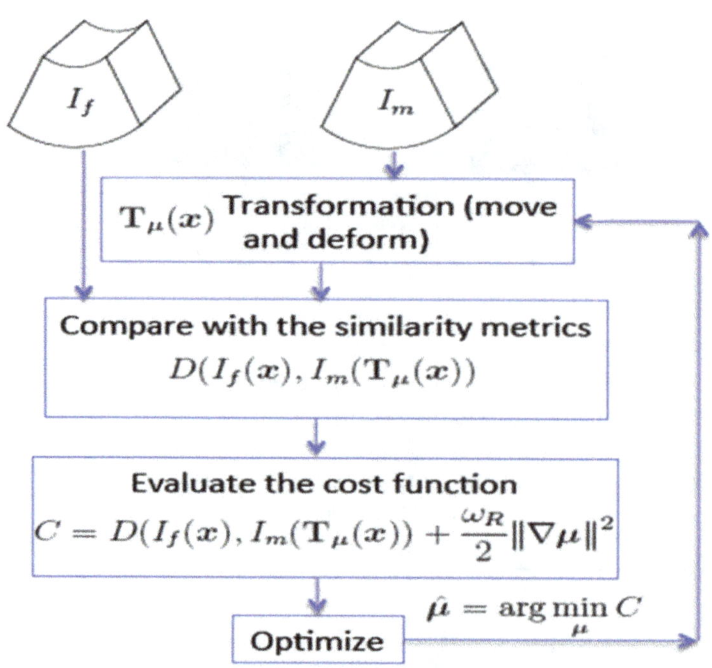

$$ICE = \left(G.H - I\right) \tag{3}$$

In Avants. *et al.* (2008), a symmetric deformable registration is presented. It calculates a transform from two different images to a common intermediate image and also ensures that the forward transform is the inverse of the backward transform. They applied a diffeomorphism $\varnothing$ of a domain Ω for transforming an image A into a new coordinate system. Thus, equation (5) indicates that, $\varnothing\left(x,1\right)$ is operated over A in a forward direction. $\varnothing\left(x,t=1\right)$ indicates a deformation map for an optimization time t $\left[t : t \in \left(0,1\right)\right]$. Here $t = 1$ represents the transformation over the full length of the geodesic. They assume two different deformation functions $\varnothing_1\, and \varnothing_2$ such that $\varnothing_2$ acts in opposite direction than $\varnothing_1$.

$$A\left(t\right) = A^{\circ}\varnothing\left(x,t\right) \tag{4}$$

$$\varnothing A = A^{\circ}\varnothing\left(x,t=1\right) = A\left(x,t=1\right) \tag{5}$$

Thus,

$$\varnothing\left(x,1\right)I = J$$

implies that,

$$\varnothing_1\left(x,t\right)I = \varnothing_2\left(z,1-t\right)J \tag{6}$$

The full forward transformation is calculated by A(0.5) ο B(0.5)−1, where ($t = 0.5$) describes a half length transformation of over the geodesic. The novelty of this method is that it reduces the ICE because diffeomorphisms are theoretically guaranteed to be invertible. Zhou and Rivaz, 2016 use an approach similar to the scheme shown in flowchart of Figure (5) with the additional application of the ICE property (Christensen, G. E. and Johnson, H. J. 2001) in the deformation block. Another novelty of their work is finding the outlier region which is basically reg ion with no correspondence between the images. Figures (7.a and b) represent two US images of (patient No-4 in BITE data base, Mercier et.al., 2012) with grade-IV glioma in the right parietal lobe. These images are taken before and after the tumor resection. After the resection of the tumor, the cavity is filled with saline water and appears as a dark region as shown in Figure (7.b), but before resection the same region appears as a hyper-echoic region. In such cases the non-corresponding region lies in the edges and in the cavity generated after resection of the tumor because of which delineation of the correct edges is not an easy task.

The cost function chosen is the $-NCC^2$ and given by,

$$D = -\sum_{i=1}^{N} \rho_i^2 \tag{7}$$

where,

$$\rho_i^2 = \frac{\left(\sum_{j=1}^{N} (V_{1j} - \overline{V_{1i}})\left(V_{2j} - \overline{V_{2i}}\right)\right)^2}{\sum_{j=1}^{N} \left(V_{1j} - \overline{V_{1i}}\right)^2 \sum_{i=1}^{N} \left(V_{2j} - \overline{V_{2i}}\right)^2} \tag{8}$$

Here, V_{1i} and V_{2i} are the ith patches of image V_1 and V_2 respectively and N is the number of pixels in each patch. Patches from both the images are chosen from the high *signal to noise ratio* (SNR) regions. The outlier regions are found from the Jacobian of NCC at every pixel and excluded from patch selection. The analytical derivation of the Jacobian is also a major contribution of the paper (Zhou, H., and Rivaz, H. 2016).

Pre Resection MR and Intraoperative US Brain Image Registration

(Trobaugh *et. al*, 2004) first introduced the concept of using US as an intraoperative modality along with preoperative MR or CT images during brain surgery. The position and the orientation of the US transducer were monitored with a tracking device in which an intraoperative US is correlated with preoperative CT or MRI images. Gronningsaeter *et. al,1996* reported the methodology and the performance of brain surgery of 8 patients using intraoperative US scanner in 3.2 to 7.5 MHz frequency range. They used color flow imaging technique which allows the detection of blood vessels. Commeau *et.al.,*1998 reported about different issues of US assisted brain surgery like brain shifting, rigidity of the target volume, the rigidity of the patient, image distortion and the tracking device error etc. Several applications

Figure 7. a. Preoperative US image with tumor, Figure 7.b. Post resection US image (1) Cystic element (2) Glioma (grade-III)(left) and saline water filled cavity(right), (3) Choroid plexus (4) Border line artifact due to blood clotting agent
(Patient No-4, BITE Database, (Mercier et.al., 2012).

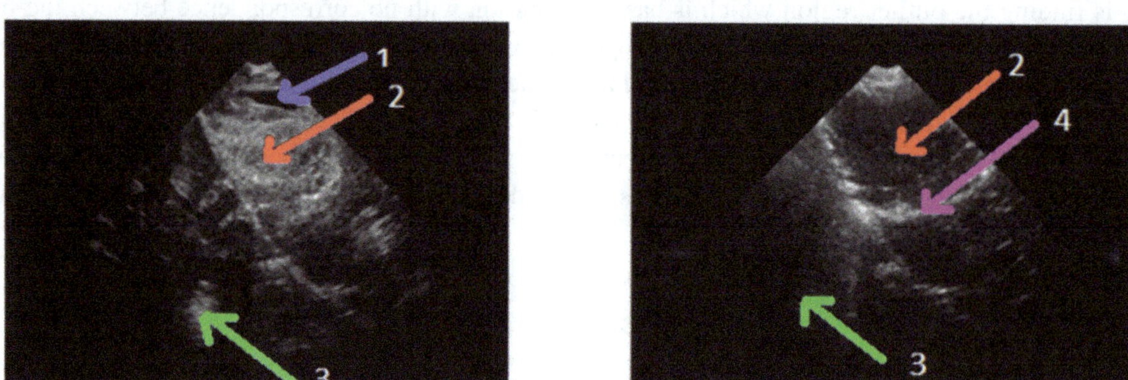

of brain surgery using neuro-navigational system are also described in the literature. Maarouf *et.al.*, 1996 validated the applicability of the US imaging as the intraoperative modality based on the clinical trial. Unsgaard *et.al*, 2002 provided a detailed clinical review on various issues like probe positioning, open tumor resection, closed tumor resection and surgical setup etc. Regarding the methodology of the registration between intraoperative US and preoperative MR images publications are found after 2000. A survey paper on medical image registration, published in 1998 by Maintz and Viergever,1998 focuses on registration between MR-CT, MR-MR, CT-CT images and also that between stereotactic and either of MR or CT images. In the registration between the MR and US images, the choice of proper similarity and dissimilarity measure is important because the statistics of two different image modalities is not similar. Roche *et.al.*, 2001 classified all the similarity measures into four groups. They are based on a) identity relationship b) affine relationship c) functional relationship and d) statistical relationship. They shows that, the CR is suitable for multimodal image registration. Table (1) shows the different types of similarity measures.

The first effort for performing US-MR multimodal image registration was made by Pagoulatos, 1999 in which a marker based phantom object was used for the generation of the images. However the first automatic rigid registration between 3D US and pre-operation MR images was proposed by Roche. *et.al*, 2001. Here automatic registration is achieved by maximizing a similarity measure which generalizes the correlation ratio. The novelty of this similarity measure is to incorporate multivariate information from the MR data using both the intensity and the gradient. This paper introduces two different variations of the CR *(CR and Bivariate CR)*.

The registration between two image frames $I_T \, and \, I_R$ is a minimization problem which is described in equation (1). Here,

$$D\left(I_T, I_R \;; \boldsymbol{u}\right) = \sum_k [I_T\left(x_k\right) - I_R\left(T(x_k)\right)]^2 \tag{9}$$

A practical limitation arises when the transformation of a point x_k crosses the dimension of the image. The point is excluded from the cost function. For considering this effect, the cost function employs a weighted sum of the distance of each pixels in a patch. When the transformation of a pixel is outside the dimension of the template image, the weight of that pixel is 0. After the application of this criterion, the cost function is written as,

$$C\left(T, f\right) = \frac{\sum_{k,l} W_{\overset{ç}{k,l}} \left[i_k - f\left(j_l\right)\right]^2}{\overset{ç}{n} \, Var\begin{pmatrix} ç \\ I \end{pmatrix}} \tag{10}$$

Here $i_k = I_T\left(x_k\right)$, $j_k = I_R\left(T(x_k)\right)$, f is a intensity mapping such that $f\left(I_R {}^\circ T\right) \approx \overset{ç}{I}$, T represents a spatial transformation, $W_{\overset{ç}{k,l}}$ are the linear interpolation weights, n is the number of points in the template and $Var\begin{pmatrix} ç \\ I \end{pmatrix}$ is the intensity variance of eight neighbor pixels of $T\left(x_k\right)$.

Table 1. Different similarity and dissimilarity measures

Name of the Similarity/ Dissimilarity Measure	*Type*	*Mathematical Expression*	*Merit/Demerit*
Sum of Squared Difference (SSD)	Identity Relationship	$SSD(I,J) = \sum_{k=1}^{N}(I(k) - J(k))^2$	Not able to cope with relative intensity changes from one image to the other
Cross Correlation	Identity Relationship	$CC(I,J) = \frac{\sum_{x=1}^{M}\sum_{y=1}^{N}(I(x,y) - \bar{I})(J(x,y) - \bar{J})}{\sum_{x=1}^{M}\sum_{y=1}^{N}(I(x,y) - \bar{I})^2 \sum_{x=1}^{M}\sum_{y=1}^{N}(J(x,y) - \bar{J})^2}$	Not able to cope with relative intensity changes from one image to the other
Absolute difference image	Identity Relationship	$ADI(I,J) = \sum_{k=1}^{N}\left\|I(k) - J(k)\right\|$ N is the number of pixels in the image.	Not able to cope with relative intensity changes from one image to the other
Correlation Coefficient	Affine Relationship	$CC(I,J) = \frac{Cov(I,J)}{\sqrt{Var(I)}\sqrt{Var(J)}}$	Not suitable for multimodal image registration. I
Correlation Ratio (Roche. *et.al* 1998, (Roche *et.al.*, 1999)	Functional Relationship	$\eta^2\left(\frac{I}{J}\right) = 1 - \frac{Var(I - \hat{\varnothing}(J))}{Var(I)}$ where $\hat{\varnothing}(J)$ is the least squares optimal nonlinear approximation of *I* in terms of *J* (Papoulis, 1991).	Suitable for multimodal image registration
Mutual Information (Maes et.al., 1997; Viola and Wells, 1997)	Statistical Relationship	$MI(I,J) = \sum_{s=1}^{255}\sum_{t=1}^{255} p(s,t)\log\left(\frac{p(s,t)}{p(i)q(j)}\right)$ For 8 bit image number of intensity level=256. $p(s,t)$ is the joint probability of intensity values s and t.	Not suitable for multimodal image registration.

In the case of an unconstrained intensity mapping f, an important result is that the optimal f at fixed T has an explicit form that is very fast to compute (Roche *et.al.*, 2001). The minimization of equation (10) may then be performed by obtaining the minima of $C(T,f)$ at fixed T. This yields the CR,

$$\eta^2_{I_T/I_R}(T) = 1 - \min_f C(T,f) \tag{11}$$

In the above, $\eta^2_{I_T/I_R}$ becomes maximum when C is minimum. The CR based method tries to predict the intensities of the US by remapping those of the MR image. Hence, the uniform regions of the original MR image remain uniform in the remapped MR image and, thus, this procedure is not able to account for the intensity variations at tissue boundaries. To enable a better prediction, a new *bivariate correlation ratio* is proposed. It uses the gradient magnitude of the MR image as an additional explanatory variable. Penny *et. al.*,2004 proposed one method for performing registration between the preoperative MR image of liver with intraoperative US images. A systematic process was

followed for searching the hepatic vessels of the liver as they are expected to move in an approximate rigid-body relationship with the liver parenchyma. By matching the hepatic vessels, this method reduces the effect of errors induced due to liver movement during MR and US image acquisition. Another major contribution of this work is the artifact removal of the US images using a two-level thresholding method. In a clinical article by Rasmussen *et.al.* in 2007 addressed the causes of reduction in the neuro-navigation accuracy such as brain shift, position of markers over the preoperative MR or fMR (functional MR) images and leakage of CSF etc. It also provided a clinical guideline for performing effective surgical planning using fMR, the Diffusion tensor imaging (DTI) and 3D US. Ji *et.al*, 2008 performed a multi-stage fiducial based registration between pre-operation MR and intraoperative US images. Here the US image is first transformed into the stationary MR imaging space. The registration scheme is explained in the Figure (8), reproduced from Ji *et.al*, 2008. It shows an IGNS system which uses a *Polaris tracking system* which for capturing the 3D world coordinates. An US trackerthe captures intraoperative US (iUS) images. The preoperative MR (pMR) images are loaded with this system in the beginning. It performs registration in the two stages. A gross level registration between the MR and US images is obtained in the first stage. The registration in the first stage is modeled as,

$$^{MR}T^{0}_{US} = {}^{MR}T^{0}_{patient} \times {}^{patient}T_{world} \times inv({}^{US_{tracker}}T_{world}) \times {}^{US\_tracker}T_{US} \tag{12}$$

where, A_{T_B} indicates a transformation from B coordinate system to the field of A coordinate system. The resulting transformation between the US and the MR images as shown in equation (12) is a combination of four different transformations. The transformation is subject to the errors from the fiducial based registration, the US scan-head calibration and possibly brain shift Ji *et.al*, 2008. For reducing this registration error in the second stage, the grossly registered US image is further reregistered with the MR volume using the relation

$$^{MR}T^{adjusted}_{US} = T^{adjusted} \times {}^{MR}T^{0}_{US} \tag{13}$$

During this step, the *normalized mutual information (NMI)* is used as a similarity measure. Powel optimization (Roche *et.al.*, 2001), (Penney *et.al.*, 2004) method was used to maximize the NMI. Nigris *et. al.*,2010 used a similarity measure, namely *local mutual information* which was earlier proposed by Karacali, 2007 They also devised the *adaptive local mutual information (ALMI)* for registration between US and MR images. An important property of the ALMI is that it saturates smoothly . This property allows the energy function to reach a stable state as the optimizer approaches an extremum.

Another important multi-resolution based approach was proposed by Nigris *et.al*, 2011 for registering preoperative MR and intraoperative US images. They proposed a new similarity metric which is related to the gradient orientation of both the reference and the test images. Let two different images I_F

Figure 8. Coordinate systems used in the image registration. Dashed arrows indicate transformations determined from registration, and are subject to adjustment through the re-registration process. Solid arrows indicate transformations determined from calibration, and are fixed. A reverse arrow means inverse transformation, obtained by matrix inversion. (This image is reproduced from Ji et.al, 2008)

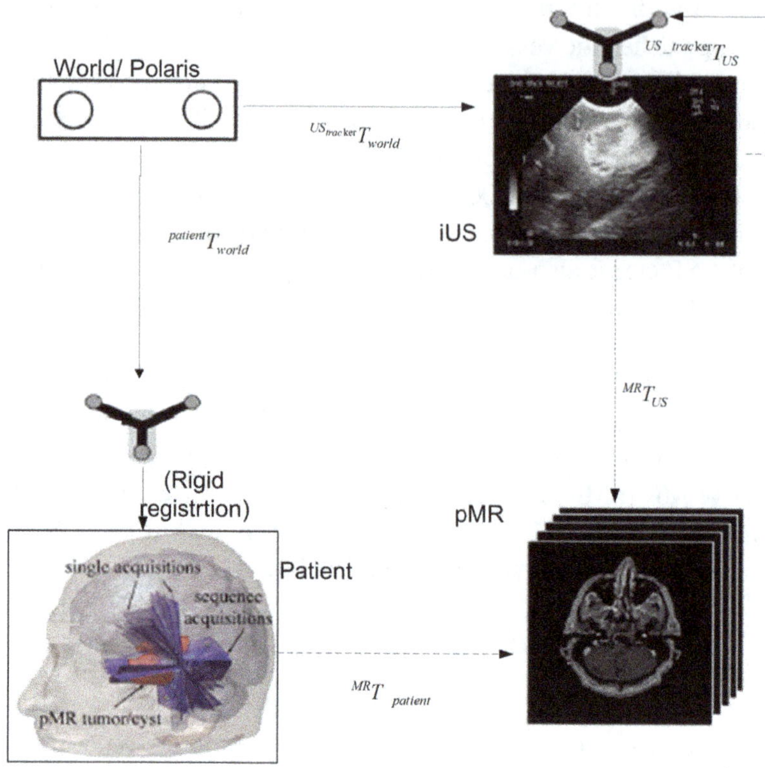

and I_M have two different gradients ∇I_F and ∇I_M respectively. The similarity metric can be defined as,

$$S\left(\nabla I_F, \nabla I_M; N\right) = \cos\left(\Delta\theta\right)^N \tag{14}$$

where $\Delta\theta$ is the inner angle between ∇I_F and ∇I_M and N is an even number representing the metric's parameter. It is a multi-resolution approach. First the images are subdivided into multiple scales i.e. from the coarsest level to the finest level. In each scale, the gradient orientations over different directions are found for all points and represented as a gradient image. Re-sampling of the gradient image is done based on some threshold value of the gradient. The threshold is calculated based on the selection of specified percentage of the total pixels. The transformation matrix is obtained by optimizing the summation of cosine of intergradient angle between two different images for all the selected pixels. Farnia *et.al.*, 2011 proposed an MR-MR and US-MR registration method on an artificial brain phantom made of PVA-C material. A brain lesion and some landmarks are artificially created by using inflatable catheters and some plastic tubes are used for representing the blood vessels. The phantom volume was scanned with both MR (Siemens 3 T scanner) and US scanner (HS 2000). To match the landmarks between US and MR images, the *coherent point drift* (CPD) (Besl, P.J. and McKay, N.D. 1992) method was applied. The CPD is a robust probabilistic multidimensional method for both rigid and nonrigid pointset registrations. It considers the alignment of two pointsets as a probability density estimation, where one point-set represents the centroids of a *gaussian mixture model* (GMM) and the other represents the data points. This algorithm iteratively fits the GMM centroids by maximizing the likelihood function. This method outperforms the *iterative closest point* (ICP) (Besl, P.J. and McKay, N.D. 1992)method. The ICP algorithm is a formulation of point set matching with a least square error minimization approach. This method is suitable for matching geometric data, parametric curves and surfaces and implicit curves and surfaces. Initially the entire data is converted in to a point set consisting of vertices of triangles representing the surface. During registration, ICP algorithm finds the best match of those points present in reference and template objects. Arbel et al., 2004 first introduced the concept of pseudo image of MR slices which has similar nature and statistics like an US image. This was essential because the statistics of MR image is different from gradient based US image. When the MR image is converted into a pseudo image, it was relatively easier to match with an US image. They uses *Automatic Non-linear Image Matching and Anatomical Labeling(ANIMAL)* package which was developed to perform non linear registration between pseudo-US preoperative image and intraoperative US image. The MR to pseudo-US conversion is combination of a segmentation and registration algorithm steps . During segmentation, the entire volume is segmented into approximately 100 anatomical structures. In an US image, only a few structures such as *ventricles, choroid plexus, white matter, cortical grey matter, sulci, and the longitudinal fissure* etc are visible. This segmentation was done manually by the experts. After performing these segmentations, the gradient of the US image is taken over the radial direction, with the US probe-tip as the origin. An intensity remapping operation is then performed on the segmented structures and on the boundaries to attain a pseudo-acoustic density simulation that is comparable to the intensity profiles of intraoperative US brain images.

Mercier *et.al.*, 2011performed two different types of registration between US and MR images. They adopted a very sophisticated multistage method for generating a pseudo-US image from a segmented MR image. The steps for forming the pseudo-US image is shown in the Figure (9), reproduced from (Mercier *et.al.* 2011). It is a better technique for the generation of pseudo-US image compared to the method proposed by Arbel *et. al.*, 2004. Mercier *et. al.*, 2012 compared the performance of registration between 3DUS and MR images by maximizing the CR and the NMI. The registration was performed using *MINC* tool in *minctracc* software . It is reported that, CR performs better than NMI as a similarity metric for US-MR registration. Rivaz *et.al.*, 2015 proposed a scheme for performing automatic MR-US nonrigid registration. It introduces the *robust patch based correlation ratio (RAPTOR)* which is invariant to the large amounts of spatial intensity in-homogeneity . This paper has many contributions like a) it measures patch based local similarity. b) it proposes an effective outlier suppression technique c) it directly performs registration between preoperative MR and post-operation US images and d) it locates corresponding anatomical landmarks between preoperative MR and post-operation US for the validation of registration results. The authors provided those landmarks online for future research work. The algorithm includes a cubic Bspline based deformation model, a novel patch based *RAPTOR* metric and *stochastics gradient descent optimization.* Rivaz and Collins, 2015 proposed one non rigid registration method between preoperative MR, preoperative ultrasound and post-resection ultrasound images. The registration between a preoperative MR and post resection US is difficult but is essential during surgery for finding the residual tumor. This task is accomplished in a consummate way by the proposed method.

First the registration between the MR and pre-resection US is done followed by a second registration between the pre- and post-resection US images. These two registrations yield two transformations. These are used to compose the transformation between the MR and post-resection US images. For performing registration between preoperative MR and intraoperative US images, an efficient RESOUND (Rivaz,H., Collins D.L. 2014) method is applied. For the second step, it uses the RAPTOR metric. This is one of the state-of-the-art models on performing registration of preoperative MR and intraoperative US or post resection US images.

In spite of these different approaches and state-of -the-art techniques, this field has a lot more to improve in the context of better similarity or dissimilarity measure, post processing, optimization etc. The present phase of the researches in this field is concentrated on the designing a suitable similarity and dissimilarity measure and mostly gradient based optimizations were adopted for increasing the speed of the iterative steps. There is space to work with this problem using better deformation models and optimization techniques which may lead to a mentionable improvement over the current state of the results.

CONCLUSION

Intraoperative US based brain surgery is becoming popular over recent times. The main reason is that it reduces the infrastructural cost for image guided neuro-surgery systems. Intraoperative US imaging is a real time modality which helps the surgeon in many aspects: i) it provides important information of different tissue structures in the brain within very short time, ii) it helps to estimate correctly the position and the edges of the brain tumor iii) it helps to find the amount of residual tumorous tissues after the surgery and. The efficiency of US as an intraoperative modality in image guided brain surgery is worth

Figure 9. Flow chart for preparation of pseudo-US image from MR image
(Mercier, L. et al, 2011)

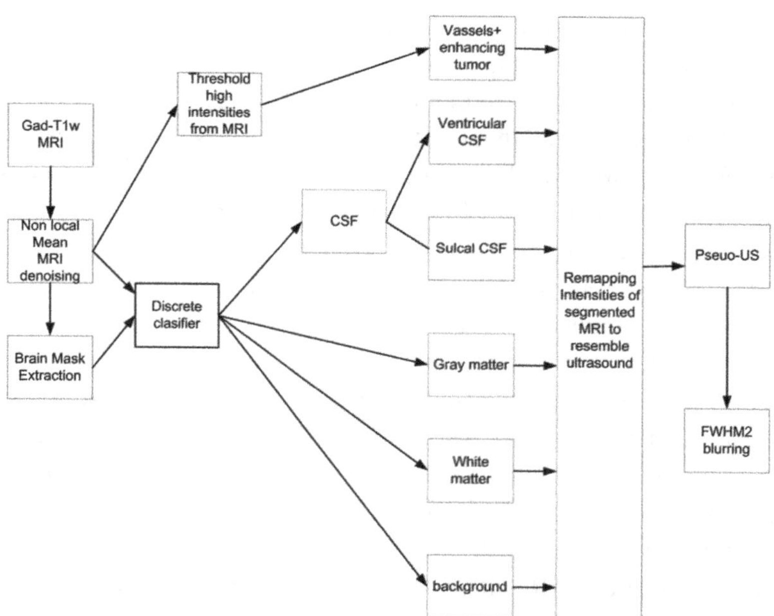

mentioning and comparable with traditional intraoperative MR imaging. US imaging is ill-reputed for its poor resolution and speckle filled images. Registering US images with MR images is challenging because of the difference in their image statistics. Another limitation of using US in brain imaging is that it can only be captured after opening the brain because ultrasound signals do not pass through the cranial bones. For these reasons, researchers in this field face difficulty in collecting data. We have provided information about the database for carrying out researches in this filed. This chapter also reviewed the state-of-the-art methods of different brain image registration techniques and approaches since 1990s.

REFERENCES

Arbel, T., Morandi, X., Comeau, R., & Collins, D.L. (2004). Automatic non-linear mri-ultrasound registration for the correction of intraoperative brain deformations. *Comput Aided Surg, 9*(4), 123–136.

Avants, B., Epstein, C., Grossman, M., & Gee, J. (2008). Symmetric diffeomorphic image registration with cross-correlation: Evaluating automated labeling of elderly and neurodegenerative brain. *Medical Image Analysis, 12*(1), 26–41. doi:10.1016/j.media.2007.06.004 PMID:17659998

Bay, H., Ess, A., Tuytelaars, T., & Van Gool, L. (2008). Speeded-up robust features (SURF). *Computer Vision and Image Understanding, 110*(3), 346–359. doi:10.1016/j.cviu.2007.09.014

Beltagy, E., Mohamed, A., & Mohamed, K. (2010). Role of intraoperative ultrasound in resection of pediatric brain tumors. *Childs Nerv Syst, 26*, 1189–1193.

Besl, P. J., & McKay, N. D. (1992, February). A Method for Registration of 3-D Shapes. *IEEE Transactions on Pattern Analysis and Machine Intelligence, 14*(2), 239–256. doi:10.1109/34.121791

Bovik, W. Z., Bovic, A.C., Sheikh, H.R., & Simoncelli, E.P. (2004). Image Quality Assessment: From Error Visibility to Structural Similarity. *IEEE Transactions on Image Processing, 13*(4), 600-612.

Brown, L. G. (1992). A Survey of Image Registration Techniques. *ACM Computing Surveys, 24*(4).

Carter, T., Tanner, C., Beechey-Newman, N., Barratt, D., & Hawkes, D. (2008). MR navigated breast surgery: method and initial clinical experience. *Proc. Int. Conf. Med. Image Comput. Comput.-Assist. Intervent.*, 356–363. doi:10.1007/978-3-540-85990-1_43

Chel, H., Nandi, D., & Bora, P. K. (2015). Image registration in presence of multiplicative noise by Particle Swarm Optimization. *2015 Third International Conference on Image Information Processing (ICIIP)*, 135-140. doi:10.1109/ICIIP.2015.7414754

Christensen, G. E., & Johnson, H. J. (2001, July). Consistent image registration. *IEEE Transactions on Medical Imaging, 20*(7), 568–582. doi:10.1109/42.932742 PMID:11465464

Coburger, J., Scheuerle, A., Thal, D. R., Engelke, J., Hlavac, M., Wirtz, C. R., & Konig, R. (2015). Linear array ultrasound in low-grade glioma surgery: Histology-based assessment of accuracy in comparison to conventional intraoperative ultrasound and intraoperative MRI. *Acta Neurochirurgica, 157*(2), 195–206. doi:10.1007/s00701-014-2314-3 PMID:25559430

Collins, D.L., & Evans, A.C. (1997). Animal: Validation and applications of nonlinear registration-based segmentation. *Int Journal of Pattern Recognition, 11*, 1271–1294.

Comeau, R. M., Fenster, A., & Peters, T. M. (1998). Intraoperative US in Interactive Image guided Neurosurgery. *Radiographics, 18*(4), 1019–1027.

El-Zahra, El-Gamal, Elmogy, & Atwan. (2016). Current trends in medical image registration and fusion. *Egyptian Informatics Journal, 17*, 99–124.

Farnia, P., Ahmadian, A., Khoshnevisan, A., Jaberzadeh, A. H., Serej, N. D., & Kazerooni, A. F. (2011). *An efficient Point Based Registration of Intra-operative Ultrasound images with MR images for computation of brain shift: A Phantom Study*. 33rd Annual International Conference of the IEEE EMBS Boston, MA.

Forsberg, D. (2013). *Robust Image Registration for Improved Clinical Efficiency Using Local Structure Analysis and Model-Based Processing*. Linköping Studies in Science and Technology. Dissertations, No. 1514.

Gronningsaeter, A., Unsgaerd, G., Ommedal, S., & Angelsen, B. A. J. (1996). Ultrasound-guided neurosurgery: A feasibility study in the 3-30 MHz frequency range. *British Journal of Neurosurgery, 10*(2), 161-168.

Hammoud, Ligon, Elsouki, Shi, Schomer, & Sawaya. (1996). Use of intraoperative ultrasound for localizing tumors and determining the extent of resection: A comparative study with magnetic resonance imaging. *Journal of Neurosurgery, 84*, 737–741.

Ji, S., Wu, Z., Hartov, A., Roberts, D. W., & Paulsen, K. D. (2008). Mutual-information-based image to patient re-registration using intraoperative ultrasound in image-guided neurosurgery. *Medical Physics, 35*(10), 4612–4624. doi:10.1118/1.2977728 PMID:18975707

Juan, L., & Gwun, O. (2009). A comparison of sift, PCA-sift and surf. *Int. J. Image Process., 3*(5), 143–152.

Kaivukangas, J., Salni, Y. L., Lakuilala, J., & Oikarinen, J. (1993). Ultrasound -Controlled Neronavigator-guided brain Surgery. *Journal of Neurosurgery, 79*, 36-42.

Karacali, B. (2007). Information theoretic deformable registration using local image information. *IJCV, Vol, 72*(3), 219–237. doi:10.1007/s11263-006-8704-0

Kim, J., & Fessler, J. A. (2004, November). Intensity-based image registration using robust correlation coefficients. *IEEE Transactions on Medical Imaging, 23*(11), 1430–1444. doi:10.1109/TMI.2004.835313 PMID:15554130

Koivukangas, J., & Kelly, P.J. (1986). Application of ultrasound imaging to stereotactic brain tumor surgery. *Annals of Clinical Research Supplement*, (47), 25-32.

Lionello, G., Sirieix, C., & Baleanin, M. (2014). An effective procedure to create a speckle pattern on biological soft tissue for digital image correlation measurements. *Journal of the Mechanical Behavior of Biomedical Materials, 39*, 1–8.

Maes, F., Collignon, A., Vandermeulen, D., Marchal, G., & Suetens, P. (1997). Multimodality image registration by maximization of mutual information. *IEEE Transactions on Medical Imaging*, *16*(2), 187–198. doi:10.1109/42.563664 PMID:9101328

Maintz, J. B. A., & Viergever, M. A. (1998). A survey of medical image registration. *Medical Image Analysis*, *2*(1), 1–36. doi:10.1016/S1361-8415(01)80026-8 PMID:10638851

McPherson, C. (n.d.). *Video lecture on "Image guided Surgery"*. Mayfield Clinic and UC Brain Tumor Center. Retrieved from www.youtube.com

Mercier, L., Araujo, D., Haegelen, C., Maestro, R. F. D., Petrecca, K., & Collins, D. L. (2013, January). Registering pre- and postresection 3-dimensional ultrasound for improved visualization of residual brain tumor. *Ultrasound in Medicine & Biology*, *39*(1), 16–29. doi:10.1016/j.ultrasmedbio.2012.08.004 PMID:23200177

Mercier, L., DelMaestro, R. F., Petrecca, K., Araujo, D., Haegelen, C., & Collins, D. L. (2012, June). On-line database of clinical MR and ultrasound images of brain tumors. *Medical Physics*, *6*(39), 3253–3261. doi:10.1118/1.4709600 PMID:22755708

Mercier, L., Fonov, V., Haegelen, C., Maestro, R.F.D., Petrecca, K., & Collins, D. L. (2012). Comparing two approaches to rigid registration of three-dimensional ultrasound and magnetic resonance images for neurosurgery. *Int J Comput Assist Radiol Surg.*, *7*(1), 125-36.

Mercier, L., Maestro, R. F. Del, Petrecca, K., Kochanowska, A., Drouin, S., Yan, C. X. B., … Collins, L. (2011). New prototype neuronavigation system based on preoperative imaging and intraoperative freehand ultrasound: system description and validation. *Int J CARS, 6*, 507–522.

Michailovich, O., & Adam, D. (2003). Robust Estimation of Ultrasound Pulses Using Outlier-Resistant De-Noising. *IEEE Transactions on Medical Imaging, 22*(3).

Michailovich, O. V., & Tannenbaum, A. (2006). De-speckling of medical ultrasound images. *IEEE Transactions on Ultrasonics, Ferroelectrics, and Frequency Control, 53*(1).

MIPAV. (2005). Labeling and Measuring Brain Components in Talairach Space. National Institutes of Health Center for Information Technology.

Moiyadi, A., Shetty, V., & Shetty, P. (2016). Direct navigated 3d ultrasound for resection of brain tumors: A useful tool for intraoperative image guidance. *Neurosurgical Focus*, *40*(3), E5. doi:10.3171/2015.12.FOCUS15529 PMID:26926063

Moore, K., & Kim, L. (2009). Primary Brain Tumors: Characteristics, Practical Diagnostic and Treatment Approaches. *Glioblastoma*, 43-75.

Morel, J.-M., & Yu, G. (2009). ASIFT: A new framework for fully affine invariant image comparison. *SIAM Journal on Imaging Sciences*, *2*(2), 438–469. doi:10.1137/080732730

Nigris, D. D., Collins, D. L., & Arbel, T. (2012). Multi-Modal Image Registration Based on Gradient Orientations of Minimal Uncertainty. *IEEE Transactions on Medical Imaging, 31*(12), 2343-2354.

Nigris, D. D., Mercier, L., Maestro, R. D., Collins, D. L., & Arbel, T. (2010). Hierarchical Multimodal Image Registration Based on Adaptive Local Mutual Information. *LNCS, 6362*, 643–651.

Pagoulatos, N., Edwards, W. S., Haynor, D. R., & Kim, Y. (1999). Interactive 3-D Registration of Ultrasound and Magnetic Resonance Images Based on a Magnetic Position Sensor. IEEE Transactions on Information Technology in Biomedicine, 3(4).

Paul, V., & William, M. W. (1997). Alignment by Maximization of Mutual Information. *International Journal of Computer Vision, 24*(2), 137–154. doi:10.1023/A:1007958904918

Pennec, X., Roche, A., Cathier, P., & Ayache, N. (2005). Non-Rigid MR/US Registration for Tracking Brain Deformations. In Multi-Sensor Image Fusion and Its Applications. CRC Press - Taylor and Francis.

Penney, G. P., Blackall, J. M., Hamady, M. S., Sabharwal, T., Adam, A., & Hawkes, D. J. (2004). Registration of freehand 3D ultrasound and magnetic resonance liver images. *Medical Image Analysis, 8*(1), 81–91. doi:10.1016/j.media.2003.07.003 PMID:14644148

Penney, G.P, Blackall, J.M., Hamady, M.S., Sabharwal, T., Adam, A., & Hawkes, D.J. (2004). Registration of freehand 3D ultrasound and magnetic resonance liver images. *Medical Image Analysis, 8*, 81–91.

Petridis, A. K., Anokhin, M., Vavruska, J., Mahvash, M., & Scholz, M. (2015). The value of intraoperative sonography in low grade glioma surgery. *Clinical Neurology and Neurosurgery, 131*, 64–68. doi:10.1016/j.clineuro.2015.02.004 PMID:25704192

Pluim, J. P. W., Maintz, J. B. A., & Viergever, M. A. (2003). Mutual information based registration of medical images: A survey. *IEEE Transactions on Medical Imaging*.

Radha, M. L. (2004). *The Essential Guide to Brain Tumors*. San Francisco, CA: National Brain Tumor Foundation.

Rasmussen, I. A. Jr, Lindseth, F., Rygh, O. M., Berntsen, E. M., Selbekk, T., Xu, J., & Unsgaard, G. et al. (2007). Functional neuronavigation combined with intra-operative 3D ultrasound: Initial experiences during surgical resections close to eloquent brain areas and future directions in automatic brain shift compensation of preoperative data. *Acta Neurochirurgica, 149*(4), 365–378. doi:10.1007/s00701-006-1110-0 PMID:17308976

Renovanz, M., Hickmann, A. K., Henkel, C., Nadji-Ohl, M., & Hopf, N. J. (2014). Navigated versus non-navigated intraoperative ultrasound: is there any impact on the extent of resection of high-grade gliomas? a retrospective clinical analysis. Journal of Neurological Surgery. Part A, Central European Neurosurgery, 75(3), 224–230.

Rivaz, H., Chen, S.J.S., & Collins, D. L. (2015). Automatic Deformable MR-Ultrasound Registration for Image-Guided Neurosurgery. *IEEE Transactions on Medical Imaging, 34*(2), 366-380.

Rivaz, H., & Collins, D. L. (2014). Near real-time robust nonrigid registration of volumetric ultrasound images for neurosurgery. *Ultrasound in Medicine & Biology, 2014*. doi:10.1016/j.ultrasmedbio.2014.08.013 PMID:25542482

Rivaz, H., & Collins, D. L. (2015, July). Deformable registration of preoperative MR, pre-resection ultrasound, and post-resection ultrasound images of neurosurgery. *International Journal of Computer Assisted Radiology and Surgery, 10*(7), 1017–1028. doi:10.1007/s11548-014-1099-4 PMID:25373447

Roche, A., Malandain, G., & Ayache, N. (1999). *Unifying maximum likelihood approaches in medical image registration.* RR-3741 1999. Retrieved from https://hal.inria.fr/inria-00072923

Roche, A., Pennec, X., Malandain, G., & Ayache, N. (2001, October). Rigid Registration of 3D Ultrasound with MR Images: A New Approach Combining Intensity and Gradient Information. *IEEE Transactions on Medical Imaging, 20*(10), 1038–1049. doi:10.1109/42.959301 PMID:11686439

Schwarz, L. A. (2007). *Non-rigid Registration Using Free-form Deformations* (Thesis). Siemens Corporate Research, Inc.

Sotiras, A., Christos, D., & Paragios, N. (2013). Deformable Medical Image Registration: A Survey. *IEEE Transactions on Medical Imaging, 32*(7), 1153–1190. doi:10.1109/TMI.2013.2265603 PMID:23739795

Sung-Hyuk, C. (2007). Comprehensive Survey on Distance/Similarity Measures between Probability Density Function. *International Journal of Mathematical Models and Methods in Applied Sciences, 1*(4), 2007.

Trobaugh, J. W., Richard, W. D., Smith, K. R., & Bucholz, R. D. (1994). Frameless stereotactic ultrasonography: Method and applications. *Computerized Medical Imaging and Graphics, 18*(4), 235-246.

Unsgaard, G., Gronningsaeter, A., Ommedal, S., & Hernes. T. A. N. (2002). Brain operations guided by real-time two-dimensional ultrasound: New possibilities as a result of improved image quality. *Neurosurgery, 51*(2), 402–412.

Unsgaard, G., Ommedal, S., Muller, T., Gronningsaeter, A., & Hernes, N.TA. (2002). Neuronavigation by intraoperative three-dimensional ultrasound: Initial experience during brain tumor resection. *Neurosurgery, 50*, 804–812.

Unsgaard, G., Selbekk, T., Brostrup, M. T., Ommedal, S., Torp, S. H., Myhr, G., & Hernes, N. T. A. et al. (2005). Ability of navigated 3D ultrasound to delineate gliomas and metastases–comparison of image interpretations with histopathology. *Acta Neurochirurgica, 147*(12), 1259–1269, discussion 1269. doi:10.1007/s00701-005-0624-1 PMID:16172831

Xie, Z., & Farin, G. E. (2004, January/February). Image Registration Using Hierarchical B-Splines. *IEEE Transactions on Visualization and Computer Graphics, 10*(1). PMID:15382700

Zhou, H., & Rivaz, H. (2016). Registration of Pre- and Postresection Ultrasound Volumes With Non-corresponding Regions in Neurosurgery. *IEEE Journal of Biomedical and Health Informatics, 20*(5).

Zitova, B., & Flusser, J. (2003). Image registration methods: A survey. *Image and Vision Computing, Vol, 21*(11), 977–1000. doi:10.1016/S0262-8856(03)00137-9

Chapter 8
Automatic Retinal Image Analysis for the Detection of Diabetic Retinopathy

Prasanna Porwal
Shri Guru Gobind Singhji Institute of Engineering and Technology, India

Samiksha Pachade
Shri Guru Gobind Singhji Institute of Engineering and Technology, India

Manesh Kokare
Shri Guru Gobind Singhji Institute of Engineering and Technology, India

Girish Deshmukh
Dr. G. A. Deshmukh Eye Clinic, India

Vivek Sahasrabuddhe
Shankarrao Chavan Government Medical College, India

ABSTRACT

Diabetic Retinopathy, a condition in the person affected by diabetes, is most common cause of blindness in the world. Recent research has given a better understanding of requirement in clinical eye care practice to identify better and cheaper ways of identification, management, diagnosis and treatment of retinal disease. The importance of diabetic retinopathy screening programs and difficulty in achieving reliable early diagnosis of diabetic retinopathy at a reasonable cost needs attention to develop computer-aided diagnosis tool. Computer aided disease diagnosis in retinal image analysis could ease mass screening of population with diabetes mellitus and help clinicians in utilizing their time more efficiently. The recent technological advances in computing power, communication systems, and machine learning techniques provide opportunities to the biomedical engineers and computer scientists to meet the requirements of clinical practice. With proper self-care, management, and medical professional support, individuals with diabetes can live a healthy and long life.

DOI: 10.4018/978-1-5225-2829-6.ch008

INTRODUCTION

Diabetes Mellitus is a metabolic disorder, characterized by hyperglycemia in which there is an excess of glucose circulating in the blood. It is also commonly known as diabetes. Insulin is the hormone secreted by pancreas responsible for maintaining blood glucose level in the body. The pancreas of the person affected with diabetes either cannot produce enough insulin, utilizes it incorrectly or both. Insulin helps the body to utilize glucose from carbohydrates in the food and facilitates it to enter into body cells for getting burned to attain energy. The body normally regulates blood glucose delicately in the fasting state in a range around 4 to 5.5 mmol/L in the plasma. Insulin helps in preventing blood glucose level from getting too high (hyperglycemia) or too low (hypoglycemia).

Hyperglycemia leads to excessive glycosylation of proteins, and this is the primary attribute of the long-term complications of diabetes. Diabetes is usually divided into two categories i.e. 'Type – I diabetes' and 'Type – II diabetes'. Type – I diabetes is characterized by the inadequacy of insulin and Type – II diabetes has attributes showing the pertinent inadequacy of insulin corresponding to insulin resistance. Insulin insufficiency – either complete or partial – is the fundamental component behind diabetes. However, different variables have an impact and can be more critical while considering treatment.

Insulin requirement depends upon a complex balance between various hormones, existing energy stores, physical activity, and resistance to insulin action in muscle, liver and adipose tissue (Worsley & Simmons, 2010). Modern lifestyle in the developing world has significantly reduced physical activity, and people tend to have an intake of high-calorie food which results in an imbalance of energy that further leads to greater obesity, insulin resistance, and Type – II diabetes. Insulin resistance is defined as the downgraded capacity of peripheral tissues and the liver to respond to insulin. This insulin resistance is frequently found in diabetes and is particularly critical in Type – II diabetes where it aggravates the secretory deformities (Scanlon et al., 2009). A person with diabetes has high blood glucose either because they are not producing enough insulin, or because the body does not respond appropriately to insulin.

Diabetes is considered the world's one of the biggest health emergencies of the 21st century. A number of people living with this condition are progressively increasing each year. According to an estimate of International Diabetes Federation (IDF, 2015), there are now 415 million people aged between 20 to 79 with diabetes worldwide. IDF estimated a further 318 million individuals with impaired glucose tolerance, which gradually increases the risk of developing the disease in the future. Also, the majority of individuals with diabetes are from developing countries like China (109 million) and India (69.2 million).

Both Type – I and Type – II diabetes is linked with long-term microvascular complications like retinopathy, nephropathy, and neuropathy. Consistent high blood glucose concentration also leads to macrovascular complications such as heart failure, stroke, disease, and peripheral vascular disease. Other health problems also continue to occur due to glycation such as diabetic foot, osteoporosis, cheiroarthropathy, and cataract. In particular diabetic retinopathy was considered as a diabetes-related health issue that research studies anticipated the time span amongst advancement and diagnosis of diabetes by backward linear regression (Worsley & Simmons, 2010).

According to a recent survey conducted by World Health Organization (WHO), healthcare costs associated with the treatment of health issues due to diabetes amounts to approximately US$ 825 billion dollars per year (NCD, 2016). Diabetes is globally significant and costly complication, and its prevalence is growing at almost epidemic levels. Furthermore, diabetic patients encounter significant decrements in daily activities and quality of life with increasing visual impairment. Hence, novel and innovative ways of identification, diagnosis, treatment and follow-up are essential in the management of this growing problem.

The most eloquent indicator of the pervasiveness of diabetic retinopathy is a span of diabetes. Given the significance of diabetic retinopathy and its impact on retina creating a visual deficiency, and also its utility in giving a window on the history of diabetes in the individuals, this chapter will concentrate on definition and classification of diabetic retinopathy, the epidemiology, automatic screening of retina by computer aided diagnosis and teleophthalmology tools.

RETINAL STRUCTURE AND FUNCTION

The human eye is a slightly asymmetrical sphere with an approximate sagittal diameter or length of 24 to 25 mm and transverse diameter of 24 mm. It has a volume of about 6.5 ccs. The visible parts of the eye (as shown in Figure 1) include the transparent cornea, the typically white sclera, colored iris, and a black-looking aperture called pupil. To the outside of the eye is a transparent white sheet called conjunctiva. A ray of light passes through the cornea, anterior chamber where the pupil and lens focus the image through vitreous humor and then incident on the retina (Modarresi & Oveisi, 2014).

The retina is semi-transparent layered tissue as shown in Figure 2, lining in the interior of the eye consisting of millions of photoreceptors. Photoreceptors enable the conversion of incoming light into a neural signal that is suitable for further processing in the visual cortex of the brain through optic nerve, tracts, and radiations. Approximate area of the retina is 1,206 square mm calculated from the expectations that the average dimension of the human eye is 24 mm from anterior to posterior poles and that 72% of the inside of the globe is retina (Kolb, Fernandez, & Nelson, 1995). By changing the size of the pupil, the amount of light entering the eye is controlled by iris by closing when the light is bright and opening when the light is dim (Hersh, 2008). Ciliary muscles in ciliary body monitor the focusing of lens automatically. For nourishment of the retina, the blood supply is primarily through the choroid

Figure 1. Anatomical structure of eye and color fundus image

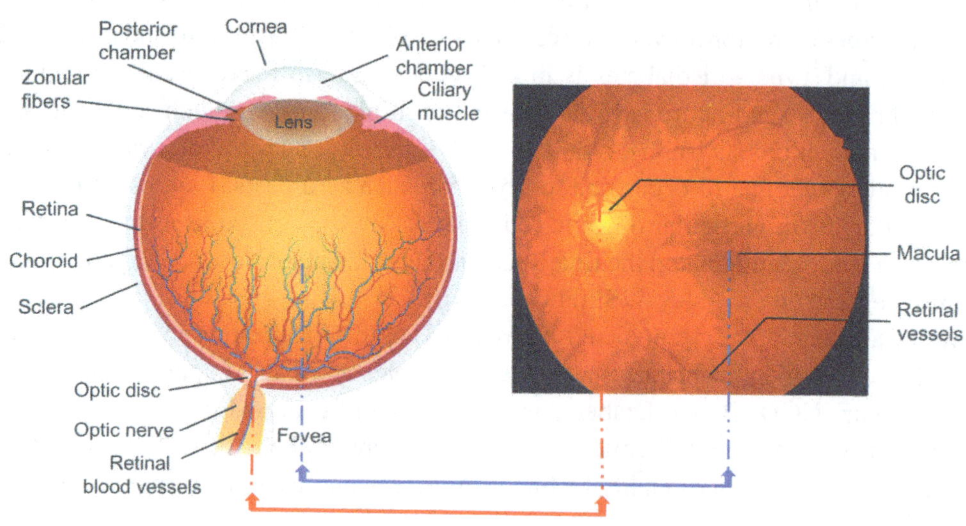

Figure 2. Illustration of layered structure of the retina

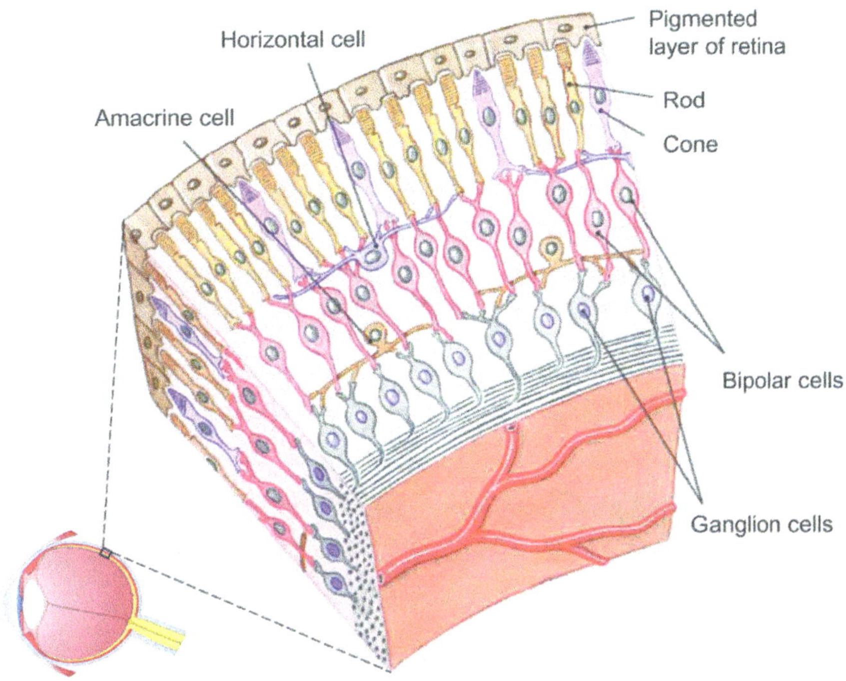

(approximately 65%) and secondarily through the retinal vasculature (about 35%) which lies on the top of the retina. The optic disc is the entry point of the main vessels which supply blood to retina and exit point for ganglion cell axons leaving the eye. The optic disc is also called as a blind spot because no photoreceptors are overlying it. There is an optic cup of variable size located at the center that can be substantial in for diagnosis of glaucoma.

The macula is a central part of approximately 6 mm diameter of the retina, having multiple layers of ganglion cells. The retina contains two types of photosensitive cells, the rods, and the cones. Cones are responsible for color vision and function in bright light, whereas rods are more sensitive than cones in dim light but do not discriminate colors. The fovea is a small pit situated close to the center of the macula. It contains the largest concentration of cones. Hence, the macula is necessary for the central, most accurate and color vision. If there is an accumulation of fluids due to leakage of blood vessels near the macular region, then this condition in diabetic retinopathy is called as diabetic macular edema.

DIABETIC RETINOPATHY AND PUBLIC HEALTH

Diabetic Retinopathy (DR) is the particular microvascular complication of diabetes and is the most common leading cause of preventable blindness in the working age population in the world (Kolb, Fernandez, & Nelson, 1995). Reports from International Council of Ophthalmology (ICO) indicate that 1 in 3 individual affected with diabetes had some form of diabetic retinopathy and also highlighted that 1 in 10 had vision-threatening DR. In India it is the sixth common cause of blindness.

DR is referred as a clinical diagnosis, depicted by the presence (see Figure 3) of one or more several retinal lesions like microaneurysms, hemorrhages, hard exudates, soft exudates. Along with these findings, there may be a presence of venous beading, retinal neovascularization which can be utilized to classify DR retinopathy in one of the two phases known as non-proliferative diabetic retinopathy (NPDR) and proliferative diabetic retinopathy (PDR) as shown in Figure 4.

Diabetic macular edema (DME) is a complication associated with DR in which retinal thickening or accumulation of fluid can occur at any stage of DR. It is classified as mild DME, moderate DME and severe DME (illustrated in Figure 5) based on the location of hard exudate or retinal thickening as mentioned in Table 2. The determination of DR and DME severity based on criteria given in Table 1 and Table 2 is used to decide the need for treatment and follow-up recommendations.

Figure 3. Clinical signs of DR

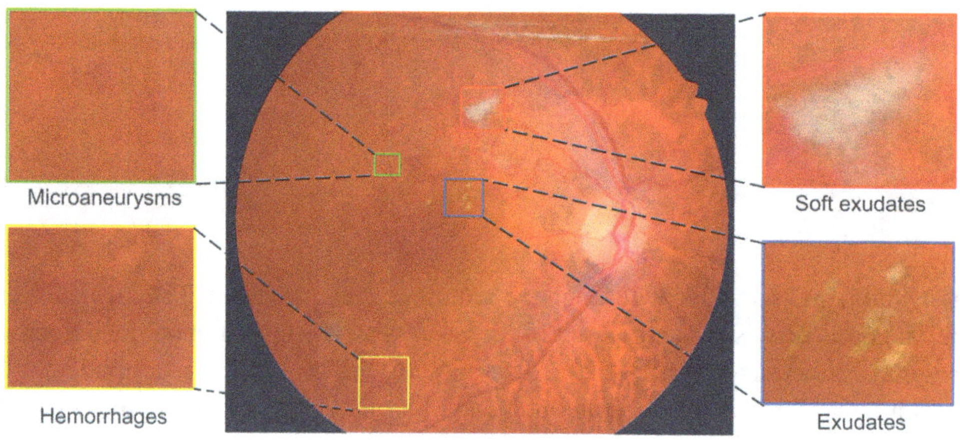

Figure 4. Stages of DR: (a) NPDR and (b) PDR

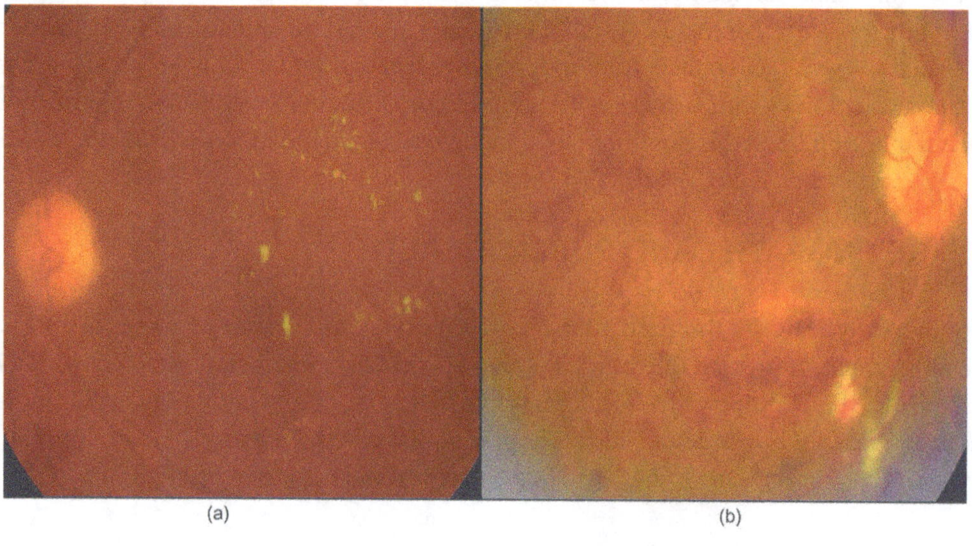

Figure 5. Classification of DME: (a) Moderate and (b) Severe

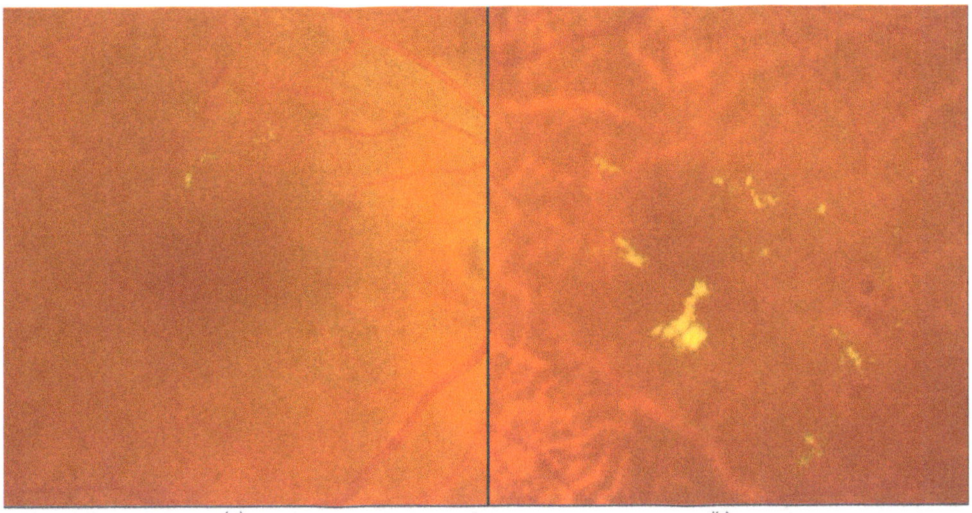

(a) (b)

Table 1. International clinical diabetic retinopathy (DR) severity scale

Disease Severity Level	Findings
No apparent retinopathy	No visible sign of abnormalities
Mild – non-proliferative diabetic retinopathy (NPDR)	Only presence of Microaneurysms
Moderate – non-proliferative diabetic retinopathy (NPDR)	More than just microaneurysms but less than severe NPDR
Severe – non-proliferative diabetic retinopathy (NPDR)	Moderate NPDR and any of the following: • > 20 intraretinal hemorrhages (each quadrant) • Venous beading (in ≥ 2 quadrants) • Intraretinal microvascular abnormalities (in ≥ 1 quadrant) • no signs of PDR
Proliferative diabetic retinopathy (PDR)	Severe NPDR and one or both of the following: • Neovascularization • Vitreous/preretinal hemorrhage

Table 2. International clinical diabetic macular edema (DME) severity scale

Mild DME	Presence of hard exudate or thickening of retina in the posterior retina but distant from center of the macula
Moderate DME	Presence of hard exudate or thickening of retina near center of the macula not including center of the macula
Severe DME	Presence of hard exudate or thickening of retina in center of the macula

A Polar coordinate system is framed based on ETDRS system that can be utilized as a landmark to image analysis techniques. According to ETDRS report (Early Treatment Diabetic Retinopathy Study Research Group, 1991), a color fundus image is divided into 10 subfields by three concentric circles with radii of 1/3-disc diameter (DD), 1DD, 2DD respectively as shown in Figure 6 that is used for DME

Figure 6. Retinal polar coordinate system with macula at center

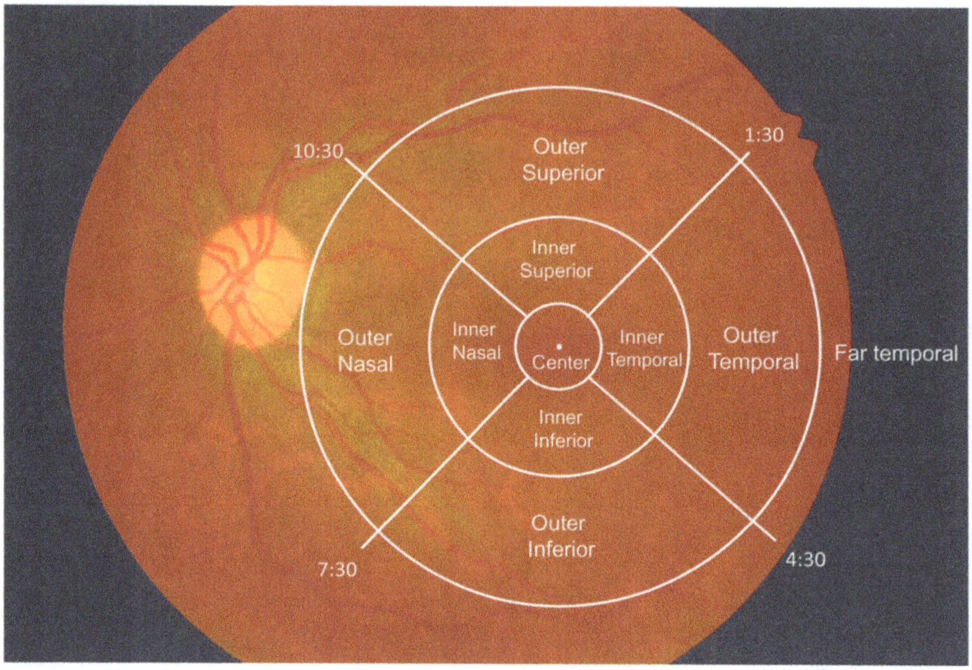

grading. These 10 sub fields are defined as: (a) central subfield called 'center' within the circle of radius 1/3 DD; (b) four inner subfields called 'inner (nasal, superior, temporal, and inferior)' located between circle of radius 1/3 DD and 1DD; (c) four outer subfields called 'outer (nasal, superior, temporal, and inferior)' located between circle of radius 1DD and 2DD; (d) subfield called 'far temporal', it is located temporal to the circle of radius 2 DD and between 1:30 and 4:30 for left eye and between 7:30 and 10:30 for right eye.

EYE SCREENING FOR DIABETIC RETINOPATHY

Due to asymptomatic nature of DR, patients are unaware of disease, which prevents an early checkup from retinal specialists that is left undetected till the visually symptomatic severe stage. A better understanding of DR progression had created awareness in research community which leads to new avenues for prevention, management, and treatment. Vision impairment due to diabetes can only be avoided by screening all the patients affected with diabetes for early detection and treatment.

At present, retinal photography and slit-lamp biomicroscopy are the two reliable media for determination of DR. Both need dilated pupils and depend on interpretation by retinal experts. On the other hand newer non-mydriatic digital retinal fundus camera is non-invasive and painless mean to screen the retina. Use of fundus camera requires basic training for the use of it but expertize is essential for slit-lamp biomicroscopy and indirect ophthalmoscopy. Moreover, fundus imaging for DR screening is cost effective and valuable health strategy that has the advantage of creating a permanent record and hence, a preferred mode of DR assessment.

Diabetic patients are suggested to do a regular biannual or annual check-up of the retina. The elimination of preventable visual impairment is mainly dependent on the pool of expert clinicians and basic health care infrastructure essential for the treatment of the eye. In the Indian subcontinent, against national eye care experts: population ratio of 1:107,000, there are various regions in which there is the ratio of 1:9000 whereas in some other parts there is only one eye care expert for 608,000 population (Raman et al., 2016). Management of such a huge population for DR screening worldwide is an important aspect, and it can be achieved by conducting large-scale screening of population with diabetes. Even if the number of eye care specialists is adequate, utilizing expertise to screen every diabetic patient is an inefficient use of resources.

The assessment process for DR includes: (a) patient history – duration of diabetes, past glycemic control, medications, ocular and systemic history, (b) a regular eye examination and screening retina of patients who had never been through the process of treatment for DR or any other eye issue, and (c) regular follow-up. The aim of a screening program is to determine patients who possibly need treatment by a retinal specialist and close monitoring and others patients who may simply be screened biannually or annually.

Screening programs rely on four parameters – target patient population to be screened for DR, actual population screened (in percent), the cost involved in making all the arrangements, and outcome of screening method in terms of sensitivity and specificity (Browning, 2010).

Figure 7. Flowchart for DR screening

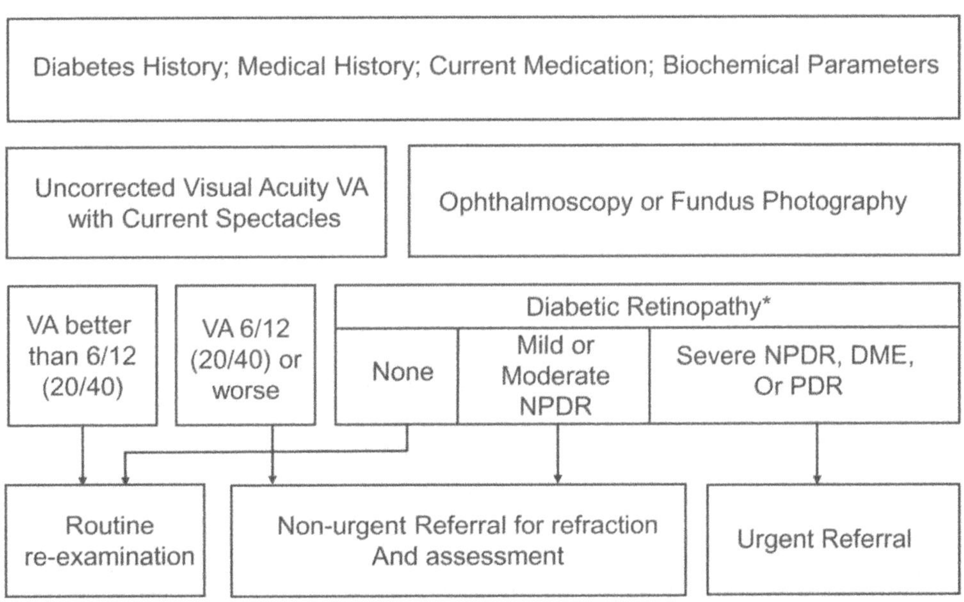

*Need to optimize medical treatment; glycemic control, hypertension and lipids.

NPDR : Non-Proliferative Diabetic Retinopathy
PDR : Proliferative Diabetic Retinopathy
DME : Diabetic Macular Edema
VA : Visual Acuity

AUTOMATIC SCREENING BY COMPUTER AIDED DIAGNOSIS SYSTEMS

Conventional health care system is manual, slow, costly and inefficient. The time when visual symptoms are observed, the recovery rate of disease is slow, and management becomes costly. The newer healthcare system primarily focuses on periodic monitoring and prevention of the disease. This, in turn, has brought down the cost of health management by ensuring timely treatment as corrective action is done in planned manner utilizing technology, paramedics, and ophthalmologists effectively. The implementation of the program is done by screening the entire risk group for DR, hence called as risk reduction program.

Tele-Diabetic Retinopathy (Tele-DR) diagnosis and digital image based referral service shown in Figure 8 can exchange the clinical data by means of a communication network, further providing significant benefits to the healthcare system. It can aid in clinical support by means of patient consultation and monitoring of patients located in the remote area utilizing mobile units and kiosk. Several feasibility studies (Mukhopadhay, Gupta & Bansal, 2014) demonstrate the usefulness of the technology combining automated image analysis tools and expert decision support systems could provide widespread screening. Digital retinal fundus images are a most preferred modality for the screening of DR. Large-scale risk reduction programs generate a huge number of fundus photographs for manual reading. Processing, managing and reading pictures for detecting abnormalities from the images acquired by screening programs is time-consuming, labor intensive, and prone to human error. Computer-aided diagnosis (CAD) tool in retinal image analysis could ease mass screening of population with diabetes mellitus and help clinicians in utilizing their time more efficiently. Such diagnostic support system (Mookiah e al., 2013) directly assists health professionals and clinicians in the task of decision-making. A medical decision

Figure 8. Model for managing and processing information in DR screening

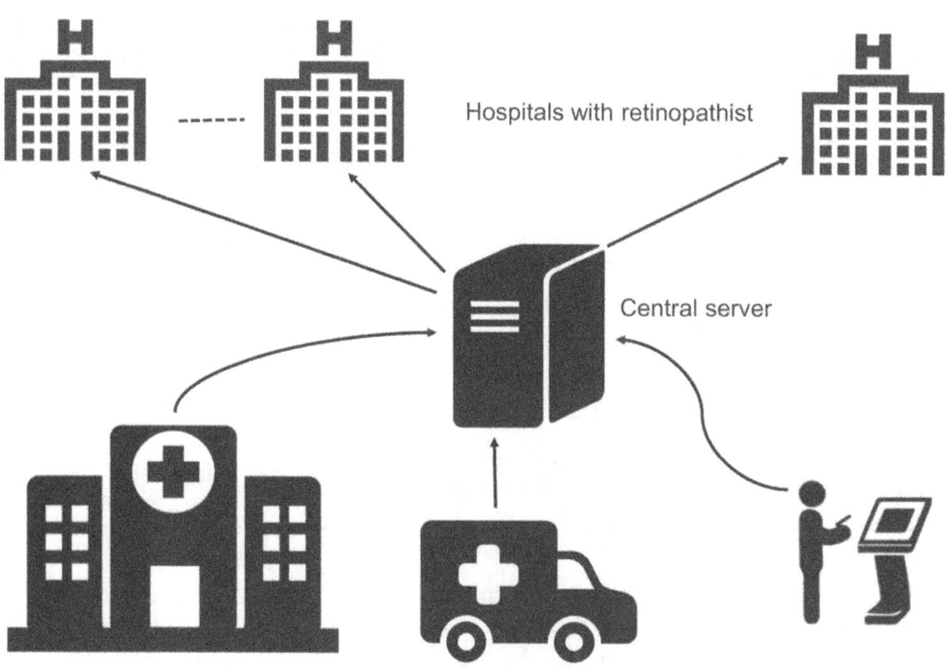

support system for DR could differentiate the healthy subjects and mild, moderate and severe DR stages of disease that will further help the treatment. Reports by CAD tools of the population can be used for planning and communicating the moderate and severe cases with priority to the retinal experts. Using adequate information as (a) patient history – duration of diabetes, past glycemic control, medications, ocular and systemic history, (b) the visual acuity test report and (c) retinal fundus examinations, diagnostic system can decide about referral of the patient to the clinician as shown in the Figure 9 and an appropriate management plan as outlined by ICO guidelines for diabetic retinopathy screening.

Patients with less than adequate retinal assessment should be referred to an ophthalmologist unless it is evident that there is no DR, or at most, only mild nonproliferative DR (i.e., microaneurysms only). In addition, persons with an unexplained visual-acuity loss should be referred.

The retinal images captured by fundus camera decouple the examination process into the disjoint tasks of image acquisition and interpretation. Interpretation of retinal images is done by automated image analysis software coupled with CAD Tool for assessment of DR as shown in Figure 9. Automated image analysis can contribute in terms of (a) image enhancement, (b) detection of normal and abnormal structures, and (c) monitoring progression of disease (Walter et al., 2002).

Image Enhancement

Images acquired from the standard examination using fundus camera often contain some artifacts, noisy, poorly contrasted and non-uniformly illuminated. Methods for artifacts and noise removal, contrast, and sharpness enhancement are required. Many approaches have been observed (Feng et al., 2007; Porwal

Figure 9. Flow of computer aided diagnosis of fundus image

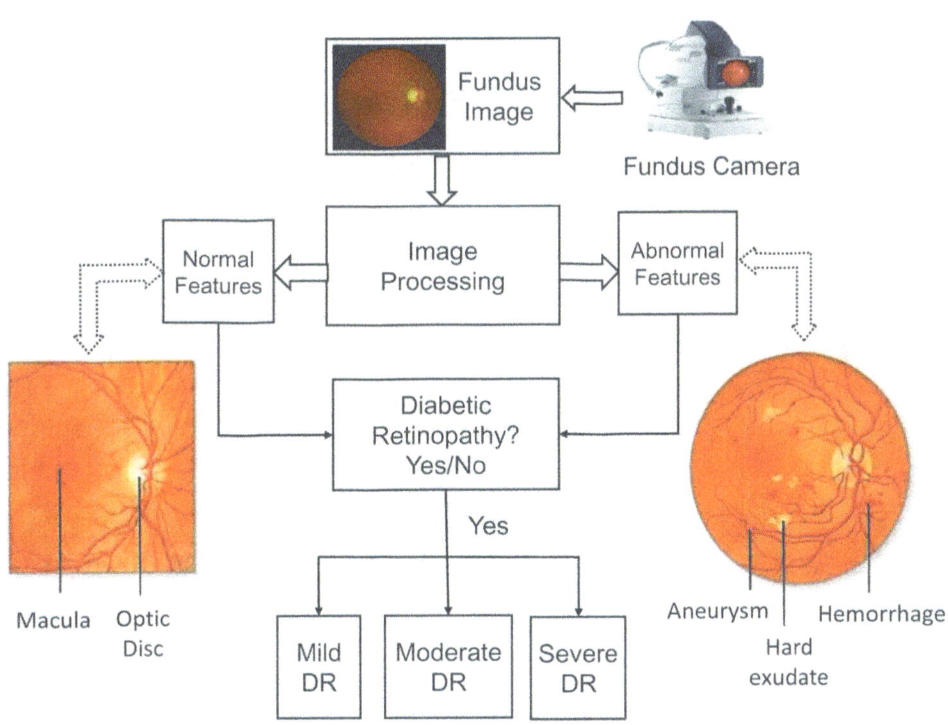

& Kokare, 2016) for contrast stretching and noise removal. Retinal image enhancement can act as aid (see Figure 10) for clinicians to interpret the fundus images. Also, it is used as a primary step toward automatic disease detection and analysis from fundus images.

Detection of Abnormalities

Manual measurements and analysis of individual abnormalities like microaneurysms, hemorrhages, hard exudates and cotton wool spots is quite difficult and time-consuming. Several attempts are made by research community for detecting them, major work is done in the automatic detection of exudates (Sopharak et al., 2008; Fleming et al., 2009; Mookiah et al., 2013) and microaneurysms (Niemeijer et al., 2010; Meysam, Mahdieh, & Alireza, 2017; Antal & Hajdu, 2012) as compared to haemorrhages (Emerson et al., 2001; Wong et al., 2006) and cotton wool spots (Niemeijer et al., 2007). It can help in reduction of examination time per patient. Along with the abnormalities, detection of normal retinal features is essential for classification of pathologies, and their location provides a clue for disease severity grading.

Figure 11 show the usual approach followed for the detection of exudate: the steps are a selection of high contrast green channel highlighting the presence of exudates, further processing by application of image enhancement technique followed by segmentation and removal of the optic disc. Furthermore, the binary exudation part is used in DME detection utilizing location information of macular region using which its grade is decided based on the international clinical standard given in Table 2. Some approaches in the literature (Giancardo et al., 2012; Akram et al., 2014; Deepak & Sivaswamy, 2012) use only macular region for segmenting lesions for analysis of the DME presence. Similarly, DR severity grading is done (Wilkinson et al., 2003; Dyck et al., 1993; Wong et al., 2006) by determining number of abnormalities in each quadrant of the image using standard given in Table 1.

Figure 10. (a) Original fundus image, and (b) image after enhancement

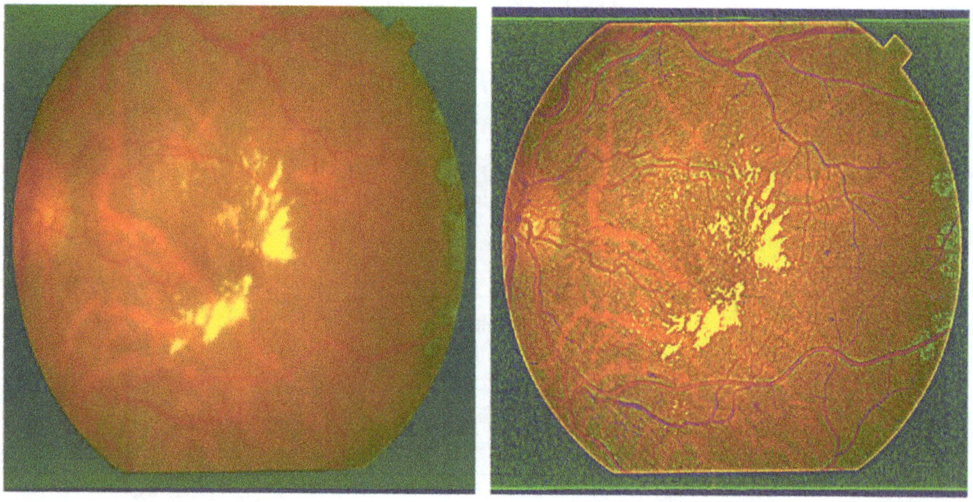

(a) (b)

Figure 11. Exudate detection from fundus image

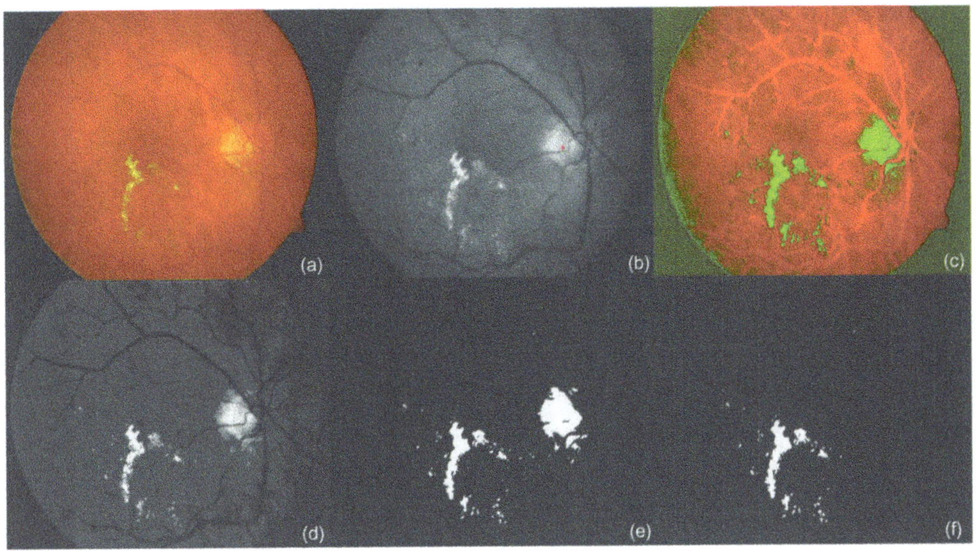

Monitoring of Disease

The assessment of disease evolution can be done by comparing medical records at different time instances that can help in observation of the turn-over effect of individual abnormality and evaluation of the effectiveness of therapeutics given to the patients. Also comparing images captured at different time instance is very time consuming and prone to observer error due to distortion in the images making it difficult to superimpose. Further, the large number of abnormalities that have to be compared make it more difficult giving rise to need of automated registration technique that can be utilized to serve the purpose. Different retinal image registration algorithms have been proposed (Chen et al., 2010; Parekar, Porwal & Kokare, 2016; Stewart, Tsai & Roysam, 2013; Chanwimaluang, Fan & Fransen, 2006) in the literature.

Retinal Vessel Width Measurement

The retinal vessels play vital role in the detection of several vascular diseases. They are only blood vessels in the body clearly visible using optical techniques that can be used to detect the regions of width change (see Figure 12). However, there are few quantitative studies (Lowell et al., 2009; Al-Diri, Hunter & Steel, 2009) of the relationships between retinal vessel features and disease due to the practical difficulties in efficiently extracting measurements that are consistent and precise.

FUTURE SCOPE

The field of retinal image analysis for detection of diabetic retinopathy is developing rapidly. Major efforts have been made for implementing CAD in clinical setup and are due in large scale trials, also awaiting final clearance from the competent authority. From the previous sections, it can be stated that

Figure 12. Retinal vessel width measurement

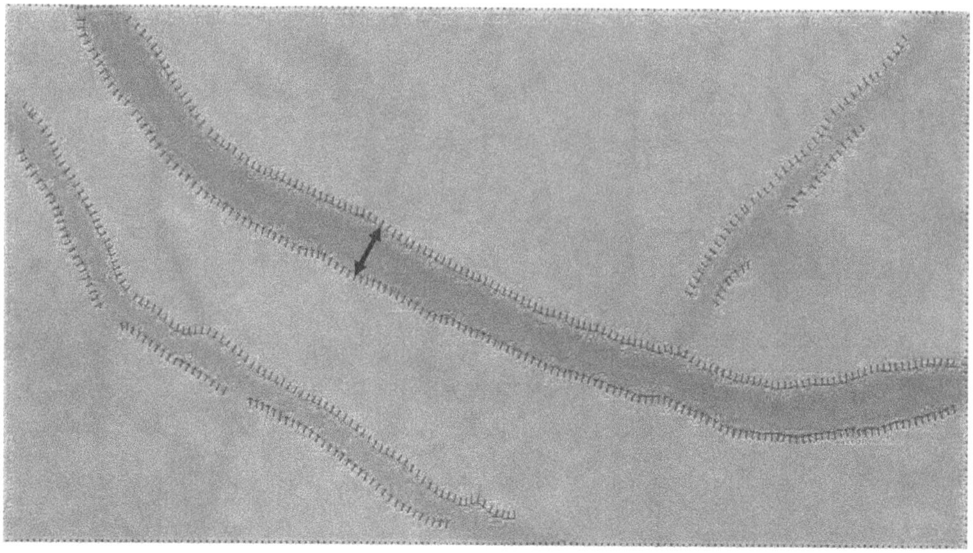

there are various avenues to utilize the technology of computer aided decision system in DR into actual clinical practice.

An approach based on detection of retinal lesions and then estimation of DR stage has always been a mainstay. Recently attention of researchers is shifting to artificial intelligence as with increased computing power, a large number of images and deep learning based approaches, lesion detection performance can improve.

Though vessel detection has been intensely focused in image analysis community, detection of vessel width changes and neovascularization that have much clinical relevance have not received proper attention. Along with DR, there are other few diseases like glaucoma, retinitis pigmentosa, hypertensive retinopathy which manifests themselves in the retina. Efforts must be made to integrate methods to detect each of the disease manifesting the retina in the single system.

CONCLUSION

The screening solution would automatically isolate abnormal cases by applying suitably calibrated detectors of disease indicators. Since the number of normal cases is expected to be greater than the abnormal, the screening process can reduce the workload of ophthalmologists, by having them examine only those cases which are hard to categorize as normal. This can also reduce the treatment costs and help to ensure treatment effectiveness amidst scale-up in the number of patients. Further, the manual analysis may be augmented by using computer-based tools. For example, an image analysis system that automatically determines if lesions are present can reduce the workload of ophthalmologists, by showing them only those cases which are abnormal and directly archiving the normal cases. With proper self-care, management, and medical professional support, individuals with diabetes can live a healthy, long life.

REFERENCES

Akram, M. U., Tariq, A., Khan, S. A., & Javed, M. Y. (2014). Automated detection of exudates and macula for grading of diabetic macular edema. *Computer Methods and Programs in Biomedicine*, *114*(2), 141–152. doi:10.1016/j.cmpb.2014.01.010 PMID:24548898

Al-Diri, B., Hunter, A., & Steel, D. (2009). An active contour model for segmenting and measuring retinal vessels. *IEEE Transactions on Medical Imaging*, *28*(9), 1488–1497. doi:10.1109/TMI.2009.2017941 PMID:19336294

Antal, B., & Hajdu, A. (2012). An ensemble-based system for microaneurysm detection and diabetic retinopathy grading. *IEEE Transactions on Bio-Medical Engineering*, *59*(6), 1720–1726. doi:10.1109/TBME.2012.2193126 PMID:22481810

Browning, D. J. (2010). Screening for diabetic retinopathy. In *Diabetic Retinopathy* (pp. 369–385). Springer New York. doi:10.1007/978-0-387-85900-2_14

Chanwimaluang, T., Fan, G., & Fransen, S. R. (2006). Hybrid retinal image registration. *IEEE Transactions on Information Technology in Biomedicine*, *10*(1), 129–142. doi:10.1109/TITB.2005.856859 PMID:16445258

Chen, J., Tian, J., Lee, N., Zheng, J., Smith, R. T., & Laine, A. F. (2010). A partial intensity invariant feature descriptor for multimodal retinal image registration. *IEEE Transactions on Bio-Medical Engineering*, *57*(7), 1707–1718. doi:10.1109/TBME.2010.2042169 PMID:20176538

Deepak, K. S., & Sivaswamy, J. (2012). Automatic assessment of macular edema from color retinal images. *IEEE Transactions on Medical Imaging*, *31*(3), 766–776. doi:10.1109/TMI.2011.2178856 PMID:22167598

Dyck, P. J., Kratz, K. M., Karnes, J. L., Litchy, W. J., Klein, R., Pach, J. M., & Melton, L. (1993). The prevalence by staged severity of various types of diabetic neuropathy, retinopathy, and nephropathy in a population-based cohort The Rochester Diabetic Neuropathy Study. *Neurology*, *43*(4), 817–817. doi:10.1212/WNL.43.4.817 PMID:8469345

Early Treatment Diabetic Retinopathy Study Research Group. (1991). Grading diabetic retinopathy from stereoscopic color fundus photographs—an extension of the modified Airlie House classification: ETDRS report number 10. *Ophthalmology*, *98*(5), 786–806. doi:10.1016/S0161-6420(13)38012-9 PMID:2062513

Emerson, M. V., Pieramici, D. J., Stoessel, K. M., Berreen, J. P., & Gariano, R. F. (2001). Incidence and rate of disappearance of retinal hemorrhage in newborns. *Ophthalmology*, *108*(1), 36–39. doi:10.1016/S0161-6420(00)00474-7 PMID:11150261

Feng, P., Pan, Y., Wei, B., Jin, W., & Mi, D. (2007). Enhancing retinal image by the Contourlet transform. *Pattern Recognition Letters*, *28*(4), 516–522. doi:10.1016/j.patrec.2006.09.007

Fleming, A. D., Goatman, K. A., Philip, S., Williams, G. J., Prescott, G. J., Scotland, G. S., & Olson, J. A. (2009). The role of haemorrhage and exudate detection in automated grading of diabetic retinopathy. *The British Journal of Ophthalmology*. PMID:19661069

Giancardo, L., Meriaudeau, F., Karnowski, T. P., Li, Y., Garg, S., Tobin, K. W. Jr, & Chaum, E. (2012). Exudate-based diabetic macular edema detection in fundus images using publicly available datasets. *Medical Image Analysis*, *16*(1), 216–226. doi:10.1016/j.media.2011.07.004 PMID:21865074

Hersh, M. A. (2008). Perception, the eye and assistive technology issues. In *Assistive Technology for Visually Impaired and Blind People* (pp. 51–101). Springer London. doi:10.1007/978-1-84628-867-8_2

International Diabetes Federation (IDF). (2015). Facts & figures. Retrieved from https://www.idf.org/about-diabetes/what-is-diabetes?language=en

Kolb, H., Fernandez, E., & Nelson, R. (1995). *Facts and Figures Concerning the Human Retina--Webvision*. The Organization of the Retina and Visual System.

Lowell, J., Hunter, A., Steel, D., Basu, A., Ryder, R., & Kennedy, R. L. (2004). Measurement of retinal vessel widths from fundus images based on 2-D modeling. *IEEE Transactions on Medical Imaging*, *23*(10), 1196–1204. doi:10.1109/TMI.2004.830524 PMID:15493688

Modarresi, M., & Oveisi, I. S. (2014, June). A Contourlet Transform Based for Features Fusion in Retina and Iris Multimodal Biometric System. In *International Workshop on Biometric Authentication* (pp. 75-90). Springer International Publishing. doi:10.1007/978-3-319-13386-7_7

Mookiah, M. R. K., Acharya, U. R., Chua, C. K., Lim, C. M., Ng, E. Y. K., & Laude, A. (2013). Computer-aided diagnosis of diabetic retinopathy: A review. *Computers in Biology and Medicine*, *43*(12), 2136–2155. doi:10.1016/j.compbiomed.2013.10.007 PMID:24290931

Mukhopadhyay, S., Gupta, A., & Bansal, R. (2014). Needs/Requirements and Design of Retinal Imaging and Image Processing Methods for Diabetic Retinopathy in the Indian Context. In *Ophthalmological Imaging and Applications* (pp. 127–134). CRC Press. doi:10.1201/b17026-8

NCD Risk Factor Collaboration. (2016). Worldwide trends in diabetes since 1980: A pooled analysis of 751 population-based studies with 4·4 million participants. *Lancet*, *387*(10027), 1513–1530. doi:10.1016/S0140-6736(16)00618-8 PMID:27061677

Niemeijer, M., Van Ginneken, B., Cree, M. J., Mizutani, A., Quellec, G., Sánchez, C. I., & Wu, X. (2010). Retinopathy online challenge: Automatic detection of microaneurysms in digital color fundus photographs. *IEEE Transactions on Medical Imaging*, *29*(1), 185–195. doi:10.1109/TMI.2009.2033909 PMID:19822469

Niemeijer, M., van Ginneken, B., Russell, S. R., Suttorp-Schulten, M. S., & Abramoff, M. D. (2007). Automated detection and differentiation of drusen, exudates, and cotton-wool spots in digital color fundus photographs for diabetic retinopathy diagnosis. *Investigative Ophthalmology & Visual Science*, *48*(5), 2260–2267. doi:10.1167/iovs.06-0996 PMID:17460289

Parekar, J., Porwal, P., & Kokare, M. (2016, October). Automatic retinal image registration using fully connected vascular tree. In *Signal and Information Processing (IConSIP), International Conference on* (pp. 1-5). IEEE. doi:10.1109/ICONSIP.2016.7857498

Porwal, P., & Kokare, M. (2016, October). A novel method to remove bright artifacts for enhancing lesion detection in retinal images. In *Signal and Information Processing (IConSIP), International Conference on* (pp. 1-5). IEEE. doi:10.1109/ICONSIP.2016.7857474

Raman, R., Gella, L., Srinivasan, S., & Sharma, T. (2016). Diabetic retinopathy: An epidemic at home and around the world. *Indian Journal of Ophthalmology*, *64*(1), 69. doi:10.4103/0301-4738.178150 PMID:26953027

Scanlon, P. H., Wilkinson, C. P., Aldington, S. J., & Matthews, D. R. (2009). *A practical manual of diabetic retinopathy management*. Academic Press.

Sopharak, A., Uyyanonvara, B., Barman, S., & Williamson, T. H. (2008). Automatic detection of diabetic retinopathy exudates from non-dilated retinal images using mathematical morphology methods. *Computerized Medical Imaging and Graphics*, *32*(8), 720–727. doi:10.1016/j.compmedimag.2008.08.009 PMID:18930631

Stewart, C. V., Tsai, C. L., & Roysam, B. (2003). The dual-bootstrap iterative closest point algorithm with application to retinal image registration. *IEEE Transactions on Medical Imaging*, *22*(11), 1379–1394. doi:10.1109/TMI.2003.819276 PMID:14606672

Tavakoli, Nazar, & Mehdizadeh. (2017). Effect of two different preprocessing steps in detection of optic nerve head in fundus images. *Proc. SPIE 10134, Medical Imaging 2017: Computer-Aided Diagnosis*. doi:10.1117/12.2254841

Walter, T., Klein, J. C., Massin, P., & Erginay, A. (2002). A contribution of image processing to the diagnosis of diabetic retinopathy-detection of exudates in color fundus images of the human retina. *IEEE Transactions on Medical Imaging*, *21*(10), 1236–1243. doi:10.1109/TMI.2002.806290 PMID:12585705

Wilkinson, C. P., Ferris, F. L., Klein, R. E., Lee, P. P., Agardh, C. D., Davis, M., & Group, G. D. R. P. (2003). Proposed international clinical diabetic retinopathy and diabetic macular edema disease severity scales. *Ophthalmology*, *110*(9), 1677–1682. doi:10.1016/S0161-6420(03)00475-5 PMID:13129861

Wong, T. Y., Klein, R., Islam, F. A., Cotch, M. F., Folsom, A. R., Klein, B. E., & Shea, S. et al. (2006). Diabetic retinopathy in a multi-ethnic cohort in the United States. *American Journal of Ophthalmology*, *141*(3), 446–455. doi:10.1016/j.ajo.2005.08.063 PMID:16490489

Wong, T. Y., Klein, R., Islam, F. A., Cotch, M. F., Folsom, A. R., Klein, B. E., & Shea, S. et al. (2006). Diabetic retinopathy in a multi-ethnic cohort in the United States. *American Journal of Ophthalmology*, *141*(3), 446–455. doi:10.1016/j.ajo.2005.08.063 PMID:16490489

Worsley, D., & Simmons, D. (2010). Diabetic retinopathy and public health. *Automated Image Detection of Retinal Pathology*, 27-66.

Zhang, X., Thibault, G., Decencière, E., Marcotegui, B., Laÿ, B., Danno, R., & Chabouis, A. (2014). Exudate detection in color retinal images for mass screening of diabetic retinopathy. *Medical Image Analysis*, *18*(7), 1026–1043. doi:10.1016/j.media.2014.05.004 PMID:24972380

Chapter 9
Selected Shape and Texture Features for Automatic Detection of Acute Lymphoblastic Leukemia

Vanika Singhal
Indraprastha Institute of Information Technology, India

Preety Singh
The LNM Institute of Information Technology, India

ABSTRACT

Acute Lymphoblastic Leukemia is a cancer of blood caused due to increase in number of immature lymphocyte cells. Detection is done manually by skilled pathologists which is time consuming and depends on the skills of the pathologist. The authors propose a methodology for discrimination of a normal lymphocyte cell from a malignant one by processing the blood sample image. Automatic detection process will reduce the diagnosis time and not be limited by human interpretation. The lymphocyte images are classified based on two types of extracted features: shape and texture. To identify prominent shape features, Correlation based Feature Selection is applied. Principal Component Analysis is applied on the texture features to reduce their dimensionality. Support Vector Machine is used for classification. It is observed that 16 shape features are able to give a classification accuracy of 92.3% and that changes in the geometrical properties of the nucleus emerge as significant features contributing towards detecting a malignant lymphocyte.

INTRODUCTION

Cancer is the world's leading cause of death. It is marked by uncontrolled cell division contributing to the abnormal growth of tissues. This affects the cellular function of the human body, ultimately leading to death (Dollinger, 2008). In 2012, there were an estimated 8.2 million deaths (comprising 57% males and 43% females) due to cancer (Cancer Research UK). According to American Cancer Society, in 2014,

DOI: 10.4018/978-1-5225-2829-6.ch009

there were an estimated 1,665,540 new cancer cases and 585,720 cancer deaths in the US alone. This includes 52380 estimated new cases (accounting for 3.1% of all new cancer cases) and 24090 estimated deaths (4.1% of all cancer deaths) due to leukemia. SEER Cancer Statistics (National Cancer Institute) say that the rates for new leukemia cases have been rising on an average of 0.2% each year over the last ten years. Leukemia can affect people of all ages though it is more common amongst children, young adults and people over 60 years of age. In leukemia, abnormal white blood cells called blasts are produced in excessive numbers which travel to other body parts. The blasts are unable to work properly and weaken the immune system (Haworth, Hepplestone, Jones, Campbell & Evans, 1981). Classification of leukemia can be divided into two groups:

- Acute or Chronic leukemia (depends on time of progression)
- Lymphoblastic or Myeloid leukemia (subject to type of white blood cells affected)

Acute leukemia progresses rapidly and requires immediate treatment. It is characterized by a surplus of abnormal cells which are not yet fully developed and do not function properly. In chronic leukemia, the number of blast cells increases slowly. Blast cells exist, but the growth of a greater number of developed cells is also present. Acute Lymphoblastic Leukemia (ALL) and Chronic Lymphoblastic Leukemia (CLL) are caused due to abnormalities in lymphocyte cells. Acute Myelogenous Leukemia (AML) and Chronic Myelogenous Leukemia (CML) are caused due to defects in myeloid cells. ALL is more common in children and accounts for about 80% of childhood leukemia (Sawyers, Denny & Witte, 1991). ALL progresses very fast and affects mostly the cells that are not yet fully developed. Early and fast diagnosis of the disease is essential, especially in the case of children, for effective recovery of the patient. The symptoms of leukemia are similar to other disorders like fever, anemia, weakness, bone pain, joint pain and for this reason, the diagnosis is very difficult.

Diagnostic procedure of ALL includes microscopic inspection of peripheral blood or bone marrow samples. Complete blood count or bone marrow biopsies are commonly used blood tests used for leukemia diagnosis (Haworth, Hepplestone, Jones, Campbell & Evans, 1981). Advanced techniques like cytogenetic testing, immunophenotyping and molecular probing are present. However, morphological evaluation of the stained blood sample is widely prevalent as an economical initial screening of ALL (Angulo &Flandrin, 2003). However, if the morphological features are partially present, it may be a difficult task for an expert hematologist too to discriminate between a healthy and malignant lymphocyte. The analysis thus becomes subjective to the skills and experience of the pathologist. Moreover, in countries with a large population and a large number of suspected cancer cases, depending on the visual diagnostic skills of a human is cumbersome and time-consuming. An automated diagnostic procedure can help in providing a fast and efficient detection of leukemia. Digital processing is also beneficial in remote analysis where only the digital image of the blood sample needs to be sent for consultation with a doctor in a different geographical location. The basic difference between normal and blast cells is based on the changes in shape, size and changes in the chromatin pattern in the nucleus (Ries, Melbert, Krapcho, Mariotto, Miller, Feuer, Clegg, Horner, Howlader, Eisner, Reichman & Edwards, 1975-2014). The normal lymphocytes are regular in shape and smaller in size as compared to blast cells. Example images of blood containing a lymphocyte and a blast cell are shown in Figures 1 and 2.

In this chapter, the authors have tried to incorporate machine vision and machine learning to develop an automated system for detection of Acute Lymphoblastic Leukemia. This chapter is an extension of a previous work where the authors worked with the Local Binary Pattern of the lymphocyte images to

Figure 1. Normal lymphocyte

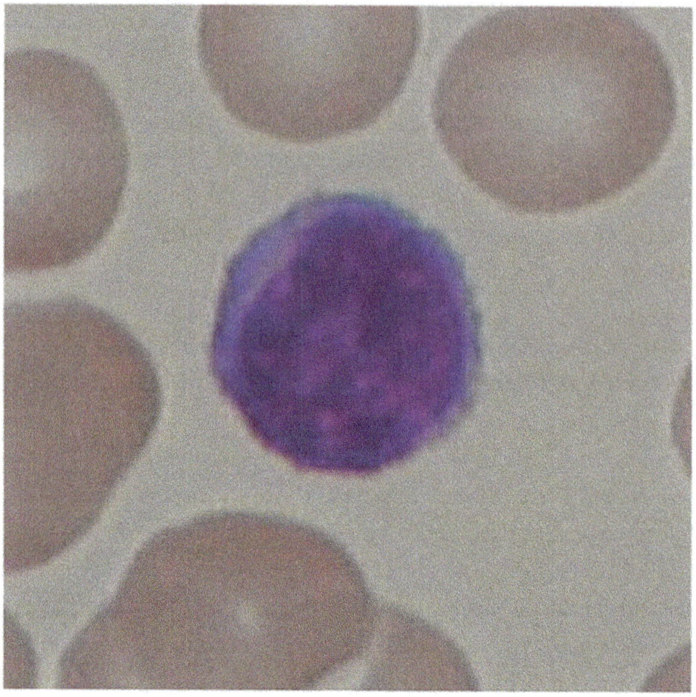

Figure 2. Blast lymphocyte

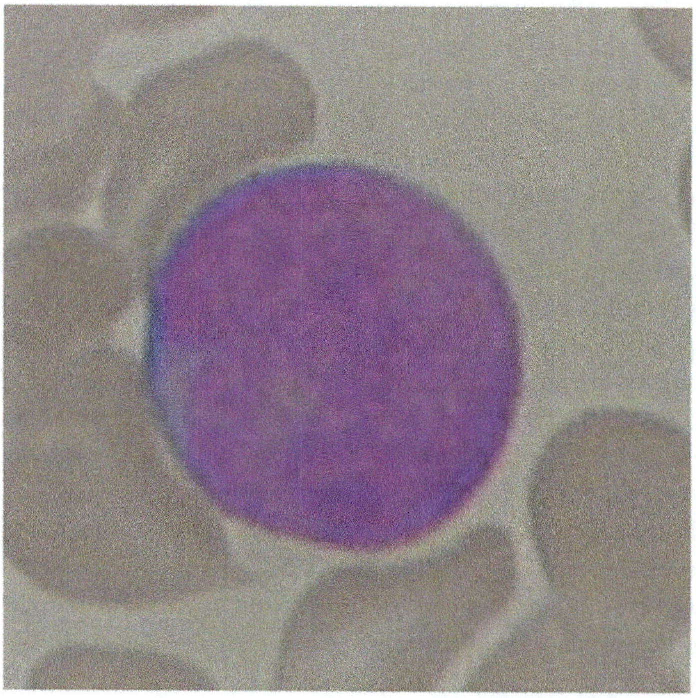

classify them based on changes in the texture of the cell (Singhal & Singh, 2014). The work is extended to extract shape and texture images from stained lymphocyte images to distinguish between a lymphocyte and a lymphoblast. Shape features are extracted from the cell, cytoplasm, and nucleus to compare changes in the geometrical structure of a normal and abnormal cell. Moreover, since it is known that leukemia causes changes in the chromatin pattern of the nucleus (Ries, Melbert, Krapcho, Mariotto, Miller, Feuer, Clegg, Horner, Howlader, Eisner, Reichman & Edwards, 1975-2014), texture features are extracted from the nucleus of the lymphocyte. Two types of texture features are used: Local Binary Pattern (LBP) (Ojala, Pietikinen & Harwood, 1994) and Gray Level Co-occurrence Matrix (GLCM) (Haralick, Shanmugam & Dinstein, 1973). Based on these features, the images of the database are classified using Support Vector Machine (Cortes & Vapnik, 1995).

The main contributions of this study are as follows: Performance comparison of top-down (shape) and bottom-up (texture features computed from pixel intensities) approaches, for differentiation between normal and blast lymphocyte.

- Identification of prominent geometrical features of the lymphocyte contributing towards ALL classification.
- Experimental results to show that while LBP features are better than GLCM features, relevant shape features outperform texture features.

The chapter discusses the process of using image processing in the detection of ALL. This includes the pre-processing steps, segmentation of lymphocyte cells and feature extraction. The experiments, results and their analysis are also presented.

PROCESS OF ALL DETECTION: LITERATURE REVIEW

The basic steps towards automatic detection of ALL in a stained blood sample image are:

- Image preprocessing
- Segmentation of white blood cells (WBC) from red blood cells (RBC) and platelets using various characteristics of the cell components
- Extraction of lymphocytes from other WBC components
- Feature extraction
- Classification into normal and blast cells. This leads to detection of leukemia as the presence of more than 20% of blast cells in blood is characterized as leukemia (Mohapatra, Patra & Satpathy, 2013)

Preprocessing

Image preprocessing is the first step in the automation process. Typically, acquisition systems used for capturing microscopic blood or bone marrow images produce good quality color images but some noise may be accumulated during this stage. The noise may render the image unsuitable for further analysis. Image enhancement is done to convert the image into a form better for further investigation. Piuri and Scotti (Piuri & Scotti, 2004) have used contrast stretching followed by the morphological opening in order to enhance only the nuclei of the cell. Dorini et al. (Dorini, Minetto & Leite, 2007) have used scale space toggle operator to solve a common leaking problem in image processing which results in a high contrast image. In (Bikhet, Darwish, Tolba & Shaheen, 2000), a median filter is used to remove noise from the blood image. Hiremath et al. (Hiremath, Bannigidad & Geeta, 2010) have used histogram equalization followed by morphological operations like erosion, reconstruction, and dilation. Global contrast stretching can also be used to enhance the area of interest in the image, which consists of white blood cell nuclei and cytoplasm (Halim, Mashor, Nasir, Mokhtar & Rosline, 2011; Hazlyna, Mashor, Mokhtar, Salihah, Hassan, Raof & Osman, 2010). Mohamed et al. (Mohamed, Far & Guaily, 2012) use linear contrast stretching and histogram equalization on a grayscale image of the blood image for enhancement.

Segmentation of WBC

Since ALL affects only the lymphocytes of the white blood cells, the WBC need to be extracted from the blood sample image for further analysis. Yampri et al. (Yampri, Pintavirooj, Daochai & Teartulakarn, 2006) use thresholding followed by erosion and dilation for segmentation. The centroid of the nucleus is then determined. Using the centroid as the center of the cell, the cell is segmented into cytoplasm and nucleus using adaptive contour technique. The scheme proposed by Dorini et al. (Dorini, Minetto & Leite, 2007) extracts nucleus using watershed transform with image forest transform. Cytoplasm is extracted using granulometric analysis technique. Rezatofighi et al. (Rezatofighi, Soltanian-Zadeh, Sharifian & Zoroofi, 2009) propose a color image segmentation method that applies Gram-Schmitt orthogonalization for WBC nucleus segmentation. Hazlyna et al. (Hazlyna, Mashor, Mokhtar, Salihah, Hassan, Raof & Osman, 2010) present a comparison between acute leukemia image segmentation using HSI and RGB color spaces and state that HSI color space is more suitable for color based segmentation as compared to RGB color space.

Segmentation can be performed on grayscale images or colored images. In (Mohamed, Far & Guaily, 2012), Otsu's thresholding technique is used to convert the preprocessed grayscale image into a monochrome image, followed by morphological opening operations in order to obtain WBC and remove unwanted small pixel groups of other blood cells. Halim et al. (Halim, Mashor, Nasir, Mokhtar & Rosline, 2011) and Lin and Hong (Lin & Hong, 2012) use region growing technique to segment the color image of blood. HSI color space is used to improve the image quality. Color map technique, image processing filters, and granulometric analysis are used to improve the quality of output image obtained from the watershed transform. Lim et al. (Lim, Mashor & Hassan, 2012) present an HSI color based segmentation method for WBC extraction. Mohapatra et al. (Mohapatra, Patra & Satpathy, 2013) use bounded box technique to extract sub-image of WBC.

Rawat et al. (Rawat, Singh, Bhadauria & Kumar, 2014) present a comparison between existing segmentation techniques. They compare the segmentation performance of global thresholding, watershed, L*a*b color space, HSV based and *k*-means clustering techniques. The best segmentation performance is reported as 82.56% for infected blood smear and 84.62% for normal cells and is obtained with *k*-means clustering technique.

Extraction of Lymphocytes

In ALL detection, since the concern is about the percentage of lymphocytes in the blood, the next step in automation of ALL detection is lymphocyte extraction. Lymphocytes can be extracted by classifying white blood cells into its subtypes. The nucleus of lymphocytes is circular in shape and has a single lobe. This information can be used to separate the lymphocytes from other WBC. Bikhet et al. (Bikhet, Darwish & Tolba, 2000) classify different types of white blood cells using a number of cell, nucleus and cytoplasm features. The method proposed by Piuri and Scotti (Piuri & Scotti, 2004) first separates the white blood cell into membrane and nucleus. Shape features extracted from membrane and nucleus, the number of lobes in the nucleus and average intensity values are used for classification. Four classifiers are used for classification of white blood cells into its subtypes and it is reported that feedforward neural network gives minimum classification error.

Yampri et al. (Yampri, Pintavirooj, Daochai & Teartulakarn, 2006) use Principal Component Analysis (PCA) technique to classify white blood cells. Hiremath et al. (Hiremath, Bannigidad, Geeta, 2010) classify white blood cells into three subtypes: lymphocytes, monocytes, and neutrophils. The proposed method uses four different combinations of seven features extracted from nucleus and cytoplasm. The combination of features which gives maximum accuracy is identified. The features used by Lin and Hong (Lin & Hong, 2012) consist of two categories: shape and texture. Distance transform and mean shift algorithm are used to find the number of lobes.

Feature Extraction

After identification of lymphocytes from various subclasses of white blood cells, the next step is to classify lymphocytes as normal or blast. For this task, features are extracted from the nucleus, cytoplasm and cell of the lymphocyte. Normal and blast cells differ in shape, size and chromatin pattern in the nucleus (Ries, Melbert, Krapcho, Mariotto, Miller, Feuer, Clegg, Horner, Howlader, Eisner, Reichman & Edwards, 1975-2014). Thus, shape and texture features of lymphocyte cell can be used for discrimination between normal and blast cells.

Asadi et al. (Asadi, Vahedi & Amindavar, 2006) proposed a method for leukemia cell classification in which Zernike moments are used as features. In (Scotti, 2005), membrane, cytoplasm, and nucleus are segmented from the sub-image of lymphocyte. The FAB (French American British) (Hassan, Bukhari, Zafar, Malik & Akhtar, 1992) method is used for selecting features that are based on the image-based morphological analysis. The FAB classification method is based on morphology and histochemical staining and classifies ALL into L1, L2 or L3 subtypes. Madhloom et al. (Madhloom, Kareem & Ariffin, 2012) have used a combination of shape features of the cell and nucleus and texture features extracted from the nucleus. In (Mohapatra, Patra & Satpathy, 2013), a combination of shape, color and three types of texture feature descriptors, viz., wavelet, Haralick, and Fourier are used to train an ensemble of classifiers. Deshmukh and Panditrao (Deshmukh and Panditrao, 2014) have determined the contour signature for detection of leukemia.

Feature Selection

All the features extracted from the lymphocyte may not be relevant in predicting a cell as normal or blast. To remove the redundancy between features and obtain a set of relevant features, feature selection is used. This is important as it improves classifier performance. In (Piuri & Scotti, 2004), forward selection method based on nearest neighbor classification has been used for feature selection. Markiewicz et al. (Markiewicz, Osowski, Marianska & Moszczynski, 2005) have used linear SVM-based feature selection method to select best 30 features from a set of shape, statistical and texture features for myeloid leukemia detection. In (Madhloom, Kareem & Ariffin, 2012), scalar feature selection is used to rank the feature set containing 15 shape and 15 texture features and top seven features are selected for further processing. Mohapatra et al. (Mohapatra, Patra &. Satpathy, 2013) have used Independent-sample test method for determining the significance of extracted features.

Classification

The features extracted from a lymphocyte image can be used to classify a cell as normal or blast. Various classifiers have been used in literature for this purpose. In (Scotti, 2005), three classifiers: linear, k-nearest neighbor and feedforward neural network (FF-NN) are used to compare the classification accuracy. FF-NN shows the minimum error rate and lymphocytes are classified with a mean error rate of 0.02%. In (Asadi, Vahedi & Amindavar, 2006), two classification methods: *k*-nearest neighbor (*k*-NN) and minimum distance mean are used for classification. It is reported that *k*-NN gives the best accuracy of 93%. Madhloom et al. (Madhloom, Kareem & Ariffin, 2012) use *k*-nearest neighbor for the purpose of classification and 92.5% accuracy is observed. In (Mohapatra, Patra & Satpathy, 2013), an ensemble of classifiers (*k*-NN, SVM, Multilayer Perceptron) is used for classification and 94.73% of accuracy is obtained.

PROPOSED METHODOLOGY

For experiments, the ALL-IDB2 database obtained from Universit Degli Studi di Milano, Italy (Labati, Piuri & Scotti, 2011) has been used. It contains 130 images of normal lymphocytes and 130 images of blast lymphocytes. Since the database consists of single cell images of lymphocytes only, segmentation of WBC and lymphocytes from other blood components need not be performed. The methodology used for automatic detection of ALL is shown in Figure 3.

The proposed method uses a combination of thresholding, morphological operations and watershed transform for WBC segmentation and provides 94.5% accuracy. Shadow C-man clustering-based technique is used in L*a*b color space for WBC segmentation.

To extract features from the image of the lymphocyte, segmentation is performed to obtain the cell, its nucleus, and cytoplasm. HSI (Hue, Saturation, Intensity) color based segmentation technique is used which provides better performance than RGB color segmentation (Hazlyna, Mashor, Mokhtar, Salihah, Hassan, Raof & Osman, 2010). Figure 4 shows the segmentation of a blood lymphocyte image into the nucleus, cytoplasm, and cell. The extracted features are described in detail in the following subsections.

The process of segmentation can be explained in the following steps:

Figure 3. Proposed methodology

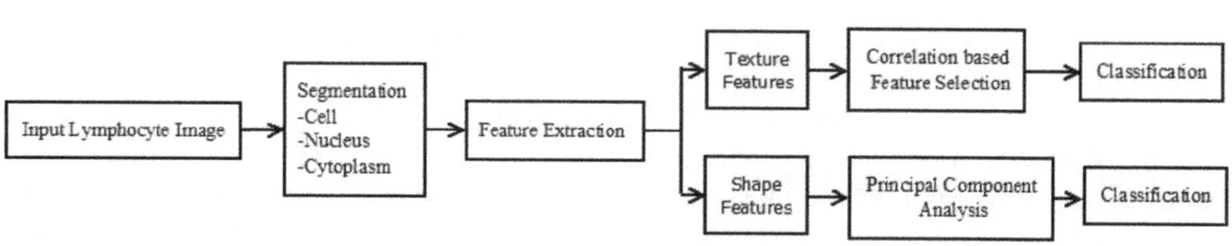

Figure 4. Segmentation of lymphocyte into cell, nucleus, and cytoplasm

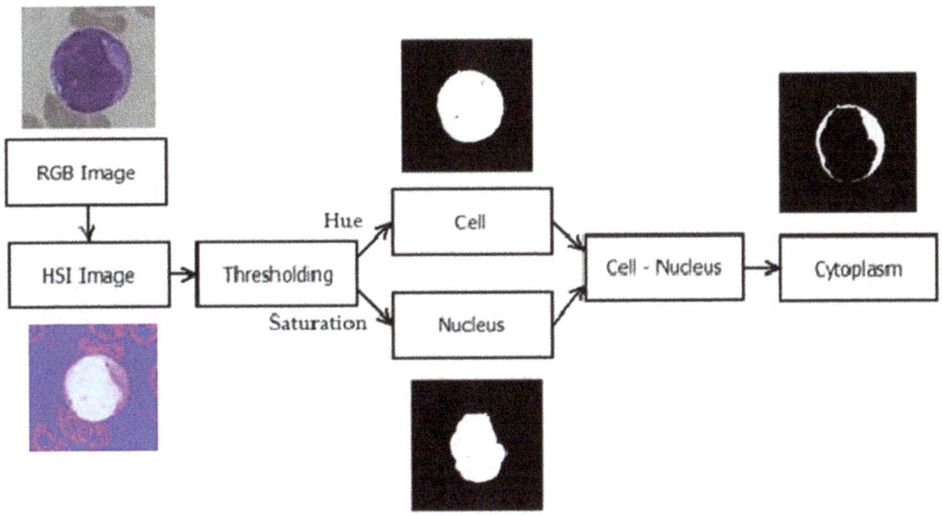

- Convert the input RGB image of the lymphocyte into HSI image format.
- Apply thresholding on the hue component of the lymphocyte image to extract the cell.
- Apply thresholding on the saturation component of the image to extract the nucleus. This gives us a binary image of the nucleus.
- Apply a median filter of size 5x5 on the resultant image to remove the noise.
- Grayscale image of the nucleus is obtained by mapping obtained binary image of the nucleus to the grayscale image of the input RGB image.
- Using cell and nucleus images, cytoplasm can be extracted by subtracting the nucleus from the cell.

Two types of features have been extracted from the image of the lymphocyte: shape and texture. These are described in the following subsections.

Shape Features

According to pathologists, shape features play a crucial role in the detection of ALL from blood microscopic images (Sawyers, Denny & Witte, 1991). Blast cells are an immature form of the normal lymphocyte cell and shape characteristics of the blast cells are different from the normal cell. Normal lymphocytes are regular and circular in shape as compared to blast lymphocytes. The cytoplasmic changes are also taken into consideration while extracting shape features.

The following shape features have been extracted from the lymphocyte:

- Area - the number of pixels in the nucleus (f_1), cell (f_{10}) and cytoplasm (f_{11}).
- Convex Area - area of the shortest convex polygon that may incorporate the nucleus (f_2) or cell (f_{14}).
- Eccentricity - a measure of the nucleus (f_3) or cell (f_{15}) being circular. It is defined as:

$$Eccentricity = \sqrt{a^2 - b^2} \quad (1)$$

where, *a, b* are the lengths of the semimajor axis and semiminor axis respectively.

- Major axis length - the number of pixels in the major axis of ellipse containing the nucleus (f_4) or cell (f_{16}).
- Minor axis length - the number of pixels in the minor axis of the ellipse containing the nucleus (f_5) or cell (f_{17}).
- Perimeter - the number of pixels around the border of the nucleus (f_6) or cell (f_{18}).
- Solidity - the ratio of the area of the nucleus (f_7) or cell (f_{19}) to their respective convex area. It is computed as:

$$Solidity = Area \,/\, Convex\ Area \quad (2)$$

- Orientation - angle between the major axis and the x -axis of nucleus or cell denoted by (f_8) and (f_{20}) respectively.
- Compactness - the measure of the roundness of the nucleus (f_9) or cell (f_{21}). It is given by:

$$Compactness = Area \,/\, Perimeter^2 \quad (3)$$

- The ratio of cytoplasm to nucleus area (f_{12}).
- The ratio of nucleus to cell area (f_{13}).

Thus, a total of 21 shape features is extracted from the segmented nucleus, cell and cytoplasm images. Some of the shape features are shown in Figure 5. To remove irrelevant features and reduce redundancy between features, feature selection technique is used. This helps in identifying the most salient features to train a classifier thereby improving the efficiency of the system. The reduced set of features provides equivalent or better results as compared to the whole dataset.

Correlation-Based Feature Selection

Correlation-Based Feature Selection (CFS) technique (Hall, 1999) is employed to identify relevant features. It works on the hypothesis that a good feature subset contains features that are highly correlated to the class, yet uncorrelated with each other. CFS has been used earlier for cancer detection by Lu et al. (Lu, Peng, Liu, Deng, Feng & Liao, 2012). While Lu et al. have applied CFS on gene expression profiles, in this chapter it is employed on geometrical features extracted from the lymphocyte. This approach avoids the cumbersome process of determining the gene array of a patient.

The CFS technique ranks features based on the extent the features are correlated to the class and other features. The merit, S_x, of a feature subset containing n features is evaluated using Equation 4.

$$S_n = \frac{n\overline{r_{cf}}}{\sqrt{n + n(n-1)\overline{r_{ff}}}} \quad (4)$$

Figure 5. Some shape features extracted from the nucleus of the lymphocyte image

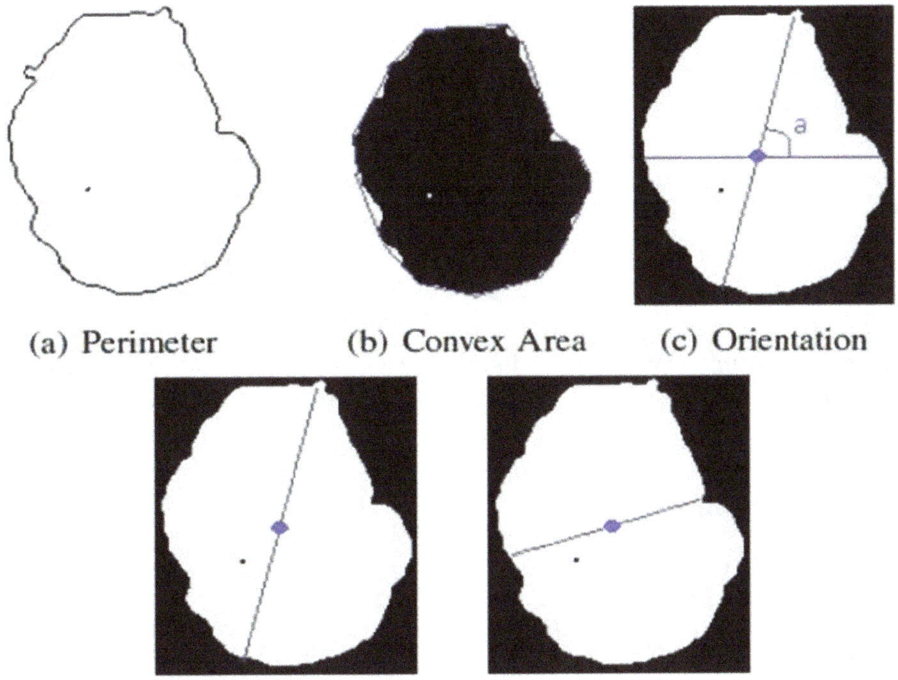

(a) Perimeter (b) Convex Area (c) Orientation

(d) Major Axis (e) Minor Axis

where, r_{cf} is the average value of correlation between features and class and r_{ff} is the average of all feature-feature correlation values.

CFS is applied on shape features to generate the feature ranking. Using the ranked features feature subsets are formed starting with the most prominent feature and keep adding features (of next highest ranking) one at a time. This gives us 21 feature subsets denoted by F_i, where $i = \{1, 2, 21\}$. For example, F_1 contains only the highest ranked feature, F_{10} contain the 10 top-ranked features and F_{21} is the complete feature set. These subsets are then used for classification. The subset which provides the best classification accuracy is selected.

Texture Features

Changes in the chromatin distribution of nucleus can be visualized from its texture which makes it an essential diagnostic feature for recognizing a blast cell. Two types of texture descriptors have been extracted from the nucleus for ALL detection:

- Local Binary Pattern (LBP)
- Gray Level Co-occurrence Matrix (GLCM)

A brief description of both types of texture features is given in the following subsections.

Local Binary Pattern

Local Binary Pattern forms labels by thresholding 3x3 neighborhood of each pixel by the center pixel value (Ojala, Pietikinen & Harwood, 1994). In the experiments, LBP features are extracted from the grayscale image of nucleus and computed as follows:

- Divide the input nucleus image into sub-images.
- For each pixel in each sub-image, threshold it with the center pixel, giving an 8-bit binary number.
- The binary number is multiplied with predefined weights starting from the top left corner. This gives a decimal number corresponding to each pixel in the sub-image. An example of this is shown in Figure 6.
- A histogram is computed over each sub-image. Histograms of all the sub-images are concatenated to form the LBP for the whole image. The LBP thus obtained can be used as a feature vector.

Gray Level Co-Occurrence Matrix

Gray Level Co-occurrence Matrix (GLCM) is a statistical texture feature proposed by Haralick et al. (Haralick & Shanmugam, 1973). For computing the GLCM of an image, it is first mapped to a smaller number of gray level values say n. The size of the obtained GLCM matrix G will then be n x n. The entry (i, j) in the GLCM, denoted by $G(i, j)$, is the number of times the gray level values i and j co-occur for a particular distance, d, and in a specific direction, α. An example of GLCM computation of an image, at distance $d = 1$ and direction $\alpha = 0°$, is shown in Figure 7.

The GLCM thus computed over a nucleus image is used for computing four features which are defined below:

Figure 6. Computation of decimal number for each pixel

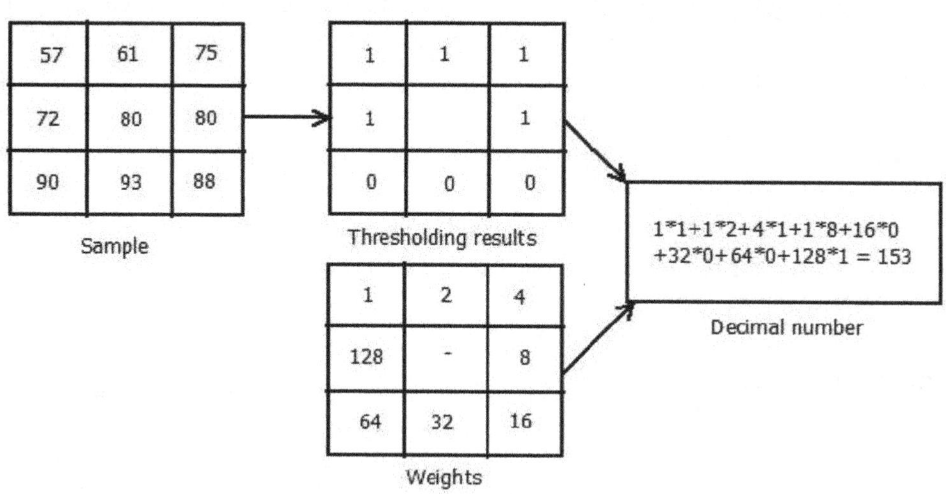

Figure 7. Computation of GLCM

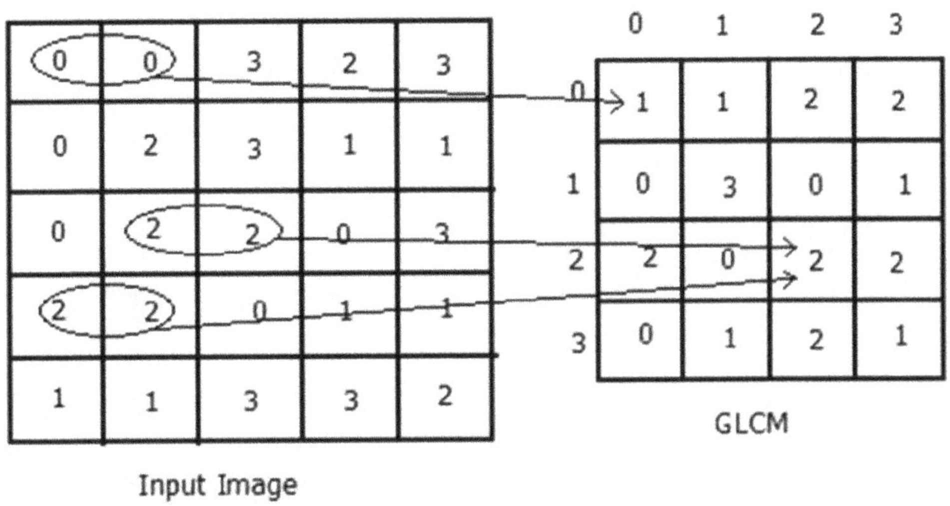

- The contrast of an image is defined as the intensity distribution between a pixel and its neighborhood, over the whole image.

$$Contrast = \sum_{i,j} | i - j |^2 G(i, j) \tag{5}$$

- Correlation provides the correlation of a pixel to its neighborhood over the whole image, defined as:

$$Correlation = \frac{\sum_{i=1}^{n} \sum_{j=1}^{n} (i - \mu_x)(j - \mu_j) G(i, j)}{\sigma_x \sigma_y} \tag{6}$$

where, μ_x, μ_y, σ_x and σ_y are the mean and variances of row and column sums of the GLCM respectively and computed as given below:

$$\mu_x = \sum_{i=1}^{n} \sum_{j=1}^{n} i G(i, j) \tag{7}$$

$$\mu_y = \sum_{i=1}^{n} \sum_{j=1}^{n} j G(i, j) \tag{8}$$

$$\sigma_x = \sqrt{\sum_{i=1}^{n}\sum_{j=1}^{n}(i-\mu_x)^2 G(i,j)} \tag{9}$$

$$\sigma_y = \sqrt{\sum_{i=1}^{n}\sum_{j=1}^{n}(j-\mu_y)^2 G(i,j)} \tag{10}$$

- Energy is computed as some of the squared elements in GLCM as given below:

$$Energy = \sum_{i,j} G(i,j)^2 \tag{11}$$

- Homogeneity is the measure of the degree of variations in an image. It is defined as:

$$Homogeneity = \sum_{i,j} \frac{G(i,j)}{1+|i-j|} \tag{12}$$

The nucleus image is divided into 16 sub-images. For each sub-image, four GLCM features are computed. The GLCM features obtained from all the sub-images are concatenated to form a feature vector of size 64. The authors have used distance $d = 1$ and directions $\alpha = [0°, 45°, 90°, 135°]$. GLCM is computed for four values of levels $n = [10, 20, 40, 60]$. Thus, a total of 16 combinations of levels and direction values are used for the experiments.

Principal Component Analysis (PCA)

Dimensionality reduction is used to reduce the size of texture feature sets used for training the classifier (Mladenic, 2006). Dimensionality reduction of texture features is done using Principal Component Analysis (PCA) (Pearson, 1901) which transforms the existing feature set into a new feature space. The top principal components include most of the variance information of the original data, thus reducing the size of the original feature space. PCA has been applied to LBP and GLCM texture features. Since the focus of this work is to maximize the recognition accuracy, principal components accounting for 99% variance are taken for classification.

Classification of Shape and Texture Features Using SVM

The authors have employed Support Vector Machine (SVM) as it has been shown in earlier research (Mohapatra, Patra & Satpathy, 2010; Mohapatra, Patra & Satpathy, 2013; Lin & Hong, 2012) that SVM is an efficient classifier for ALL detection. Sequential Minimal Optimization (Cortes & Vapnik, 1995) with the Pearson VII Universal Kernel (PUK) (Ustun, Melssen & Buydens, 2006), from WEKA (Hall, Frank, Holmes, Pfahringer, Reutemann & Witten, 2009) has been used for training the SVM classifier. Experiments were performed using RBF (Wang, Chen & Chen, 2003) and Polynomial kernel (Mejia-Guevara, Morales & Kuri, 2007) also, but the PUK kernel generated the best results.

For the kernel, the cost parameter C is optimized using k-fold cross-validation parameter selection. To choose C, the available data is first divided into k subsets. Then, the cross-validation errors using different values for C are computed. The value of C providing minimum error is selected for training the SVM classifier. Classification has been done on the following feature sets:

- 21 shape features and feature subsets formed using CFS ranked shape features.
- LBP features and principal components of LBP features (LBP-PCA).
- GLCM features and principal components of GLCM features (GLCM-PCA).

The classification results are compared to determine an optimal set of features which is reduced in size and gives comparable classification results.

EXPERIMENTS AND RESULT ANALYSIS

The ALL-IDB2 database obtained from Universit Degli Studi di Milano, Italy (Labati, Piuri & Scotti, 2011) has been used for experiments. It contains 130 images of normal lymphocytes and 130 images of blast lymphocytes. All the images are in *.jpg* format and have a resolution of 257 x 257. Shape and texture features are extracted from the segmented images of the nucleus, cell, and cytoplasm, as discussed earlier. The feature space is reduced through feature selection (for shape features) or PCA (for texture features). The reduced feature sets are classified using SVM. The evaluation metrics used and the results of classification are described in the following subsections.

Evaluation Metrics

The confusion matrix shown in Table 1 is used to compute four evaluation metrics (Scotti, 2010): Misclassification, Sensitivity, Specificity, and Accuracy. While it is desired that the accuracy of the system be high, it is also important that the sensitivity of the classifier be maximum so that no blast cell is missed out. Misclassification should be minimized. Specificity should also be high as classifying a normal cell as a lymphocyte may ring false alarms and the patient might be unduly subjected to further tests.

- Misclassification - is the total number of misclassified lymphocytes:

$$Misclassification = FP + FN \tag{13}$$

- Sensitivity - is the probability of correctly identifying a blast cell. It is given by:

Table 1. Confusion matrix

Actual class/Predicted Class	Blast	Normal
Blast	True Positives (TP)	False Negatives (FN)
Normal	False Positives (FP)	True Negatives (TN)

$$Sensitivity = \frac{TP}{TP + FN} \tag{14}$$

- Specificity - is the probability of correctly classifying a normal cell:

$$Specificity = \frac{TN}{TN + FP} \tag{15}$$

- Accuracy is given by:

$$Accuracy = \frac{TP + TN}{TP + FP + TN + FN} \tag{16}$$

Shape Features

Classification for all the feature subsets F_1 .. F_{21} using the PUK kernel of SVM is done and the results are shown in Figure 8. It is observed from results that the best classification accuracy of 92.30% is obtained using subset F_{16}. The number of misclassified cells using F_{16} is only 20. Sensitivity and specificity values for this feature set are 91.53% and 93.07% respectively. F_{16} outperforms the complete feature set F_{21} in all evaluation metrics. Thus, it can be argued that F_{16} is a near-optimal set of shape features which can be used for leukemia classification as it exhibits reasonable evaluation metrics and feature length.

Figure 8. Performance of PUK kernel over shape feature subsets

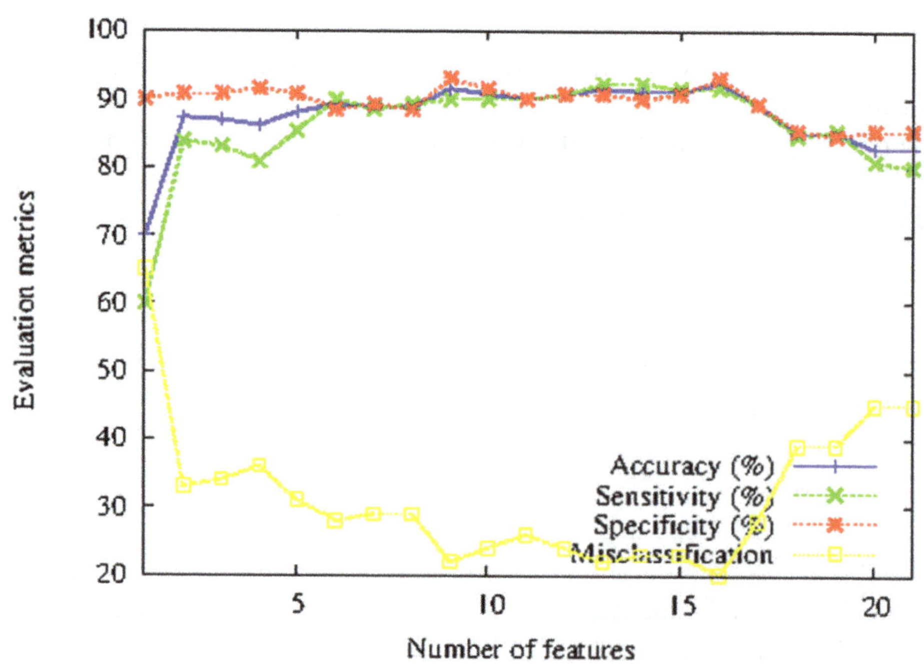

Texture Features

As discussed in the previous section, LBP and GLCM texture features are extracted from the grayscale image of the nucleus. Results obtained using both are discussed in the following subsections.

LBP Features

4096 LBP feature descriptors have been computed for each nucleus contained in the lymphocyte images in the database. Classification results using SVM over LBP texture descriptors are shown in Table 2. Since the dimensionality of the texture features is very large, PCA is applied on the LBP descriptors. It is found that 46 principal components account for nearly 99% of the total variance. The classification results using the reduced set of 46 principal components are shown in Table 2. It can be seen that the accuracy is improved from 73.84% to 90.38%. Specificity also increases while the number of misclassifications is reduced. However, there is a slight degradation in the sensitivity of the system.

GLCM Features

As discussed earlier, 64 GLCM features are computed for each of the 16 different combinations of the number of levels and directions for each grayscale nucleus image. After experimenting with all combinations, it is seen that the best results are obtained with the number of levels $n = 60$ and direction $\alpha = 0°$. GLCM features for this level and direction are classified using SVM and results are given in Table 2. It can be seen from results that maximum classification accuracy of 84.61% is obtained. Sensitivity and specificity are 84.61% and 93.07% respectively. The number of misclassified cells is 29.

On application of PCA on GLCM feature vector, 15 principal components, accounting for 99% of total variability in data are used for classification. As can be seen, while accuracy and sensitivity are only marginally affected, misclassification increases, thus degrading specificity.

Comparative Analysis of Shape and Texture Features

A comparison of shape and texture features is shown in Table 3. It can be observed from results that while LBP texture features perform considerably better than GLCM features, their performance is slightly degraded as compared to the shape features. Moreover, while the LBP-PCA feature set consists of 46 features, only 16 shape features give good classification results. The accuracy of selected shape features is 92.3% while that of LBP-PCA features is 90.38%. The sensitivity of shape features is also higher, though specificity is slightly on the lower side as compared to LBP-PCA features.

Table 2. Classification results of texture features

Feature set	No. of features	Accuracy (%)	Sensitivity (%)	Specificity (%)	Misclassification
LBP	4096	73.84	98.46	49.23	68
LBP-PCA	46	90.38	84.61	96.15	25
GLCM	64	84.61	84.61	93.07	29
GLCM-PCA	15	79.61	83.84	75.38	53

Table 3. Comparison of results of shape and texture features

Feature set	No. of features	Accuracy (%)	Sensitivity (%)	Specificity (%)	Misclassification
F_{16}	16	92.3	91.53	93.07	20
LBP-PCA	46	90.38	84.61	96.15	25
GLCM-PCA	15	79.61	83.84	75.38	53

The features contained in F_{16} are shown in Table 4 in order of their prominence. Analyzing the features, it is observed that nucleus and cell features play an important part while most features of the cytoplasm are redundant. The majority of the features in F_{16} are related to the nucleus. The ratio of nucleus to cell area emerges as the most prominent feature. Observing the features, it can be argued that most changes take place in the geometry of the nucleus and cell.

State-of-Art

Published research on detection of ALL has majorly used sample images from various hospitals while in this chapter the ALL-IDB2 database has been used. Thus, the results cannot be compared with results reported in the literature. However, the observed performance figures are presented mainly for completeness of this research (refer Table 5). Madhloom et al. (Madhloom, Kareem & Ariffin, 2012) have used 30 features and reported a classification accuracy of 92.5%. Mohapatra et al. (Mohapatra, Patra & Satpathy, 2013) have used 32 features and have reported a classification accuracy of 94.73% using

Table 4. Features in feature subset F_{16} in order of their prominence

Feature	Description
f_{13}	Ratio of nucleus to cell area
f_1	Area of nucleus
f_{18}	Perimeter of cell
f_7	Solidity of nucleus
f_9	Compactness of nucleus
f_{10}	Area of cell
f_4	Major axis length of nucleus
f_{14}	Convex area of nucleus
f_{11}	Area of cytoplasm
f_6	Perimeter of nucleus
f_{12}	Ratio of cytoplasm to nucleus area
f_5	Minor axis length of nucleus
f_{16}	Minor axis length of cell
f_2	Convex area of nucleus
f_{17}	Minor axis length of cell
f_3	Eccentricity of nucleus

Table 5. Comparison of research in ALL detection

Author	Features	Number of features	Classifier	Accuracy (%) / Mean error
Madhloom, Kareem & Ariffin, 2012	Shape and texture	30	*k*-NN	92.5
Mohapatra, Patra & Satpathy, 2013	Shape and texture	32	Ensemble SVM	94.73 91.43
Asadi, Vahedi & Amindavar, 2006	Zernike moments	Moment order 15	*k*-NN	93
Scotti, 2005	Shape	23	FF-NN	0.0133
Proposed	Shape	16	SVM	92.3

an ensemble of classifiers (*k*-NN, MLP, and SVM), which is computationally cumbersome. They also mention a classification accuracy of 91.43% when only SVM is used as a classifier. However, in their sample images, while extracting lymphocytes, they have assumed that only lymphocytes are present along with RBC. This might not be the case and other types of leukocytes may also be present. Lymphocytes constitute only 30% of the leucocytes.

In (Scotti, 2005), 23 shape features have been extracted and an error rate of 0.0133 is reported. However, the database is small and the results need to be validated on a larger database. The shape feature vector yields comparable recognition accuracy and is limited in size. Asadi et al. (Asadi, Vahedi & Amindavar, 2006) report an accuracy of 93%. However, their database consists of images of four different types of leukemia. Moreover, the images are computer generated holograph images.

In (Bhattacharjee & Saini, 2015), ALL-IDB dataset is used for experiments. The images are preprocessed using contrast enhancement and quality adjustment techniques. Canny filter followed by morphological operations are used for segmentation of the lymphocyte cell and the nucleus of the blood microscopic images. After segmentation, shape features including area, perimeter, circularity and form factor are extracted. Four classifiers *k*-NN, SVM, Artificial Neural Networks (ANN) and *k*-means clustering are used for classifying a cell as normal or blast. Best Specificity of 95.23% is obtained using the *k*-NN classifier.

The proposed system is able to achieve 92.3% accuracy with only 16 features. Minimizing the number of features results in faster detection. This can be beneficial in hospitals where the number of suspected cases is large and time is crucial.

CONCLUSION

In this chapter, the authors have used shape and texture features for automatic detection of Acute Lymphoblastic Leukemia. Shape features are extracted from segmented images of the nucleus, cell, and cytoplasm. Correlation based Feature Selection is applied on shape features and classification is done to obtain the subset containing the most prominent features. It is observed that a set of 16 most prominent features provide a classification accuracy of 92.30%. Two types of texture feature: LBP and GLCM are used for classification. PCA is applied to them to reduce their dimensionality. It is seen that LBP features perform better than GLCM texture features but not better than the shape features. It can be concluded that a small set of shape features is able to provide reasonably accurate results. A reduced feature set will help minimize processing time detection time of ALL. As future work, other texture variants and shape features can be explored to achieve better classification accuracy.

REFERENCES

Angulo, J., & Flandrin, G. (2003). Microscopic image analysis using mathematical morphology: application to hematological cytology. In A. Mendez-Vilas (Ed.), Science, Technology and Education of Microscopy: An overview (pp. 304–312). Academic Press.

Asadi, M., Vahedi, A., & Amindavar, H. (2006) Leukemia Cell Recognition with Zernike Moments of Holographic Images. *Proceedings of the 7th Nordic Signal Processing Symposium*, 214-217. doi:10.1109/NORSIG.2006.275226

Bhattacharjee, R., & Saini, L. M. (2015) Robust Technique for the Detection of Acute Lymphoblastic Leukemia. *IEEE Power, Communication and Information Technology Conference*, 657-662. doi:10.1109/PCITC.2015.7438079

Bikhet, S., Darwish, A., Tolba, H., & Shaheen, S. (2000) Segmentation and classification of white blood cells. *IEEE International Conference on Acoustics, Speech, and Signal Processing,* 2259-2261. doi:10.1109/ICASSP.2000.859289

Cancer Research UK. (n.d.). *Worldwide cancer statistics*. Retrieved from http://www.cancerresearchuk.org

Cortes, C., & Vapnik, V. (1995). Support Vector Networks. *Machine Learning, 20*(3), 273–297. doi:10.1007/BF00994018

Deshmukh, A., & Panditrao, A. (2014). Automated leukemia detection using contour signature in blood microscopic images. *International Journal of Research in Computer and Communication Technology,* 304-308.

Dollinger, M., Ko, A., & Rosenbaum, E. (2008). *Everyone's guide to cancer therapy*. Riverside: Andrew's McMeel Publishing.

Dorini, L., Minetto, R., & Leite, N. (2007) White blood cell segmentation using morphological operators and scale-space analysis. *XX Brazilian Symposium on Computer Graphics and Image Processing,* 294-304. doi:10.1109/SIBGRAPI.2007.33

Halim, N., Mashor, M., Nasir, A. S. A., Mokhtar, N. R., & Rosline, H. (2011) Nucleus segmentation technique for acute Leukemia. *IEEE 7th International Colloquium on Signal Processing and its Applications*, 192-197. doi:10.1109/CSPA.2011.5759871

Hall, M., Frank, E., Holmes, G., Pfahringer, B., Reutemann, P., & Witten, I. H. (2009). The WEKA Data Mining Software: An Update. *SIGKDD Explor. Newsl., 11*(1), 10–18. doi:10.1145/1656274.1656278

Hall, M. A. (1999). *Correlation-based Feature Selection for Machine Learning* (Ph.D. thesis). The University of Waikato, Hamilton, New Zealand.

Haralick, R., Shanmugam, K., & Dinstein, I. (1973). Textural Features for Image Classification. *IEEE Transactions on Systems, Man, and Cybernetics*, *SMC-3*(6), 610–621. doi:10.1109/TSMC.1973.4309314

Hassan, K., Bukhari, K., Zafar, A., Malik, M., & Akhtar, M. (1992). Acute leukemia in children. French-American-British (FAB) classification and its relation to clinical features. *JPMA. The Journal of the Pakistan Medical Association*, *42*, 29–31. PMID:1573762

Haworth, C., Hepplestone, A., Jones, P. M., Campbell, R., & Evans, M. P. D. (1981). Routine Bone Marrow Examination in the Management of Acute Lymphoblastic Leukemia of childhood. *Journal of Clinical Pathology*, *34*(5), 483–485. doi:10.1136/jcp.34.5.483 PMID:6941970

Hazlyna, H. N., Mashor, M., Mokhtar, N., Salihah, A. A., Hassan, R., Raof, R., & Osman, M. (2010). Comparison of acute leukemia Image segmentation using HSI and RGB color space. *10th International Conference on Information Sciences Signal Processing and their Applications*, 749-752. doi:10.1109/ISSPA.2010.5605410

Hiremath, P., Bannigidad, P., & Geeta, S. (2010). Automated Identification and Classification of White Blood Cells (Leukocytes) in Digital Microscopic Images. *IJCA*, 59-63.

Labati, R., Piuri, V., & Scotti, F. (2011). All-IDB: The acute lymphoblastic leukemia image database for image processing. *18th IEEE International Conference on Image Processing*, 2045-2048. doi:10.1109/ICIP.2011.6115881

Lim, H., Mashor, M., & Hassan, R. (2012). White blood cell segmentation for acute leukemia bone marrow images. *International Conference on Biomedical Engineering*, 357-361. doi:10.1109/ICoBE.2012.6179038

Lin, S., & Hong, Y. (2012). Differential count of white blood cell in noisy normal blood smear. *7th IEEE Conference on Industrial Electronics and Applications*, 1784-1789.

Lu, X., Peng, X., Liu, P., Deng, Y., Feng, B., & Liao, B. (2012). A novel feature selection method based on CFS in cancer detection. *IEEE 6th International Conference on Systems Biology*, 226-231.

Madhloom, H., Kareem, S., & Arifin, H. (2012). A Robust Feature Extraction and Selection Method for the Recognition of Lymphocytes versus Acute Lymphoblastic Leukemia. *International Conference on Advanced Computer Science Applications and Technologies*, 330-335. doi:10.1109/ACSAT.2012.62

Markiewicz, T., Osowski, S., Marianska, B., & Moszczynski, L. (2005). Automatic recognition of the blood cells of myelogenous leukemia using SVM. *IEEE International Joint Conference on Neural Networks*, 4, 2496-2501. doi:10.1109/IJCNN.2005.1556295

Mejia-Guevara, I., Morales, A., & Kuri, F. (2007). MP-Polynomial Kernel for Training Support Vector Machines. In *CIARP of Lecture Notes in Computer Science* (Vol. 4756, pp. 584–593). Springer.

Mladenic, D. (2006). Feature Selection for Dimensionality Reduction. In *Subspace, Latent Structure and Feature Selection* (Vol. 3940, pp. 84–102). Berlin: Springer. doi:10.1007/11752790_5

Mohamed, M., Far, B., & Guaily, A. (2012). An efficient technique for white blood cells nuclei automatic segmentation. *IEEE International Conference on Systems, Man, and Cybernetics*, 220-225. doi:10.1109/ICSMC.2012.6377703

Mohapatra, S., Patra, D., & Satpathy, S. (2010). Image analysis of blood microscopic images for acute leukemia detection. *International Conference on Industrial Electronics, Control Robotics*, 215-219. doi:10.1109/IECR.2010.5720171

Mohapatra, S., Patra, D., & Satpathy, S. (2013). An ensemble classifier system for early diagnosis of acute lymphoblastic leukemia in blood microscopic images. *Neural Computing & Applications*, 1–18.

Ojala, T., Pietikinen, M., & Harwood, D. (1994). Performance evaluation of texture measures with classification based on Kullback discrimination of distributions. *Proceedings of the 12th IAPR International Conference on Pattern Recognition*, 582-585. doi:10.1109/ICPR.1994.576366

Pearson, K. (1901). On Lines and Planes of Closest Fit to Systems of Points in Space. *Philosophical Magazine*, *11*(1), 559–572. doi:10.1080/14786440109462720

Piuri, V., & Scotti, F. (2004). Morphological classification of blood leucocytes by microscope images. *IEEE International Conference on Computational Intelligence for Measurement Systems and Applications*, 103-108. doi:10.1109/CIMSA.2004.1397242

Rawat, J., Singh, A., Bhadauria, H. S., & Kumar, I. (2014). Comparative analysis of segmentation algorithms for leukocyte extraction in the acute Lymphoblastic Leukemia images. *International Conference on Parallel, Distributed and Grid Computing*, 245-250. doi:10.1109/PDGC.2014.7030750

Rezatofighi, S., Soltanian-Zadeh, H., Sharifian, R., & Zoroofi, R. (2009). A New Approach to White Blood Cell Nucleus Segmentation Based on Gram-Schmidt Orthogonalization. *International Conference on Digital Image Processing*, 107-111. doi:10.1109/ICDIP.2009.19

Ries, L. A. G., Melbert, D., Krapcho, M., Mariotto, A., Miller, B. A., Feuer, E. J., . . . Edwards, B. K. (Eds.). (1975-2004). *SEER Cancer Statistics Review*. National Cancer Institute. Retrieved from http://seer.cancer.gov/csr/1975-2004/

Sawyers, C. L., Denny, C. T., & Witte, O. N. (1991). Leukemia and the disruption of normal hematopoiesis. *Cell*, *64*(2), 337–350. doi:10.1016/0092-8674(91)90643-D PMID:1988151

Scotti, F. (2005). Automatic morphological analysis for acute leukemia identification in peripheral blood microscope images. *IEEE International Conference on Computational Intelligence for Measurement Systems and Applications*, 96-101. doi:10.1109/CIMSA.2005.1522835

Scotti, F. (2010). *ALL-IDB, Acute Lymphoblastic Leukemia Image Database for Image Processing*. Retrieved from http://www.dti.unimi.it/fscotti/all/results.php

Singhal, V., & Singh, P. (2014). Local Binary Pattern for Automatic Detection of Acute Lymphoblastic Leukemia. *Twentieth National Conference on Communications*, 1-5. doi:10.1109/NCC.2014.6811261

Ustun, B., Melssen, W., & Buydens, L. (2006). Facilitating the application of Support Vector Regression by using a universal Pearson VII function based kernel. *Chemometrics and Intelligent Laboratory Systems*, *81*(1), 29–40. doi:10.1016/j.chemolab.2005.09.003

Wang, J., Chen, Q., & Chen, Y. (2003). RBF Kernel Based Support Vector Machine with Universal Approximation and its Applications. In F. Yin, J. Wang, & C. Guo (Eds.), Lecture Notes in Computer Science: Vol. 3173. Advances in Neural Networks (pp. 512–517). Springer.

Yampri, P., Pintavirooj, C., Daochai, S., & Teartulakarn, S. (2006). White Blood Cell Classification based on the Combination of Eigen Cell and Parametric Feature Detection. *IEEE Conference on Industrial Electronics and Applications*, 1-4. doi:10.1109/ICIEA.2006.257341

Chapter 10
Automated Method of Analysing Sputum Smear Tuberculosis Images Using Multifractal Approach:
Automated Analysis of Sputum Smear Tuberculosis Images

Ebenezer Priya
Sri Sairam Engineering College, India

Srinivasan Subramanian
Anna University, India

ABSTRACT

In this chapter, an attempt has been made to automate the analysis of positive and negative Tuberculosis (TB) sputum smear images using multifractal approach. The smear images (N=100) recorded under standard image acquisition protocol are considered. The images are subjected to multifractal analysis and the corresponding spectrum parameters are extracted. Most significant parameters are selected based on the principal component analysis. Further, these parameters are subjected to classification using support vector machine classifier with different kernels. Results demonstrate that the multifractal analysis is capable of discriminating positive and negative TB images. The values of apex, broadness and aperture of the singularity spectrum are higher for TB positive than negative images and are statistically significant. The performance estimators obtained in the classification process show that the polynomial kernel performs better. It appears that this method of texture analysis could be useful for automated analysis of TB using digital sputum smear images.

DOI: 10.4018/978-1-5225-2829-6.ch010

INTRODUCTION

World Health Organization (WHO) has declared Tuberculosis (TB) a global emergency, as it is an air-borne infectious disease. TB is a major cause of illness and death in many countries, especially in Asia and Africa (WHO Tuberculois fact, 2010). TB is caused by Mycobacterium tuberculosis which is an Acid Fast Bacillus (AFB). The bacilli most frequently infect the lungs causing pulmonary tuberculosis.

There are several diagnostic techniques which include both invasive and non-invasive procedures. Smear microscopy, culture and chest radiography are the less expensive non-invasive diagnostic procedures (Sotaquira, Rueda, & Narvaez, 2009). Among the non-invasive tests, microscopic examination of stained sputum smears still remains a cornerstone for the diagnosis of pulmonary tuberculosis throughout the world (Steingart, Henry, Ng, Hopewell, Ramsay, Cunningham, Urbanczik, Perkins, Aziz, & Pai, 2006). The diagnostic method of smear microscopy involves manual examination which is labour intensive and may lead to high false negative rate. Further, repeated tests are needed to be performed for early detection of the disease (Crnčević-Urek, Stipić-Marković, Kardum-Skelin, Stipić, Crnek-Kunstelj, & Urek, 2002). Hence there is a need to automate the diagnostic process for improvement in the sensitivity and accuracy of the test. It also entails substantial reduction in the labour workload despite large number of images analyzed (Veropoulos, Campbell, Learmonth, Knight, & Simpson, 1998).

The smear images are obtained by either using a fluorescence microscope for auramine stained smear or a bright field microscope for Ziehl–Neelsen stained sputum smear (Khutlang, Krishnan, Whitelaw, & Douglas, 2010). Mobile phone based microscopy systems enable greater access to high quality health care monitoring system especially for TB patients. This system support the WHO's Directly Observed Treatment, Short course program, which guide TB eradication efforts (Breslauer, 2009).

Several image analysis techniques have been reported for the automatic identification and classification of sputum smear samples. Existing methods are based on colour and shape analysis of TB images. The shape of the bacillus alone is not a discriminable feature because the bacilli may be faint, occluded, obscured by cells or remnants, or inside macrophages. This imparts a hazy outline to the bacilli, which may cause oversights in recognition (Veropoulos, Campbell, Learmonth, Knight, & Simpson, 1998; Forero, Cristobal, & Desco, 2006). Also colour alone cannot distinguish the stained areas from the fine bacteria because colour spectrum of bacilli is quite wide making it indistinguishable from debris (Tadrous, 2010).

During the past decade, results from numerous published articles have shown the ability of texture analysis algorithms to extract diagnostically meaningful information from medical images (Lopes & Betrouni, 2009). But texture analysis of microscope images faces problem which depends on the level of observation (magnification of the microscope) (Beil, Irinopoulou, Vassy, & Wolf, 1995). This problem of scaling is overcome by the fractal-based texture analysis as fractal is invariant to geometrical changes which includes view point changes and non-rigid deformations of the texture surface (Xu, Ji, & Fermuller, 2009). Fractal is shown to be a tool that describes the fractal geometry and allows capturing that is not available in traditional geometrical representation of shapes (Lopes & Betrouni, 2009).

An extension of fractal is the multifractal approach that offers appropriate tools to overcome limitations arising from the fractal geometry. The multifractal approach reveals distinct distributions of pixels and detects variations within the image. It is capable of describing image features both from local and global point of view (Stojic, Reljin, & Reljin, 2006). Multifractal approach provides a spectrum of fractal dimensions characterizing the image and potentially gives more information about the image compared to the single fractal dimension (Nilsson, 2007). The multifractal spectrum reflects the real features of the image more accurately as it concerns with the probability of pixel distribution. Recently, multifractal analysis has found wide applications in the field of medical diagnosis such as characterization of EEG, ECG signals, brain images, mammography and microscopic images (Lopes & Betrouni, 2009; Soares, Freire, Pereira, Janela, & Seabra, 2009; Hemsley & Mukundan, 2009).

The multifractal behaviour leads to singularity and generalized dimension spectra. There are numerous parameters that can be derived from these spectra which quantitatively analyze the image. Principal Component Analysis (PCA) reduces dimensionality of data set consisting of a large number of interrelated variables, and retains the variation present in the dataset as much as possible. The transformed new set of variables are the principal components that are uncorrelated and are ordered so that the first few retain most of the variation present in all of the original variables (Jolliffe, 2002). PCA is widely employed in feature reduction and clustering techniques (Huang, Velliste, & Murphy, 2003; Tasoulis, Doukas, Maglogiannis, & Plagianakos, 2010).

Classifiers are used in discriminating pathological condition from the normal. Classifier such as Support Vector Machine (SVM) is a machine learning technique based on statistical theory. It seeks for an optimal separating hyperplane, where the margin is maximal. An important and unique feature of this approach is that the solution is based only on those data points which are at the margin (Vapnik, 2013). SVM has currently proved effective in clinical classification (Lenseigne, Brodin, Jeon, Christophe, & Genovesio, 2007; Karvelis, Fotiadis, Georgiou, & Sakaloglou, 2009).

In this chapter, to enhance the need of automation, multifractal analysis is performed to extract spectrum parameters from both positive and negative TB sputum smear images. Significant features are derived from the spectrum parameters using PCA and are further subjected to classification using SVM.

BACKGROUND

TB affects people living in dense urban communities and are prone to have a high probability of becoming infected and develop active disease. Hence, the risk of becoming infected and ill with TB remains higher among people living in congregated institutions, such as social shelters, prisons, youth correctional facilities, nursing homes for elderly people, day nurseries and schools. People with HIV/Acquired Immunodeficiency Syndrome (AIDS) are also susceptible to TB (Palomino, Leao, & Ritacco, 2007).

The causative agent of TB is Mycobacterium Tuberculosis which is a rod-shaped, non-spore forming aerobic bacterium. Being an airborne infection, TB predominantly affects lungs causing pulmonary TB. Other organs such as the lymphatics, pleura, bones and joints or meninges are also equally affected leading to extrapulmonary tuberculosis (Knechel, 2009).

Tuberculosis global fact (WHO Global Tuberculosis Control 2011) states that TB is among the three greatest causes of death among women aged between fifteen and forty four, and nearly 320,000 women died from this contagious disease in 2010. Bhaumik & Biswas (2012) have estimated two million new cases of TB annually within India's borders. The notion of a TB free India, the stated vision of the nation's decades old Revised National Tuberculosis Control Program seems to be remote. The increase in morbidity and mortality made the global plan Stop TB strategy initiated between 2006 and 2015 and to allocate a fund of fifty six billion US dollars. This is a three-fold increase in investment compared to 2005 (WHO Tuberculosis facts 2007). The importance of TB control can be realized by observing the amount spent and to be spent to stop TB.

TB can be diagnosed by both invasive and non-invasive methods. Non-invasive clinical diagnosis of pulmonary TB is performed through clinical attributes or symptoms, chest radiography, tissue-based screening, culture and microscopic examination of sputum specimen. Several attempts have been made to diagnose TB with clinical inferences and demographic studies. Probable diagnosis is suggested based on the values of several important attributes and clinical symptoms (Asha, Natarajan, & Murthy, 2010). Elveren and Yumusak (2011) aimed to present a study on diagnosing tuberculosis with the help of multi-layer neural networks trained with genetic algorithm on patient's epicrisis reports. Though there is symptom based identification, the survey conducted by Ruiz-Manzano et al (2008) suggests that TB cannot be identified from these nosological entities on the basis of clinical signs and symptoms alone.

Knechel (2009) investigated the first laboratory test performed to detect active tuberculosis in a patient with abnormal finding on chest radiograph. Patil & Udupi (2011) estimated texture features using gray level co-occurrence matrix technique from the active shape model based segmented lung images. Although abnormal findings on a chest radiograph may suggest tuberculosis, it is not a specific, sensitive method for the diagnosis of TB (Ruiz-Manzano, Blanquer, Calpe, Caminero, Caylà, Domínguez, García, & Vidal, 2008).

Tadrous (2010) proposed the first tissue-based acid fast bacilli screening algorithm for use in ZN-stained tissues. Osman et al (2012) extracted geometrical features and affine moment invariants from the tissue images. These features are fed to hybrid multi-layered perceptron network to discriminate between TB bacilli and non-TB bacilli. But the histopathologic diagnosis of mycobacterial infection on tissue section is expensive.

Lewis et al (2012) determined the diagnostic accuracy of an automated hardware-software integrated system. The authors used culture as the gold standard and compare it with microscopist's performance. It presented a similar specificity and positive predictive value but with a low sensitivity. Rulaningtyas et al (2015) came out with automatic scanning microscope and an automatic identification of TB bacilli procedure in tissue slides. The identification of TB bacilli seems to produce better results for sputum smear slide with normal staining, but did not work well in over staining and less staining tissue slide.

The mycobacterium tuberculosis can be cultured to detect TB. Clinicians must wait for culture results as long as two months, as this bacillus takes 5 - 20 hours to duplicate (Forero, Cristobal, & Desco, 2006). Thus culture examination is not used to guide a clinical decision when there are much faster techniques such as the sputum smear microscopy. Young et al (2014) used state-of-the-art proteomic approaches to discover urinary diagnostic biomarkers associated with pulmonary TB that distinguish active TB disease from non-TB which contribute in the development of new TB diagnostic tests.

Sputum smear microscopy has several operational advantages over others as a diagnostic tool and has an important role in the follow up of TB treatment (Raof, Mashor, Ahmad, & Noor, 2011). Problems reported with manual screening process especially for screening of the negative slides are labor-intensive and time consuming. This calls for an automated TB diagnosis where large number of cases can be handled quickly with the same accuracy. Costa et al (2008) reasoned to incorporate microscopy for sputum smear diagnosis because of its non-invasive nature.

Many attempts have been made to enable the image captured by a camera that is attached to the microscope, to be viewed through the computer screen. Moreover, human eye has considerable sharpness in discriminating fine detail consisting of high frequency information, but is not sensitive to low frequency or slowly varying image information (Wu, Merchant, & Castleman, 2010). Thus computerized automated techniques are developed to meet the challenges involved in identifying the TB objects (bacilli and outliers) from the sputum smear images.

Several image processing and pattern recognition algorithms have also been developed in order to carry out automatic TB bacilli detection in auramine and ZN-stained sputum smear images. Identification of TB bacilli based on shape and color was also proposed (Forero, Cristobal, & Desco, 2006; Khutlang, Krishnan, Whitelaw, & Douglas, 2010). Purwanti & Widiyanti (2012) attempted to automatically identify TB bacilli in sputum using image processing and learning vector quantization techniques.

Filho et al (2015) proposed scalar selection technique to select input variables for the segmentation classifiers from four color spaces. Goyal et al (2015) implemented tubeness filtering in conjunction with Otsu thresholding and connected component for the automatic detection of mycobacterium tuberculosis from stained sputum smear images. Panicker et al (2016) presented a comprehensive review on the different image processing methods attempted by various researchers working in the field of TB automation.

Recently fractal analysis has been proposed as an additional to histogram analysis which can capture the spatial distribution in a better way (Xu, Ji, & Fermuller, 2009). Histogram analysis is used to perform intensity distribution in the images. The drawback is that the histogram analysis gives only global variations. To perform both local and global intensity distribution, multifractal analysis is performed.

Mandelbrot (1967) introduced the concept of fractals which was later extended to multifractals which is used for modeling and analyzing different complex shapes and signals. The basic idea of multifractal analysis deals with a set of measures which are labeled statistically to obtain efficient texture analysis for the same singularity in different scales. It is a technique which quantitatively evaluates intensity distribution and represents it in different scales of singularity and generalized dimension spectra. These are invariant to geometrical scale changes and have wide-spread application in texture segmentation and classification (Novianto, Guimaraes, Suzuki, Maeda, & Anh, 1999). The multifractal analysis provides precise quantitative description on the inhomogeneous information, especially the intensity distribution within an image.

A review of fractal and multifractal analysis by Lopes & Betrouni (2009) described the implementation of various algorithms including their pros and cons. Fractals look at the geometry of the patterns present whereas multifractals look at the arrangement of the patterns. The multifractal spectrum can be used to describe and compare spatial patterns of any continuous variable (Saravia, 2014, Ţalu, 2012). Several studies have shown the possibilities offered by multifractal analysis in image processing, in particular in classification of complex textures (Harrar & Khider, 2014). A study by Pantic et al (2014) proved fractal and GLCM analysis to be helpful in distinguishing normal from pathological tissue.

Feature selection techniques are employed to select the most significant features. It is also desirable to keep the number of features used as low as possible to get a better generalization property of the classifier (Wahlby, Lindblad, Vondrus, Bengtsson, & Bjorkesten, 2002; Iqbal, Valous, Sun, & Allen, 2011). PCA has been widely used to identify and summarize many inter-relationships that exist among individual variables. PCA technique has been investigated previously by researchers for signal and image processing (Malhi & Gao, 2004). Such analyses were employed in assessing the chest wall movement in pathologies like chronic obstructive pulmonary disease, emphysema, cystic fibrosis and muscular dystrophy.

PCA explores overall rank orders for treatment and relationship between outcomes with classes of asthma medication (Jenkins, Thien, Wheatley, & Reddel, 2005). Mina et al (2009) estimated the level of unconsciousness based on Principal Component Analysis from the EEG waveforms captured in intensive care unit and operating room. Principal component analysis-enhanced cosine radial basis function neural network for epilepsy and seizure detection has been performed by Ghosh-Dastidar et al (2008). The authors concluded that the analysis employing PCA is superior and reported with high classification accuracy for epilepsy diagnosis.

The classification process involves grouping objects into pre-defined classes or finding the class to which an object belongs. The task of classification plays an important role for domain practitioners using medical images especially in the process of decision making (Uwimana & Ruiz 2008). Lotte et al (2007) in their review on the different classification algorithms for EEG based Brain – Computer Interfaces have concluded that SVM reached the best results in several synchronous experiments, both in its linear and non-linear form. Samanta & Nataraj (2009) applied particle swarm optimization in combination with a proximal support vector machine for machinery fault detection.

The time domain vibration signals of a rotating machine with normal and defective bearings were processed for feature extraction and the features extracted from original and pre-processed signals were used as inputs to the SVM classifier for detection of machine condition. The authors concluded that results of the PSO based approach performed better when compared to Genetic algorithm and PCA based approaches. Yan et al (2008) combined SVM with k-nearest neighbor technique for text classification and proved that the combined method of classification proved better than the two methods when performed individually

AUTOMATED ANALYSIS OF SPUTUM SMEAR TB IMAGES

Image Acquisition

The sputum smear slides used were prepared by smearing the sputum specimen on a clean slide. The air dried smears were then fixed to the slide by passing the slides through a low flame two to three times. The slides were flooded with Auramine O stain to bind the cell wall of the acid fast bacilli and left for 10 minutes. Then the slides were decolorized with acid alcohol and washed with running water. To get a contrast background the slides were counter stained with potassium permanganate. Then the slides were rinsed with water and air dried before viewing under the microscope. The fluorescence-stained slides were prepared at the South African National Health Laboratory Services, Groote Schuur Hospital in Cape Town.

The images (N=100) were captured using a camera in monochrome binning mode attached to a 20x objective fluorescence microscope of 0.5 numerical aperture. The camera (AxioCam HR) has a resolution of 4164 x 3120 with a pixel size 6.45 μm (h) x 6.45 μm (v).

The acquired images suffer from non-uniform illumination, and hence these images are pre-processed by non-uniform illumination correction technique (Priya, Srinivasan, & Ramakrishnan, 2014). The pre-processed sputum smear images of size 256 x 256 pixels are considered for multifractal based texture analysis.

Typical Representation of TB Image

Typical representative images of TB positive and negative sputum smear images are shown in Figures 1 and 2 respectively. In general, the objects present in sputum smear images are called as bacilli and non-bacilli. The TB positive image shows the presence of rod-shaped bright foreground objects (bacilli) on a dark background. The negative images show scanty or absence of bacilli. The non-bacilli objects are categorized into outliers and overlapping bacilli. The presence of outliers can be due to poor or non-specific staining of the smear slides or due to overlapping bacilli. The overlapping bacilli exist when

Figure 1. Typical TB positive sputum smear image

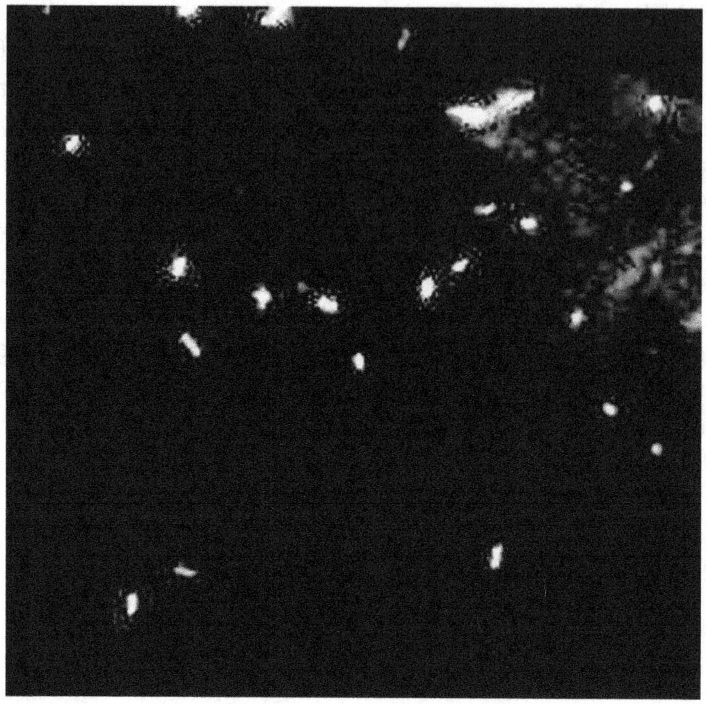

Figure 2. Typical TB negative sputum smear image

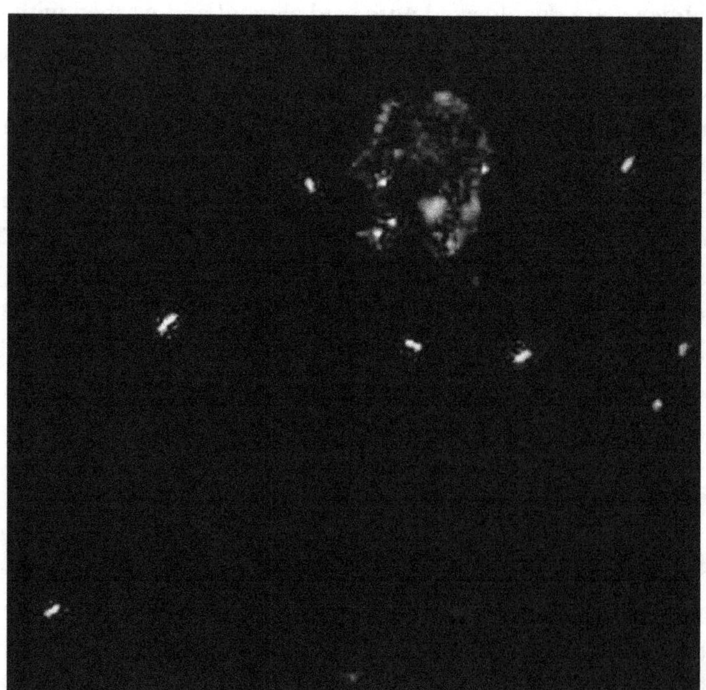

there is a conglomeration of bacilli in the image. The outliers present in the sputum smear images do not have uniform morphology and the only objects that have uniform morphology are the disease causative agent called as TB bacilli.

Thus in a sputum smear image distinguishing bacilli from outliers cannot be effectively done by manual intervention. Hence automated procedures aid in demarcation of TB positive from negative smear images. The multifractal analysis attempted in this chapter serve as an automated procedure which captures the repetitive patterns in the image, as the TB causing bacilli has a uniform rod shape. Also the multifractal analysis quantifies the scale invariant, self-similar structure that is persistent in medical diagnostic images (Fetterhoff, Kraft, Sandler, Opris, Sexton, Marmarelis, Hampson, & Deadwyler, 2015).

Multifractal Analysis

Multifractals are the structures characterized by fractal dimension that varies with the observed scale. To find global and local variations, multifractal analysis is performed based on box counting approach. In this method, the image is covered by a grid of boxes of size ε. The probability distribution of pixels in an ith box is measured as

$$P_i\left(\varepsilon\right) = \frac{N_i\left(\varepsilon\right)}{\sum_i N_i} \tag{1}$$

where $N_i\left(\varepsilon\right)$ is the of number of pixels in the ith box and $\sum_i N_i$ is the total number of pixels in all boxes. The probability $P_i\left(\varepsilon\right)$ scales with different exponents for each box as

$$P_i\left(\varepsilon\right) \sim \varepsilon^{\alpha_i} \tag{2}$$

where α_i is the singularity or Holder exponent which describes the local singularity degree of probability measure $P_i\left(\varepsilon\right)$. Number of boxes for which P_i's has singularity strengths between α and $\alpha + d\alpha$ has scaling relation defined as:

$$N_{\alpha_i}\left(\varepsilon\right) \sim \varepsilon^{-f(\alpha_i)} \tag{3}$$

where $f\left(\alpha_i\right)$ represents the spectrum of fractal dimension that characterize the singularity scaling α_i as shown in Figure 3. The low and high probability distribution of pixels are denoted by $\alpha_{\max}$ and $\alpha_{\min}$. The width $\left(\Delta\alpha = \alpha_{\max} - \alpha_{\min}\right)$ or broadness may be considered as an indicator of symmetry of the singularity spectrum. Right skewed spectrum (low left aperture) corresponds to fine structures present in the image whereas left skewed spectrum (low right aperture) corresponds to smooth looking structures in the image. Left aperture $\left(\alpha_0 - \alpha_{q+}\right)$ and right aperture $\left(\alpha_{q-} - \alpha_0\right)$ of the spectrum represents low

Figure 3. Multifractal singularity spectrum

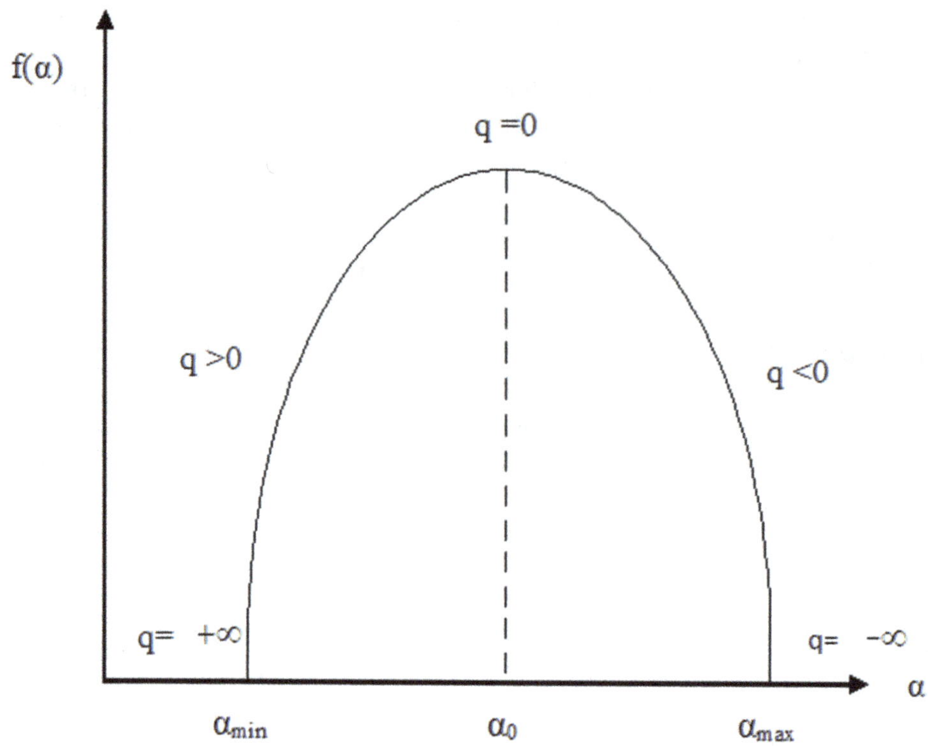

and high fractal exponents (Miranda, Montero, Alves, González, & Vázquez, 2006; Munoz-Diosdado & Del Rio-Correa 2006).

The probability to cover the object of interest for every box i, also called the partition function, is obtained for different q which varies from $-\infty$ to $+\infty$. The value of q resembles a microscope for exploring different regions in the image, i.e., at different scales. Partition function of multifractal is defined as,

$$\chi_q(\varepsilon) = \sum_i P_i^q \tag{4}$$

where P_i is the probability measure with different q values which enlarges different regions of the singular measurement (Dathe, Tarquis, & Perrier, 2006). The function evaluates all possible singularities for all the q values of distribution. The parameter q enlarges different regions of the singular measurement. Large positive q values $(q > 1)$ correspond to low intensity regions of the image, i.e. dark regions. Large negative q values $(q < 1)$ correspond to high intensity regions, i.e., white regions and for $q = 1$ the original measure is replicated (Takahashi, Murata, Narita, Hamada, Kosaka, Omori, Takahashi, Kimura, Yoshida, & Wada, 2006; Lopes & Betrouni 2009).

The linear range of partition function is the scaling range. The partition function plot also called as bi-logarithmic plot represents the probability distribution of pixel intensities in the image both locally and globally for different box sizes and at different scales (q values).

Increase in box sizes produces less number of non-empty boxes and for the maximum size of the box, the measure (number of non-empty box) at different scales remains the same. Positive values of q represent zoom out and negative values of q represent zooming in. Hence for negative q values and at different box sizes, lines of negative slopes are arrived at; and similarly for positive q values lines of positive slopes are derived.

The mass exponent τ is derived from the slope of the partition function as

$$\tau\left(q\right)=\frac{\ln \chi_q}{\ln \varepsilon}\ \tau\left(q\right)=\frac{\ln \chi_q}{\ln \varepsilon}\ .\ \tau\left(q\right)=\frac{\ln \chi_q}{\ln \varepsilon} \tag{5}$$

The multifractal is also characterized in terms of generalized dimension, D_q which correspond to the scaling exponents for the qth moment of the measure. The relationship between singularity exponent, α and spectrum of fractal dimension, $f\left(\alpha\right)$ can be determined by the Legendre transform

$$\alpha=\frac{d\tau\left(q\right)}{dq}\ \alpha=\frac{d\tau\left(q\right)}{dq}\ .\ \alpha=\frac{d\tau\left(q\right)}{dq} \tag{6}$$

$$f\left(\alpha\right)=\alpha q-\tau\left(q\right) \tag{7}$$

The mass exponent τ and the generalized dimension D_q are related as

$$\tau\left(q\right)=\left(q-1\right)D_q\ \tau\left(q\right)=\left(1-q\right)D_q\ .\ \tau\left(q\right)=\left(1-q\right)D_q \tag{8}$$

where D_q for all q values is defined as:

$$D_q=\frac{1}{q-1}\lim_{\varepsilon\to 0}\frac{\ln \chi_q}{\ln \varepsilon} \tag{9}$$

The curve D_q is sigmoidal and non-increasing for positive q values representing the multifractal nature. The generalized dimensions D_0, D_1 and D_2 correspond to the capacity (fractal or box counting), information (or Shannon) and correlation dimension respectively. The lower and the upper limiting generalized dimensions are $D_{-\infty}$ and $D_{+\infty}$ respectively (Stosic & Stosic 2006; Miranda, Montero, Alves, González, & Vázquez, 2006; Landini 2011).

Extraction of Multifractal Features

Multifractal analysis is performed for the considered images by choosing box size varying from 1 to 256 pixels in steps of 2^k in the image, where $1 < k < 8$ is chosen. This is to avoid artifacts occurring at the borders of the image. The upper limit of the box size is the image size and the lower limit is the pixel unit. The multifractal features are extracted from the sputum smear image using the most popular box counting procedure. The global and local variations in the image are found by considering grid of boxes at different scaling factor q. The scaling factor behaves similar to a microscope that is used to explore the regions of the image. The range of scaling factor for the considered images is limited to ± 10, since α value remains constant for $|q| > 10$. The α represents the local distribution in the image and in turn signifies the image homogeneity. The intensity distribution of the image thus forms a smooth concave or bell shaped function called a multifractal spectrum. The multifractal spectrum is figured out as the data or graph showing the behaviour of the patterns amplified in certain ways (orderly fashion) in the image. The distribution of α in the image frames the global distribution $f(\alpha)$. The value of α at $q = -10$ is α_{max} and at $q = +10$ is α_{min} which is at the right and left extreme of the spectrum and the corresponding $f(\alpha)$ values are represented as $f(\alpha_{max})$ and $f(\alpha_{min})$. The maximum and minimum value of $f(\alpha)$ are referred to as f_{max}, f_{min} and their difference is Δf. The Hurst exponent, $\alpha(0)$ represents the apex of the spectrum. Since the scaling range is linear for the q values from 0 to 2, the corresponding D_q values alone are considered for the analysis.

The statistical inference of these parameters is presented in Table 1. Standard deviation of the parameters is high for TB negative images. Increase in mean values for TB positive images is due to the presence of large intensity variations in them.

All the multifractal parameters presented in the table are statistically significant except f_{min}, D_{q-} and $D_{q(q=0)}$. Due to occurrence of rare events like spots or debris in both TB positive and negative images, these parameters which represent the rareness measure are statistically insignificant.

The singularity spectrum obtained for a typical TB positive and negative image presents a single hump-shaped curve as shown in Figures 4 and 5.

It is observed that the width of the spectrum for positive images is greater than the negative images. The broadness of the spectrum in the positive images represents large range of gray levels which is due to the presence of numerous tiny rod-shaped bacilli. The decrease in spectrum range in negative images is due to small range of gray values that are present in the debris.

Negative images have lower maxima than positive images at the apex which is due to the high concentration of lower intensity values representing the objects other than bacilli.

Figures 6 and 7 show the averaged singularity spectrum of $f(\alpha)$ and α with error bars representing the standard deviation. It is observed that the error bars are distinctly seen over the entire spectrum and do not overlap, which is be due to multifractal scaling exhibited by the sputum smear images. Since the objects other than bacilli do not have a uniform morphology in TB negative images, the error bar corresponding to f(α) is of higher range (0.08 to 0.27) for negative images than positive images (0.06 to 0.16).

Table 1. Statistical inference of multifractal parameters for TB positive and negative images

S.no	Multifractal Parameters	Mean with SD†		p value
		TB Positive Images (N=50)	TB Negative Images (N=50)	
	Singularity Spectrum Parameters			
1.	Left extreme, $\left(\alpha_{\min}\right)$	0.88 ± 0.10	0.97 ± 0.16	0.0001*
2.	Right extreme, $\left(\alpha_{\max}\right)$	2.41 ± 0.16	2.20 ± 0.15	0.0001*
3.	Width, $\left(\Delta\alpha = \alpha_{\max} - \alpha_{\min}\right)$	1.53 ± 0.10	1.22 ± 0.17	0.0001*
4.	Apex, $\left(\alpha\left(0\right)\right)$	2.03 ± 0.10	1.89 ± 0.13	0.0001*
5.	Right aperture, $\left(\alpha_{q-}\alpha_{0}\right)$	0.38 ± 0.07	0.31 ± 0.05	0.0001*
6.	Left aperture, $\left(\alpha_{0} - \alpha_{q+}\right)$	1.14 ± 0.07	0.91 ± 0.16	0.0001*
7.	Minimum of $f\left(\alpha\right)$, $\left(f_{\min}\right)$	0.26 ± 0.14	0.48 ± 0.25	0.9035
8.	Maximum of $f\left(\alpha\right)$, $\left(f_{\max}\right)$	1.73 ± 0.06	1.67 ± 0.09	0.0001*
9.	Difference, $\left(\Delta f = f_{\max} - f_{\min}\right)$	1.47 ± 0.14	1.19 ± 0.25	0.0006*
	Generalized Dimension Spectrum Parameters			
10.	Lower limit, $\left(D_{q-\left(q=-10\right)}\right)$	1.16 ± 0.08	1.23 ± 0.13	0.0045
11.	Capacity dimension, $\left(D_{q\left(q=0\right)}\right)$	0.80 ± 0.03	0.79 ± 0.02	0.6210
12.	Information dimension, $\left(D_{q\left(q=1\right)}\right)$	0.67 ± 0.04	0.54 ± 0.09	0.0001*
13.	Correlation dimension, $\left(D_{q\left(q=2\right)}\right)$	0.58 ± 0.05	0.41 ± 0.10	0.0001*
14.	Upper limit, $\left(D_{q+\left(q=+10\right)}\right)$	0.46 ± 0.05	0.31 ± 0.07	0.0001*

† - standard deviation * - statistically significant

Figure 4. Singularity spectrum of typical TB positive image

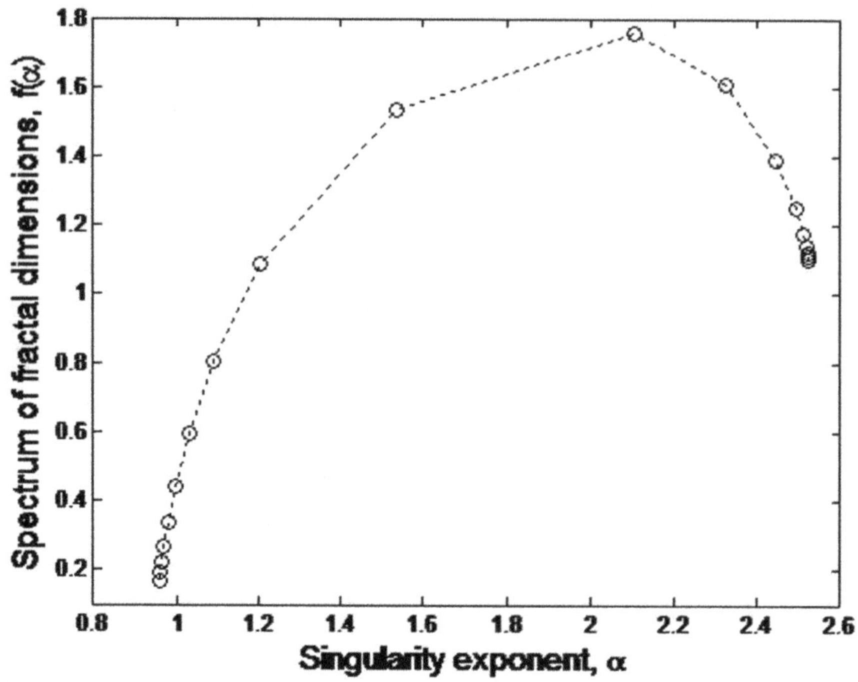

Figure 5. Singularity spectrum of typical TB negative image

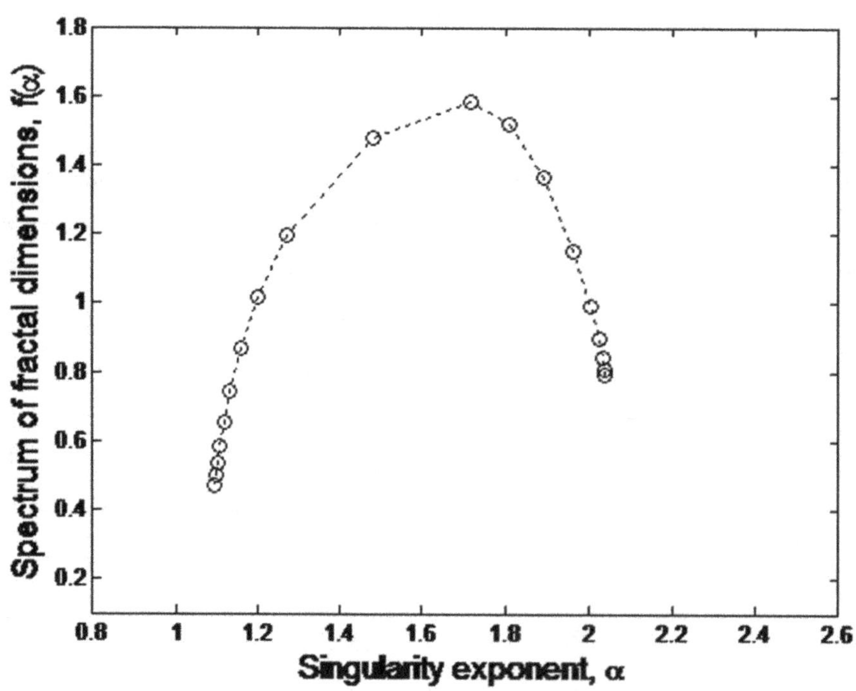

Figure 6. Error bar plot of averaged singularity spectrum of the TB positive smear images

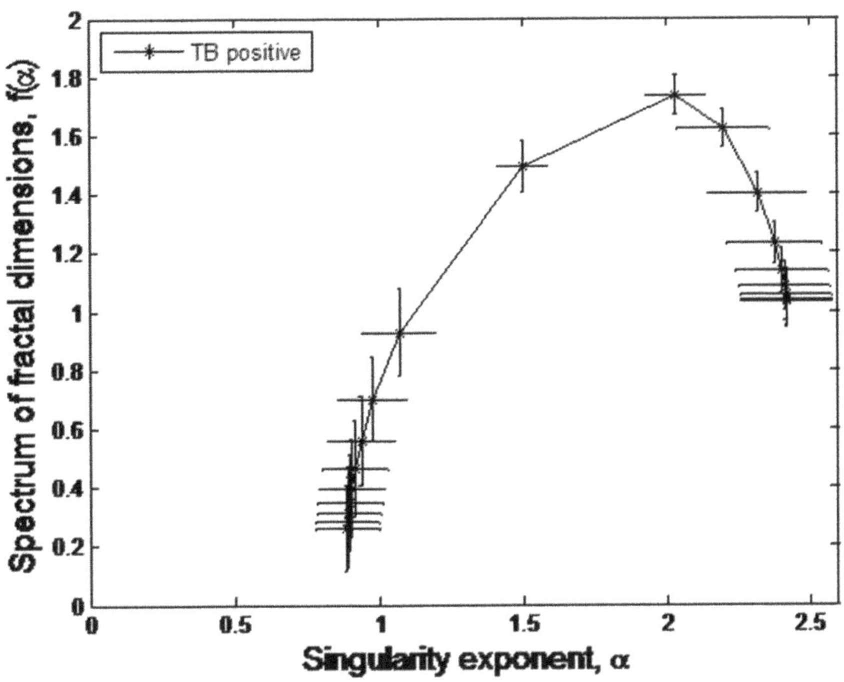

Figure 7. Error bar plot of averaged singularity spectrum of the TB negative smear images

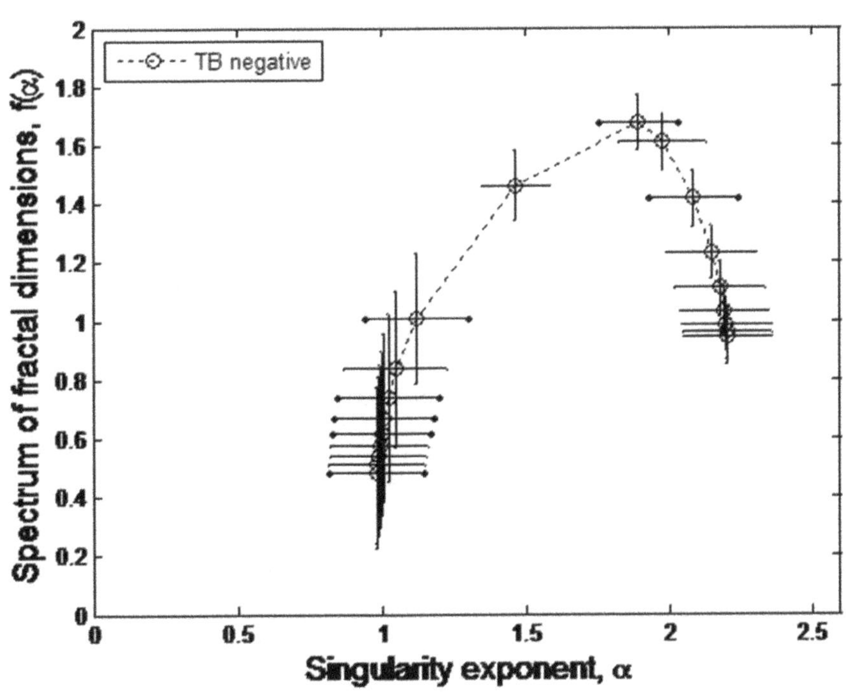

Further, the left and right sides of $f(\alpha)$ spectrum exhibit asymmetry with aperture $(\alpha_0 - \alpha_{q+})$ greater than $(\alpha_{q-} - \alpha_0)$. This left skewed spectrum is due to the heterogeneity nature of the images. Even though both positive and negative images are left skewed, the left aperture is greater in TB positive than negative images. This represents the large group of low fractal exponents α corresponding to fine structures of bacilli in the considered TB positive images.

The average value of generalized fractal dimension D_q for both TB positive and negative smear images are presented in Figure 8. The sigma-shaped spectrum passes through 0.8 at $q = 0$ and reach minimum and maximum values at $q >> 1$ and $q << 1$ respectively. The capacity or fractal dimension D_0 for $q = 0$ is identical for TB positive and negative images. The measure D_{q+} is lower for TB negative images than positive due to high concentration of low intensity values representing spots and debris.

The fourteen multifractal parameters calculated from the singularity and the generalized dimension spectra are further subjected to PCA.

Figure 8. Variation of D_q with q for the average values of all the TB positive and negative smear images

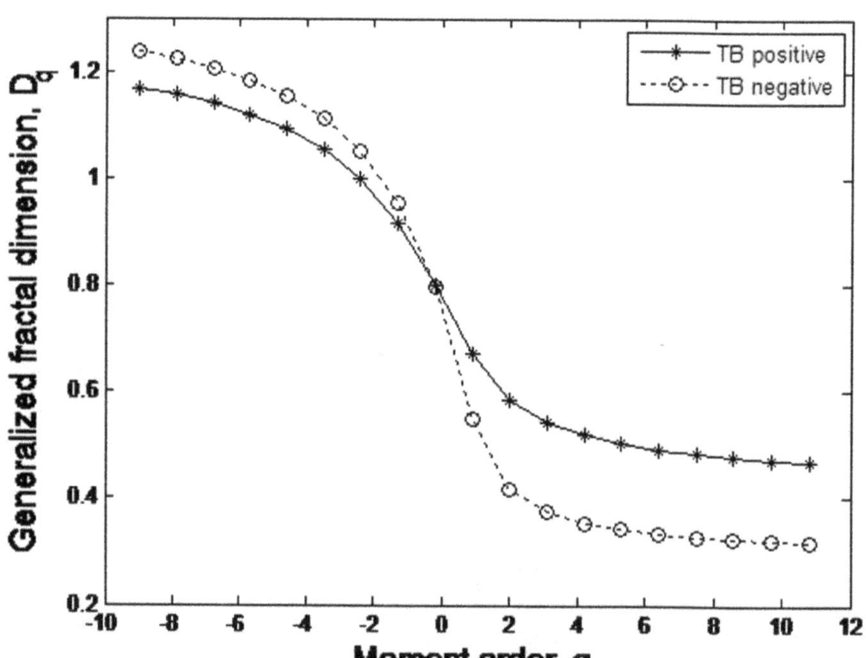

Principal Component Analysis

PCA uncovers combinations of original variables which describe the dominant patterns and the main trends in the data. It is based on the statistical representation of a random variable. The mean μ_x and the covariance matrix C_x for a random vector population $x = \left(x_1, \ldots, x_n\right)^T$ are given by

$$\mu_x = E\left(x\right) \tag{10}$$

$$C_x = E\left\{\left(x - \mu_x\right)\left(x - \mu_x\right)^T\right\} \tag{11}$$

The components of C_x, denoted by C_{ij}, represent the covariance between the random variable components and x_i. The component C_{ii} is the variance of the x_i component. The variance of a component indicates the spread of the component values around its mean value. The eigenvectors e_i and the corresponding eigenvalues λ_i are the solutions obtained from the covariance matrix of the equation

$$C_x e_i = \lambda_i e_i \text{ for } i = 1, \ldots, n \tag{12}$$

Eigenvectors are ordered in descending eigenvalues with the first eigenvector having the direction of largest variance of the data to find directions in which the data set has the most significant amount of energy. By transforming the data vector x, y is obtained from a matrix A consisting of eigenvectors of the covariance matrix as the row vectors represented as:

$$y = A(x - \mu_x) \tag{13}$$

which is a point in the orthogonal coordinate system defined by the eigenvectors. Components of y are the coordinates in the orthogonal base. The original data vector x can be reconstructed from y using:

$$x = A^T y + \mu_x \tag{14}$$

The original vector x was projected on the coordinate axes defined by the orthogonal basis. The original vector was then reconstructed by a linear combination of the orthogonal basis vectors.

Representing only a few basis vectors of the orthogonal basis instead of using all the eigenvectors of the covariance matrix which are the principal components, the matrix having the first K eigenvectors as rows is denoted by A_K and a similar transformation can be created for which

$$y' = A_K \left(x - \mu_x\right) \tag{15}$$

$$x' = A_K^T y' + \mu_x \tag{16}$$

The original data vector is projected on the coordinate axes having the dimension K and transforming the vector back by a linear combination of the basis vectors. This minimizes the mean-square error between the data and this representation with given number of eigenvectors (Ghosh-Dastidar, Adeli, & Dadmehr, 2008; Aguado, Montoy, Borras, Seco, & Ferrer, 2008).

Among the fourteen multifractal parameters, five most significant parameters are selected using PCA. The selection of the parameters was based on the highest magnitude of eigenvalues in the first principal component.

The percentage variances of the significant principal components are shown in Table 2. It is observed that the first five principal components contribute to 95% of the variance. Since the first principal component PC1 alone contributes to maximum variance, the significant features are selected from PC1 based on their magnitude.

The contributions of most significant parameters to the magnitudes of first two principal components for TB positive and negative images are shown in Figures 9 and 10 respectively. The significant parameters selected have a decreasing order of magnitude with the highest for $\alpha_{\min}$. The remaining parameters are ranked as $\Delta\alpha$, D_{q+}, $D_{q(q=1)}$ and $D_{q(q=2)}$.

It is observed that the angle between $\alpha_{\min}$ (left extreme) and $\Delta\alpha$ (width) is small. The angles between the D_q's (generalized dimensions) also exhibit similar observation. This is because of the high correlation that exists between these parameters. It is also observed that the angles between the singularity and generalized dimension spectra vectors are very large. This shows the independent nature of these parameters and the existence of low correlation between them. The magnitude of projection of the vectors over the other also represents similar correlation among the vectors.

The orientation of the vectors $\alpha_{\min}$ and $\Delta\alpha$ differ greatly among the positive and negative images and they symbolizes inhomogeneity with them. The five most significant parameters derived using PCA are used as input feature vectors to the SVM classifier.

Table 2. Contribution of the principal components in the percentage variance for TB positive and negative images

Principal Components	% Variance	
	TB Positive	TB Negative
PC1	54.3	38.8
PC2	19.5	29.3
PC3	11.3	16.0
PC4	6.4	7.7
PC5	4.3	4.5

Figure 9. Variation in component magnitudes of selected multifractal parameters with the first two principal components for TB positive images

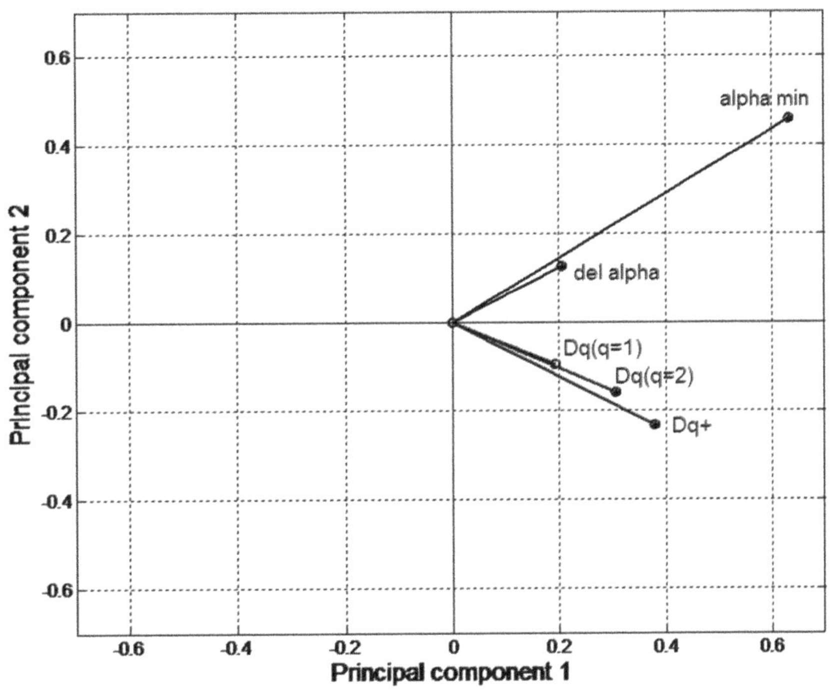

Support Vector Machines

The SVM is a linear classifier in the parameter space, but it becomes a non-linear classifier as a result of the non-linear mapping of the space of the input patterns into the high dimensional feature space. Figure 11 depicts the basic architecture of support vector machine classification. The number of support vectors, weights and bias in classifying the output is shown the figure.

For the set of training vectors belonging to two separate classes,

$$D = \left\{ \left(x^1, y^1\right), \ldots, \left(x^l, y^l\right) \right\} \tag{17}$$

for $x \in R^n$ and $y \in \left\{1, -1\right\}$ with a hyperplane

$$\left\langle w, x \right\rangle + b = 0 \tag{18}$$

where w is the vector of hyperplane coefficients and b is a bias term so that the periphery between the hyperplane and the nearest point is maximized (Hsu & Lin 2002).

Figure 10. Variation in component magnitudes of selected multifractal parameters with the first two principal components for TB positive images

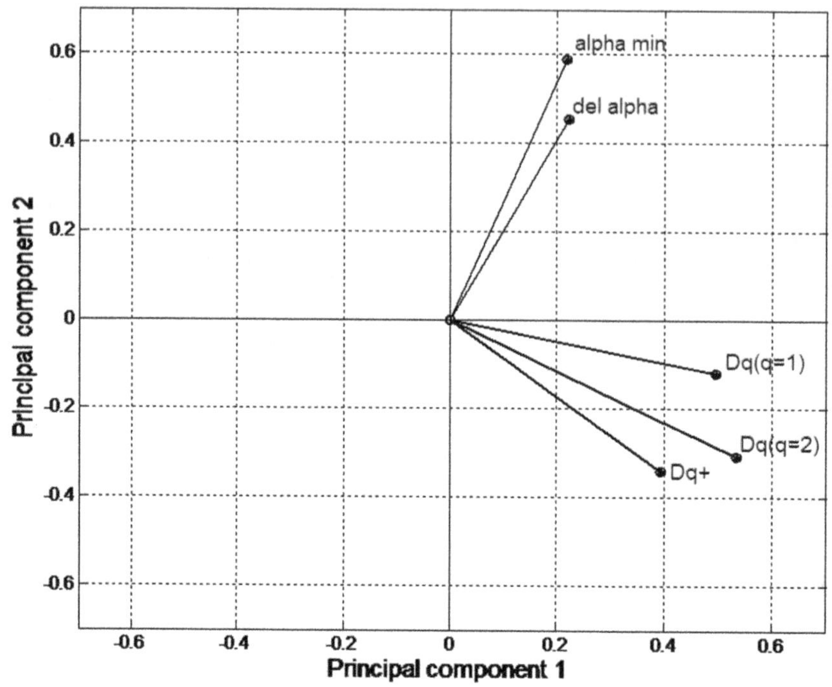

Figure 11. Basic architecture of support vector classification

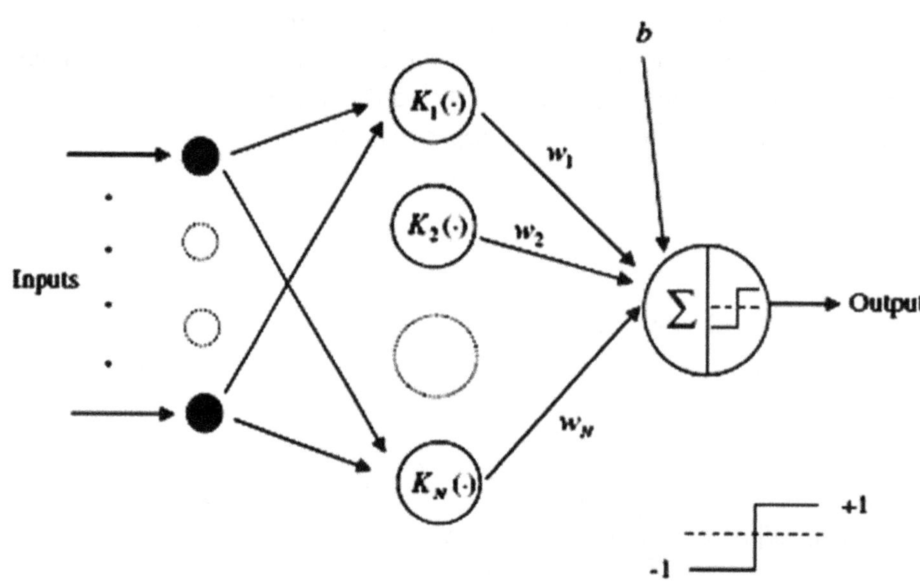

It is appropriate without loss of generality to consider a canonical hyperplane where the parameters w and b are constrained by $\min_i \left|\left\langle w, x^i \right\rangle + b\right| = 1$.

A separating hyperplane in canonical form satisfy the following constraint,

$$y^i \left|\left\langle w, x^i \right\rangle + b\right| \geq 1 \text{ where } i = 1, \ldots, l \quad (19)$$

The distance $d\left(w, b; x\right)$ of a point x from the hyperplane $\left(w, b\right)$ is,

$$d\left(w, b; x\right) = \frac{\left|\left\langle w, x^i \right\rangle + b\right|}{\left\| w \right\|} \quad (20)$$

The optimal hyperplane is obtained by maximising the margin ρ

$$\rho\left(w, b\right) = \min_{x^i : y^i = -1} d\left(w, b; x^i\right) + \min_{x^i : y^i = 1} d\left(w, b; x^i\right) = \frac{2}{\left\| w \right\|} \quad (21)$$

Hence the hyperplane that optimally separates the data is the one that minimises

$$\varphi\left(w\right) = \frac{1}{2}\left\| w \right\|^2 \quad (22)$$

The solution to the optimization problem is given by the saddle point of the Lagrange functional

$$\varphi\left(w, b, \alpha\right) = \frac{1}{2}\left\| w \right\|^2 - \sum_{i=1}^{l} \alpha_i \left(y^i \left[\left|\left\langle w, x^i \right\rangle + b\right|\right] - 1 \right) \quad (23)$$

where α and α_i are the Lagrange multipliers. The Lagrange functional has to be minimized with respect to w, b and maximized with respect to $\alpha \geq 0$ and is given by

$$w^* = \sum_{i=1}^{l} \alpha_i y_i x_i \quad (24)$$

$$b^* = -\frac{1}{2}\left\langle w^*, x_r + x_s \right\rangle \quad (25)$$

where x_r and x_s are support vectors from each class.

The classifier produces a real valued output between -1 and 1 when the classifier is queried within the margin, where no training data resides. From the Kuhn-Tucker condition

$$\alpha_i(y^i[|\langle w, x^i\rangle + b|] - 1) = 0 \text{ for } i = 1,...,l \tag{26}$$

and hence only the points x^i which satisfy

$$y^i[|\langle w, x^i\rangle + b|] = 1 \tag{27}$$

will have non-zero Lagrange multipliers. These points are termed Support Vectors (SV). If the data is linearly separable all the SV will lie on the margin and hence the number of SV can be very small. Hence SVM can be used to summarize the information contained in a data set by the SV produced.

In the case where a linear boundary is inappropriate the SVM can map the input vector x into a high dimensional feature space z. By choosing a non-linear mapping a priori, the SVM constructs an optimal separating hyperplane in this higher dimensional space.

The parameters selected using PCA are classified by linear, quadratic, Radial Basis Function (RBF) and polynomial kernels of the classifier. The optimal order of the polynomial kernel and optimal width of the RBF kernel employed in SVM classifier is chosen for obtaining maximum values of the performance estimators.

The chosen parameters by PCA are used to classify the TB images by SVM. The performance analysis of the classifier is estimated for linear, quadratic, RBF and polynomial kernels. Further, to improve the classifier performance the width of the RBF and the order of the polynomial kernel are varied for which the Receiver Operating Characteristic (ROC) curve is obtained. Figures 12 and 13 show the ROC curves corresponding to various widths of RBF and order of polynomial kernels respectively. Results demonstrate that RBF kernel performs better for a width of 2.6 and polynomial for an order 3, as maximum values are obtained for the sensitivity, specificity and accuracy.

Classifier Performance

The performance of the classifier was tested using various estimators such as sensitivity, specificity and accuracy. Sensitivity indicates the proportion of true positive of all the positive classes in the dataset. Specificity is related to true negatives of all the negative cases in the dataset. Sensitivity = TP / (TP+FN) and Specificity = TN / (TN+FP). The Positive Predictive Value (PPV) and Negative Predictive Value (NPV) are the proportion of true positives out of all positive results and of true negatives out of all negative results respectively. Accuracy predicts the classifier performance in global sense.

Table 3 shows the performance analysis of the classifier for different kernels. It is observed that polynomial kernel presents similar value of sensitivity, specificity and accuracy. Based on accuracy, polynomial kernel seems to perform better than the linear, quadratic and RBF kernels for classification.

Further sub analysis was performed on the parameters $\alpha_{\min}$, the left extreme and $\Delta\alpha$, the width which exhibit high correlation among the singularity spectrum parameters. The graphical illustration of the sub analysis performed on the considered parameters using polynomial kernel is shown in Figure 14. The figure illustrates the training vectors, classified parameters and the number of support vectors

Figure 12. Receiver Operating Characteristic curves for different width values in RBF kernel

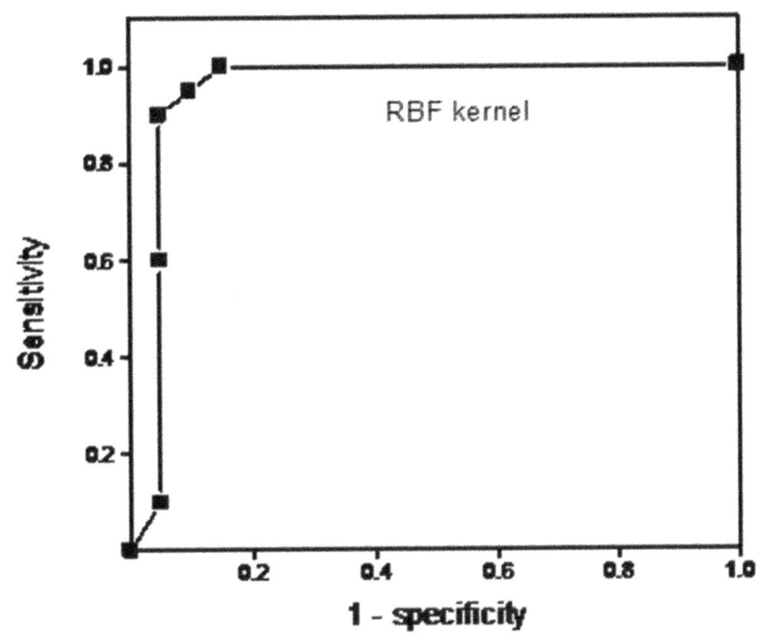

Figure 13. Receiver Operating Characteristic curves for different width values in polynomial kernel

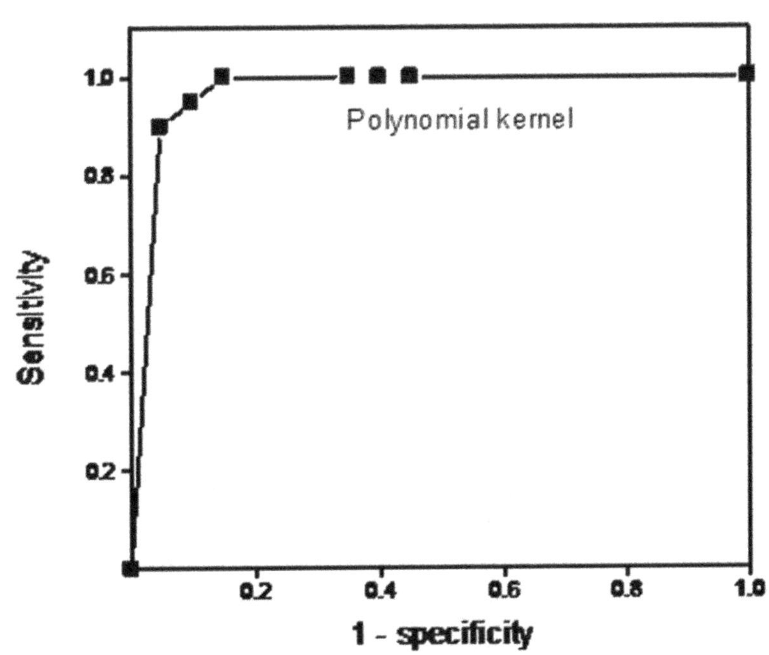

Table 3. Performance analysis of the classifier for different kernels

Kernel Types	Sensitivity (%)	Specificity (%)	Accuracy (%)	PPV (%)	NPV (%)
Linear	95	90	93	90	95
Quadratic	90	95	93	95	90
RBF	95	90	93	90	95
Polynomial	95	95	95	95	95

Figure 14. Representative sub analysis of left extreme (α_{min}) and width $(\Delta\alpha)$ parameters using SVM for polynomial kernel of order 3

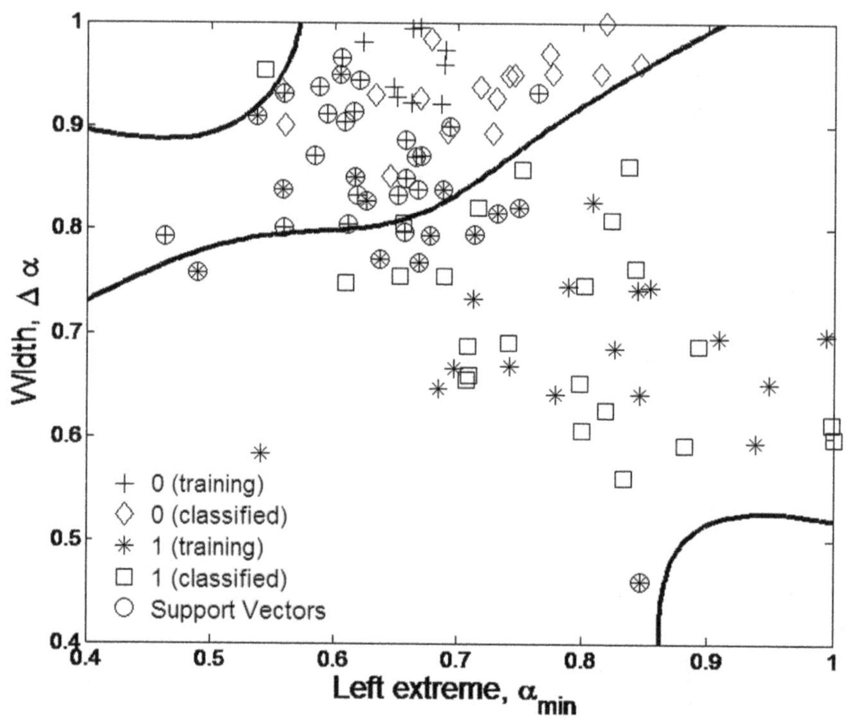

used for classification. It is observed that polynomial kernel is more efficient in utilizing the dataset for training procedure with less number of support vectors. Hence it could be concluded that, the polynomial kernel of order 3 provides better classification of TB sputum smear images compared to other kernels using SVM based classification.

The performance of SVM classifier is compared with the state-of-art approach namely the radial basis function neural network classifier. It is observed that for seven number of hidden layer neurons the neural network classifier is able to perform with a higher accuracy. The comparison performance measures of the classifiers are presented in Table 4. Results demonstrate that the accuracy of neural network is low, as the network performance in generalizing new situation is low.

Table 4. Performance analysis of the radial basis function neural network and support vector machine classifier

Classifier	Performance measures				
	Sensitivity (%)	Specificity (%)	Accuracy (%)	PPV (%)	NPV (%)
RBFNN	85	80	82.5	85	84.2
SVM	95	95	95	95	95

The proposed algorithm is analyzed by comparing it with the literature on the automation procedures in identification and classification of TB images as presented in Table 5.

There are some observations made from the literatures reported with high accuracy. Sotaquira et al (2009) reported a specificity of 99.13%, by discarded the artifacts present in the images. In order to completely characterize the algorithm the authors need to analyze large number of patients. Khutlang et al (2010) used additional prior shape information in the second stage of one class pixel classifier. Osman et al (2009) analyzed the identification of TB bacilli in tissue section which is invasive method and also the histopathologic diagnosis is expensive. Veropoulos et al (1998) discarded images with numerous

Table 5. Performance analysis of various automation procedures in TB detection

Features & Classifier (Authors With Year)	Performance Measures		
	Sensitivity (%)	Specificity (%)	Accuracy (%)
Methods Proposed for Conventional Microscope			
Color channels, size filters, adaptive thresholding (Costa et al 2008)	76.65	False positive rate: 12%	
Color space, first derivative of histogram (Sotaquira et al 2009)	90.90	99.13	95.70
Shape descriptors & pixels classifier (Khutlang et al 2010)	97.77	99.13	98.55
Color channel thresholding & pixel classifier (Morales-Carbajal et al 2010)	86.08	92.39	Not declared
Geometric & HMLP (Osman et al 2010)	100	96.19	98.07
Color space & decision tree (Zhai et al 2010)	100	94	> 80
Color space parameters (Nayak et al 2010)	Success rate: 93.5%		
Morphological & improved ELM (Osman et al 2012)	93.20	79.10	88.33
ANN as pixel classifier (Ayas & Ekinci 2014)	76.82	63.78	66.28
SVM as pixel classifier (Ayas & Ekinci 2014)	86.71	60.15	66.13
Random forest as pixel classifier (Ayas & Ekinci 2014)	75.71	77.33	76.95
Color space & SVM (Filho et al 2015)	93.75	92.75	93.25
Methods Proposed for Fluorescence Microscope			
Shape descriptors & BPNN (Veropoulos et al 1998)	93.53	98.79	97.57
Color thresholding & GMM clustering, Bayesian (Forero et al 2006)	97.89	94.67	Not declared
HU moments, photometric, geometric, HoG & SVM (Chang et al 2012)	83.90	88	78.40
Shape based descriptors & pixel classifier (Santiago-Mozos et al 2014)	73.53	99.99	Not declared

presence of bacilli clusters, as this hinders the separation process and this improved the classification accuracy to 97.57%.

ADVANTAGES AND LIMITATIONS OF MULTIFRACTAL ANALYSIS

One of the advantages of multifractal is that they require fewer conditions on data than more classical statistics such as autocorrelation and variograms. These usually require isotropy and stationarity but multifractal can be used with anisotropic data and are inherently non-stationary (Saravia, 2014).

Fractal and multifractal geometries allow researchers and physicians the early detection and diagnosis of diseases, based on the analyses of medical data and images. Its advantage is that it characterizes the local scale properties in addition to the global properties. It helps in examining the complex patterns found in biological and medical practice compared to traditional Euclidean geometry (Ţalu, 2012).

One of the practical issues when estimating multifractal is the choice of box size. Boxes of large size may contain empty space outside the object and therefore underestimate its complexity. But if boxes are too small they will not guarantee a sensible range of scale and the resulting unaccounted boxes would lead to an underestimation. Also the boundaries of irregular objects resemble fractals at low resolutions, but appear smooth (Euclidean) at very high resolutions (Lopes & Betrouni, 2009, Landini, 2011).

SOLUTIONS AND RECOMMENDATIONS

As a replacement to histogram, multifractal analysis is used by Xu et al (2009 & 2006) for texture analysis. Multifractal analysis has been recognized as a powerful tool in characterizing textures. Several studies have shown the possibilities offered by multifractal analysis in image processing, especially in most cases the mode of multifractal spectrum is used for classification of complex textures.

Box-counting method is one of the empirical algorithms for calculating the fractal dimension. Multifractal analysis using the box-counting method reveals the bimodal character observed for some textures. The box-counting method characterizes the texture that is more difficult to emphasize in the multimodal nature.

FUTURE RESEARCH DIRECTIONS

The automated analysis, carried out in this chapter to identify the presence or absence of pulmonary tuberculosis, is performed for auramine-stained sputum smear images. This methodology could be used to potentially quantify bacilli in ZN smears as a surrogate marker of prognosis or cure in TB patient. Further, the image level classification can be extended to slide level classification so that 10 to 100 images are analyzed per slide. Also, severity analysis depends on the number of bacilli present in an image which could be performed.

CONCLUSION

Any person with active tuberculosis is capable of infecting on average between 10 and 15 people every year (WHO Tuberculois fact, 2010). Therefore, early detection of the disease is vital for monitoring, treatment and for the control of TB. Although many diagnostic methods have been developed, acid fast bacilli smear microscopy is still considered as the gold standard to identify highly contagious patients (Palomino, Leao, & Ritacco, 2007). Thus performing automated analysis is essential for mass screening of this disorder.

In this chapter, an attempt has been made to automate the analysis of digital TB images using multifractal approach. Parameters corresponding to multifractal spectrum are extracted from the sputum smear images. The most significant of them are selected based on PCA. Further, these parameters are subjected to classification using SVM classifier and the performance analysis was studied.

Results demonstrate that the multifractal parameters are able to differentiate TB positive and negative images. It is observed that the multifractal singularity spectrum obtained for the TB negative images has lower maxima, narrow spectrum range and lower left aperture compared to positive images. The lower maxima signifies the high concentration of low intensity values representing the spots and debris and the narrow spread of the spectrum signifies the small range of gray values in the negative images. The greater left aperture in positive images corresponds to low fractal exponents which represents fine structures of bacilli in these images. The singularity spectrum and the spectrum of generalized fractal dimension represent the multifractality nature of the sputum smear images. It was observed that SVM classifier with polynomial kernel presented relatively higher sensitivity, specificity and accuracy. It appears that the proposed methodology seems to be useful for automated analysis of TB sputum smear images.

ACKNOWLEDGMENT

The authors acknowledge Dr.Tania S. Douglas and Mr.Sriram Krishnan of Medical Imaging Research Unit, University of Cape Town, South Africa for the thought worthy discussions during acquisition of sputum smear images.

REFERENCES

Aguado, D., Montoya, T., Borras, L., Seco, A., & Ferrer, J. (2008). Using SOM and PCA for analysing and interpreting data from a P-removal SBR. *Engineering Applications of Artificial Intelligence*, *21*(6), 919–930. doi:10.1016/j.engappai.2007.08.001

Asha, T., Natarajan, S., & Murthy, K. N. B. (2010, July). Notice of Retraction Diagnosis of tuberculosis using ensemble methods. *3rd IEEE International Conference on Computer Science and Information Technology (ICCSIT)*, 8, 409-412.

Ayas, S., & Ekinci, M. (2014). Random forest-based tuberculosis bacteria classification in images of ZN-stained sputum smear samples. *Signal, Image and Video Processing, 8*(1), 49–61.

Beil, M., Irinopoulou, T., Vassy, J., & Wolf, G. (1995). A dual approach to structural texture analysis in microscopic cell images. *Computer Methods and Programs in Biomedicine*, *48*(3), 211–219. doi:10.1016/0169-2607(96)81866-9 PMID:8925647

Bhaumik, S., & Biswas, T. (2012). India makes tuberculosis a notifiable disease. *Canadian Medical Association Journal*, *184*(10), E519–E520. doi:10.1503/cmaj.109-4213 PMID:22641684

Breslauer, D. N., Maamari, R. N., Switz, N. A., Lam, W. A., & Fletcher, D. A. (2009). Mobile Phone Based Clinical Microscopy for Global Health Applications. *PLoS ONE*, *4*(7), e6320. doi:10.1371/journal.pone.0006320 PMID:19623251

Chang, J., Arbelaez, P., Switz, N., Reber, C., Tapley, A., Davis, J. L., & Malik, J. et al. (2012). Automated tuberculosis diagnosis using fluorescence images from a mobile microscope. *Medical Image Computing and Computer-Assisted Intervention.*, *15*(3), 345–352. PMID:23286149

Costa, M. G., Costa Filho, C. F., Sena, J. F., Salem, J., & de Lima, M. O. (2008, August). Automatic identification of mycobacterium tuberculosis with conventional light microscopy. *30th Annual International Conference of the IEEE Engineering in Medicine and Biology Society*, 382-385. doi:10.1109/IEMBS.2008.4649170

Crnčević-Urek, M., Stipić-Marković, A., Kardum-Skelin, I., Stipić, J., Crnek-Kunstelj, V., & Urek, R. (2002). Induced Sputum: A Method for Cytologic Analysis of Bronchial Specimens. *Acta Clinica Croatica*, *41*(2), 89–93.

Dathe, A., Tarquis, A. M., & Perrier, E. (2006). Multifractal analysis of the pore-and solid-phases in binary two-dimensional images of natural porous structures. *Geoderma*, *134*(3), 318–326. doi:10.1016/j.geoderma.2006.03.024

Elveren, E., & Yumuşak, N. (2011). Tuberculosis disease diagnosis using artificial neural network trained with genetic algorithm. *Journal of Medical Systems*, *35*(3), 329–332. doi:10.1007/s10916-009-9369-3 PMID:20703557

Fetterhoff, D., Kraft, R. A., Sandler, R. A., Opris, I., Sexton, C. A., Marmarelis, V. Z., & Deadwyler, S. A. et al. (2015). Distinguishing cognitive state with multifractal complexity of hippocampal interspike interval sequences. *Frontiers in Systems Neuroscience*, *9*, 130. doi:10.3389/fnsys.2015.00130 PMID:26441562

Filho, C. F. F. C., Levy, P. C., Xavier, C. de M., Fujimoto, L. B. M., & Costa, M. G. F. (2015). Automatic identification of tuberculosis mycobacterium. *Research on Biomedical Engineering*, *31*(1), 33–43. doi:10.1590/2446-4740.0524

Forero, M. G., Cristóbal, G., & Desco, M. (2006). Automatic identification of Mycobacterium tuberculosis by Gaussian mixture models. *Journal of Microscopy*, *223*(2), 120–132. doi:10.1111/j.1365-2818.2006.01610.x PMID:16911072

Ghosh-Dastidar, S., Adeli, H., & Dadmehr, N. (2008). Principal component analysis-enhanced cosine radial basis function neural network for robust epilepsy and seizure detection. *IEEE Transactions on Bio-Medical Engineering*, *55*(2), 512–518. doi:10.1109/TBME.2007.905490 PMID:18269986

Global Tuberculosis Control. (2011). WHO Report.

Goyal, A., Roy, M., Gupta, P., Dutta, M. K., Singh, S. & Garg, V. (2015). Automatic Detection of Mycobacterium tuberculosis in Stained Sputum and Urine Smear Images. *Archives of Clinical Microbiology, 6*(3-5), 1-4.

Harrar, K., & Khider, M. (2014). Texture analysis using multifractal spectrum. *International Journal of Modeling and Optimization, 4*(4), 336–341. doi:10.7763/IJMO.2014.V4.396

Hemsley, A., & Mukundan, R. (2009, December). Multifractal measures for tissue image classification and retrieval. *11th IEEE International Symposium on Multimedia, 2009. ISM'09*, 618-623. doi:10.1109/ISM.2009.94

Hsu, C. W., & Lin, C. J. (2002). A comparison of methods for multiclass support vector machines. *IEEE Transactions on Neural Networks, 13*(2), 415–425. doi:10.1109/72.991427 PMID:18244442

Huang, K., Velliste, M., & Murphy, R. F. (2003, June). Feature reduction for improved recognition of subcellular location patterns in fluorescence microscope images. In *Biomedical Optics 2003* (pp. 307–318). International Society for Optics and Photonics.

Iqbal, A., Valous, N. A., Sun, D. W., & Allen, P. (2011). Parsimonious classification of binary lacunarity data computed from food surface images using kernel principal component analysis and artificial neural networks. *Meat Science, 87*(2), 107–114. doi:10.1016/j.meatsci.2010.08.014 PMID:21062668

Jenkins, C. R., Thien, F. C. K., Wheatley, J. R., & Reddel, H. K. (2005). Traditional and patient-centred outcomes with three classes of asthma medication. *The European Respiratory Journal, 26*(1), 36–44. doi:10.1183/09031936.05.00144704 PMID:15994387

Jolliffe, I. (2002). *Principal component analysis*. John Wiley & Sons, Ltd.

Karvelis, P. S., Fotiadis, D. I., Georgiou, I., & Sakaloglou, P. (2009, September). Enhancement of the classification of multichannel chromosome images using support vector machines. *Annual International Conference of the IEEE Engineering in Medicine and Biology Society*, 3601-3604. doi:10.1109/IEMBS.2009.5333757

Khutlang, R., Krishnan, S., Whitelaw, A., & Douglas, T. S. (2010). Automated detection of tuberculosis in Ziehl-Neelsen-stained sputum smears using two one-class classifiers. *Journal of Microscopy, 237*(1), 96–102. doi:10.1111/j.1365-2818.2009.03308.x PMID:20055923

Knechel, N. A. (2009). Tuberculosis: Pathophysiology, clinical features, and diagnosis. *Critical Care Nurse, 29*(2), 34–43. doi:10.4037/ccn2009968 PMID:19339446

Landini, G. (2011). Fractals in microscopy. *Journal of Microscopy, 241*(1), 1–8. doi:10.1111/j.1365-2818.2010.03454.x PMID:21118245

Lenseigne, B., Brodin, P., Jeon, H. K., Christophe, T., & Genovesio, A. (2007, April). Support vector machines for automatic detection of tuberculosis bacteria in confocal microscopy images. *4th IEEE International Symposium on Biomedical Imaging: From Nano to Macro*, 85-88. doi:10.1109/ISBI.2007.356794

Lewis, J. J., Chihota, V. N., van der Meulen, M., Fourie, P. B., Fielding, K. L., Grant, A. D., & Churchyard, G. J. et al. (2012). Proof-Of-Concept Evaluation of an Automated Sputum Smear Microscopy System for Tuberculosis Diagnosis. *PLoS ONE*, *7*(11), e50173. doi:10.1371/journal.pone.0050173 PMID:23209666

Lopes, R., & Betrouni, N. (2009). Fractal and multifractal analysis: A review. *Medical Image Analysis*, *13*(4), 634–649. doi:10.1016/j.media.2009.05.003 PMID:19535282

Lotte, F., Congedo, M., Lécuyer, A., Lamarche, F., & Arnaldi, B. (2007). A review of classification algorithms for EEG-based brain–computer interfaces. *Journal of Neural Engineering*, *4*(2), R1–R13. doi:10.1088/1741-2560/4/2/R01 PMID:17409472

Malhi, A., & Gao, R. X. (2004). PCA-based feature selection scheme for machine defect classification. *IEEE Transactions on Instrumentation and Measurement*, *53*(6), 1517–1525. doi:10.1109/TIM.2004.834070

Mandelbrot, B. B. (1967). How long is the coast of Britain. *Science*, *156*(3775), 636–638. doi:10.1126/science.156.3775.636 PMID:17837158

Mina, T., Behzad, A., & Rassoul, A. (2009). Assessment of depth of anes-thesia using principal component analysis. *J Biomedical Science and Engineering*, *96*(2), 9–15.

Miranda, J. G. V., Montero, E., Alves, M. C., González, A. P., & Vázquez, E. V. (2006). Multifractal characterization of saprolite particle-size distributions after topsoil removal. *Geoderma*, *134*(3), 373–385. doi:10.1016/j.geoderma.2006.03.014

Morales-Carbajal, C., Bravo-Zanoguera, M. E., Vera-Perez, M., Arriola, H., Lopez-Avitia, R., & Reyna-Carranza, M. A. (2010). *Identification of tuberculosis bacillus in direct smears with low image quality. Pan American Health Care Exchange*. PAHCE.

Muñoz-Diosdado, A., & Del Río-Correa, J. L. (2006, August). Further study of the asymmetry for multifractal spectra of heartbeat time series. *Engineering in Medicine and Biology Society, 2006. EMBS'06. 28th Annual International Conference of the IEEE*, 1450-1453. doi:10.1109/IEMBS.2006.260166

Nayak, R., Shenoy, V. P., & Galigekere, R. R. (2010). A new algorithm for automatic assessment of the degree of TB-infection using images of ZN-stained sputum smear. *Proceedings of International Conference on Systems in Medicine and Biology (ICSMB)*, 294–299. doi:10.1109/ICSMB.2010.5735390

Nilsson, E. (2007). *Multifractal-based image analysis with applications in medical imaging*. Umea, Sweden: Umea Univ.

Novianto, S., Guimaraes, L., Suzuki, Y., Maeda, J., & Anh, V. V. (1999). Multiwindowed approach to the optimum estimation of the local fractal dimension for natural image segmentation. *International Conference on Image Processing*, 3, 222-226. doi:10.1109/ICIP.1999.817105

Osman, M. K., Mashor, M. Y., & Jaafar, H. (2010). Detection of mycobacterium tuberculosis in Ziehl Neelsen stained tissue images using Zernike moments and hybrid multilayered perceptron network. *Proceedings of IEEE International Conference on Systems Man and Cybernetics*, 4049-4055. doi:10.1109/ICSMC.2010.5642191

Osman, M. K., Mashor, M. Y., & Jaafar, H. (2012). Performance comparison of extreme learning machine algorithms for mycobacterium tuberculosis detection in tissue sections. *Journal of Medical Imaging and Health Informatics*, *2*(3), 307–312. doi:10.1166/jmihi.2012.1100

Palomino, J. C., Leao, S. C., & Ritacco, V. (2007). *Tuberculosis 2007. From basic science to patient care*. Institute of Tropical Medicine.

Panicker, R. O., Soman, B., Saini, G., & Rajan, G. (2016). A Review of Automatic Methods Based on Image Processing Techniques for Tuberculosis Detection from Microscopic Sputum Smear Images. *Journal of Medical Systems, 40*(17), 1-13.

Pantic, I., Dacic, S., Brkic, P., Lavrnja, I., Pantic, S., Jovanovic, T., & Pekovic, S. (2014). Application of fractal and grey level co-occurrence matrix analysis in evaluation of brain corpus callosum and cingulum architecture. *Microscopy and Microanalysis*, *20*(05), 1373–1381. doi:10.1017/S1431927614012811 PMID:24967845

Patil, S. A., & Udupi, V. R. (2011). Geometrical and texture features estimation of lung cancer and TB images using chest X-ray database. *International Journal of Biomedical Engineering and Technology*, *6*(1), 58–75. doi:10.1504/IJBET.2011.040453

Priya, E., Srinivasan, S., & Ramakrishnan, S. (2014). Retrospective Non-Uniform Illumination Correction Techniques in Images of Tuberculosis. *Microscopy and Microanalysis*, *20*(05), 1382–1391. doi:10.1017/S1431927614012896 PMID:25115957

Purwanti, E., & Widiyanti, P. (2012). Using learning vector quantization method for automated identification of mycobacterium tuberculosis. *Indonesian Journal of Tropical and Infectious Disease*, 3(1), 26-29.

Raof, R. A. A., Mashor, M. Y., Ahmad, R. B., & Noor, S. S. M. (2011). *Image Segmentation of Ziehl-Neelsen Sputum Slide Images for Tubercle Bacilli Detection*. INTECH Open Access Publisher.

Ruiz-Manzano, J., Blanquer, R., Calpe, J. L., Caminero, J. A., Caylà, J., Domínguez, J. A., & Vidal, R. et al. (2008). Diagnosis and treatment of tuberculosis. *Archivos de Bronconeumologia*, *44*(10), 551–566. PMID:19006636

Rulaningtyas, R., Suksmono, A. B., Mengko, T. L. R., & Saptawati, P. (2015). Identification of mycobacterium tuberculosis in sputum smear slide using automatic scanning microscope. *AIP Conference Proceedings*, *1656*, 060011. doi:10.1063/1.4917142

Samanta, B., & Nataraj, C. (2009). Application of particle swarm optimization and proximal support vector machines for fault detection. *Swarm Intelligence*, *3*(4), 303–325. doi:10.1007/s11721-009-0028-6

Santiago-Mozos, R., Fernandez-Lorenzana, R., Perez-Cruz, F., & Artes-Rodriguez, A. (2008). On the uncertainty in sequential hypothesis testing. *Proceedings of IEEE International Symposium on Biomedical Imaging: From Nano to Macro*, 1223-1226. doi:10.1109/ISBI.2008.4541223

Saravia, L. A. (2014). mfSBA: Multifractal analysis of spatial patterns in ecological communities. *F1000 Research*, *3*, 14. doi:10.12688/f1000research.3-14.v2 PMID:25324962

Soares, F., Freire, M. M., Pereira, M., Janela, F., & Seabra, J. (2009, August). Towards the detection of microcalcifications on mammograms through multifractal detrended fluctuation analysis. *2009 IEEE Pacific Rim Conference on Communications, Computers and Signal Processing*, 677-681. doi:10.1109/PACRIM.2009.5291288

Sotaquira, M., Rueda, L., & Narvaez, R. (2009). Detection and quantification of bacilli and clusters present in sputum smear samples: a novel algorithm for pulmonary tuberculosis diagnosis. *Proceedings of International Conference on Digital Image Processing*, 117-121. doi:10.1109/ICDIP.2009.59

Steingart, K. R., Henry, M., Ng, V., Hopewell, P. C., Ramsay, A., Cunningham, J., & Pai, M. et al. (2006). Fluorescence versus conventional sputum smear microscopy for tuberculosis: A systematic review. *The Lancet Infectious Diseases*, *6*(9), 570–581. doi:10.1016/S1473-3099(06)70578-3 PMID:16931408

Stojić, T., Reljin, I., & Reljin, B. (2006). Adaptation of multifractal analysis to segmentation of microcalcifications in digital mammograms. *Physica A: Statistical Mechanics and its Applications, 367*, 494-508.

Stosic, T., & Stosic, B. D. (2006). Multifractal analysis of human retinal vessels. *IEEE Transactions on Medical Imaging*, *25*(8), 1101–1107. doi:10.1109/TMI.2006.879316 PMID:16895002

Tadrous, P. J. (2010). Computer-Assisted Screening of Ziehl-Neelsen–Stained Tissue for Mycobacteria. *American Journal of Clinical Pathology*, *133*(6), 849–858. doi:10.1309/AJCPMR3BLVBH8THV PMID:20472842

Takahashi, T., Murata, T., Narita, K., Hamada, T., Kosaka, H., Omori, M., & Wada, Y. et al. (2006). Multifractal analysis of deep white matter microstructural changes on MRI in relation to early-stage atherosclerosis. *NeuroImage*, *32*(3), 1158–1166. doi:10.1016/j.neuroimage.2006.04.218 PMID:16815037

Ţălu, Ş. (2012). Mathematical methods used in monofractal and multifractal analysis for the processing of biological and medical data and images. *ABAH Bioflux*, *4*(1), 1–4.

Tasoulis, S. K., Doukas, C. N., Maglogiannis, I., & Plagianakos, V. P. (2010, August). Classification of apoptosis using advanced clustering techniques on digital microscopic images. *2010 Annual International Conference of the IEEE Engineering in Medicine and Biology*, 5565-5568. doi:10.1109/IEMBS.2010.5626777

Tuberculosis Facts. (2007). Stop TB Partnership, World Health Organization.

Uwimana, E., & Ruiz, M. E. (2008). Integrating an automatic classification method into the medical image retrieval process. *AMIA ... Annual Symposium Proceedings / AMIA Symposium. AMIA Symposium*, *2008*, 747. PMID:18999165

Vapnik, V. (2013). *The nature of statistical learning theory*. Springer Science & Business Media.

Veropoulos, K., Campbell, C., Learmonth, G., Knight, B., & Simpson, J. (1998). The automated identification of tubercle bacilli using image processing and neural computing techniques. In ICANN 98 (pp. 797-802). Springer London. doi:10.1007/978-1-4471-1599-1_123

Wählby, C., Lindblad, J., Vondrus, M., Bengtsson, E., & Björkesten, L. (2002). Algorithms for cytoplasm segmentation of fluorescence labelled cells. *Analytical Cellular Pathology, 24*(2-3), 101-111.

World Health Organization (WHO). (2010). *Tuberculosis Fact Sheet No. 104*. WHO.

Wu, Q., Merchant, F., & Castleman, K. (2010). *Microscope image processing*. Academic Press.

Xu, Y., Huang, S., Ji, H., & Fermuller, C. (2009). Combining powerful local and global statistics for texture description. In *IEEE Conference on* In *Computer Vision and Pattern Recognition*, 573-580.

Xu, Y., Ji, H., & Fermuller, C. (2006). A projective invariant for textures. *IEEE Computer Society Conference on Computer Vision and Pattern Recognition*, *2*, 1932-1939.

Xu, Y., Ji, H., & Fermüller, C. (2009). Viewpoint invariant texture description using fractal analysis. *International Journal of Computer Vision*, *83*(1), 85–100. doi:10.1007/s11263-009-0220-6

Yan, A., Wang, Z., & Cai, Z. (2008). Prediction of human intestinal absorption by GA feature selection and support vector machine regression. *International Journal of Molecular Sciences*, *9*(10), 1961–1976. doi:10.3390/ijms9101961 PMID:19325729

Young, B. L., Mlamla, Z., Gqamana, P. P., Smit, S., Roberts, T., Peter, J., & Blackburn, J. et al. (2014). The identification of tuberculosis biomarkers in human urine samples. *The European Respiratory Journal*, *43*(6), 1719–1729. doi:10.1183/09031936.00175113 PMID:24743962

Zhai, Y., Liu, Y., Zhou, D., & Liu, S. (2010). Automatic identification of mycobacterium tuberculosis from ZN-stained sputum smear: algorithm and system design. *Proceedings of IEEE International Conference on Robotics and Biomimetrics*, 41-46. doi:10.1109/ROBIO.2010.5723300

KEY TERMS AND DEFINITIONS

Hyperplane: A subspace of a vector space having dimension one less than the dimension of the vector space that maximizes the margin between the two classes of data sets.

Kernel Function: A transformation of the input data in the original space that return inner products in the feature space to treat/process it more easily.

Multifractal Analysis: It investigate datasets by describing the degree of regularity and (statistical) distribution from global quantities.

Mycobacterium Tuberculosis: The causative agent of tuberculosis which is a rod-shaped, non-spore forming aerobic bacterium belonging to an acid fast species.

Non-Uniform Illumination: Variation in brightness across an image that mainly lie in the low frequency band due to indecorous microscope optics.

Principal Components Analysis: A procedure for identifying smaller number of uncorrelated variables that account for most of the variance in a set of observed variables.

Pulmonary Tuberculosis: A bacterial contagious disease developed with lung as local foci and characterized by the growth of tubercles especially in the lungs.

Sputum Smear Images: Images captured by a camera of the sputum sample spread and stained on a glass slide for TB treatment monitoring and diagnosis under a microscope.

Support Vectors: Support vectors are the very small subset of training samples that lie closest to the decision surface or boundary that supports it.

Section 3

Virtual Reality and Telemedicine in Patient Care

Different related topics to Biomedical Engineering are covered in this section, which includes virtual reality in rehabilitation and development of wireless control Iontophoretic Drug Delivery System.

Chapter 11
Rehabilitation and Medical Assistant Technique in Virtual Reality

Greeshma Sharma
DRDO, India

ABSTRACT

In the modern world, Virtual Reality (VR) has been accepted by the researcher as a state-of-the-art neuropsychological assessment tool in clinical research. Owing to the two prominent VR attributes i.e. immersivity and interactivity, VR is being used as an assessment tool as well as a training module. Combining cognitive knowledge with existing VR technology can propel VR to achieve a quantum leap in the rehabilitation sector. In addition, it offers potential radical modifications in the traditional way of neuropsychological assessment in the clinical settings, by improving ecological validity of the existing tests. Subsequently, features of VR facilitate customisation of an individual's treatment plan with the informed gradual progression of the challenge. This chapter explains VR as an innovative platform in the sector of medical & others such as military and sports for assessment as well as for training.

INTRODUCTION

Clinical psychologists/cognitive scientists are struggling to keep up with the changing times and the corresponding advancements in technology. The modus operandi followed by a cognitive psychologist is in a dire need for a paradigm shift, involving the re-evaluation of prior trivia and formation of assumptions. For example, in the field of psychology, the changes are observed for mind theory as in mentalist, to behaviourism, and now connectionism frameworks. On the other hand, in the field of psychiatry, understanding of psychiatric disorders and the subsequent investigation in molecular biology paves the way for another "paradigm shift" (Meyer, 1996). Relatively, the growth and transformation of a neuropsychologist with respect to embracing the "paradigm shift" have not been significant. According to Dodrill (1997), clinical neuropsychologists claim to use knowledge of constructs for the paper-pencil tests which were developed a century ago (such as Binet test of Intelligence dated in 1900). This suggests

DOI: 10.4018/978-1-5225-2829-6.ch011

that still psychologists are struggling with the old tested methods that might not be applicable to the present generation. On the contrary, development of other streams such as neuroradiology could have been limited to radioisotope brain scans if they had not maintained pace with the technological development. On the same note, Sternberg (1997) sufficed the evidence presented by Dodrill (1997). He explained that present standardised tests slightly differed from tests that were constructed over a century ago. For example, Wechsler Adult Intelligence Scale (WAIS) has created its modification in versions like paper-pencil tests to computerised tests, but not in its constructs. As a consequence, there is a requirement to change in ideas rather than the introduction of new measures.

There are two major limitations faced by psychologist's apprehensions of using modern day technology (Parsons, 2015). First, present neuropsychological assessment procedures corresponds to technology that has hardly changed since the first scales were developed in the early 1900s. Second, the role of neuropsychologist has changed with the progress of other associated streams such as psychiatry, imaging modality and they are more focused towards more ecologically valid predictions.

These limitations can be overcome by embracing current technology and the solution as provided by Bilder (2011). He suggests the evolution of clinical neuropsychology in three ways. In Neuropsychology 1.0 (1950–1979), dysfunction was diagnosed through localisation and this era was pre neuroimaging. It failed to develop ecologically oriented assessments. In Neuropsychology 2.0 (1980-present), the computer automated neuropsychological assessments were invented. These assessments were more affected by neuroimaging advancements and subsequently rather than focusing on differential diagnosis, it characterised cognitive strengths and weaknesses. However, computerised test battery has some advantages over traditional paper-pencil tests such as increased standardisation of administration and accuracy of timing presentation etc. (Sternberg, 1997). The limitation with the Neuropsychology 1.0 and 2.0 is that, the clinical neuropsychologists are required to provide the normative description of everyday functioning. There is limited generalisation of results in approximating real world function; therefore, there is a need to establish ecological validity in the neuropsychological assessment which focuses on either (or both) verisimilitude and veridicality (Chaytor & Schmitter-Edgecombe, 2003). Verisimilitude signifies that method for the data collection should be similar to the real-life task of open environment whereas Veridicality implies that the test results should reflect and predict real-world phenomena (Chaytor & Schmitter-Edgecombe, 2003; Parsons, 2011a). Major challenges faced by administrating paper -pencil tests is that transferring verisimilitude approach from the lab setting to the applied frameworks of the clinical framework would be difficult (Rabin et al., 2007). Furthermore, by adding instruments resembling everyday activities would not suffice the modernisation of computer technology which is the major drawback of the current neuropsychological testing. Thus, progress in such kind of assessment is slower than expected. Although, present psychologist tests have an adequate predictive value but the traditional tests may not replicate the situation of every day. The aforestated limitations are overcome by Neuropsychological Assessment 3.0 which involves the use of virtual environments.

The virtual environments is an advanced computer interface that permits humans to become immersed within a computer-created simulation. It imbibes the concept of Virtual reality (VR) with key properties of immersivity and interactivity. By adding technical values in the existing systems, VR offers opportunities to build test with the ingenious gadgets. Particularly, VR technology adding to its characteristics includes trackers and head mounted displays (HMDs) for immersion as well as data gloves or joysticks for interaction. Integration of different sensors and high-fidelity devices (like trackers, position and motion sensors etc.) makes the virtual environment visually near realistic, thus enabling it to considerably bridge the gap created by the dogma followed by conservative psychologists. Evolution of VR began with 2D environment Java applet, which was upgraded by usage of python. Later 3D environment with meaningful interaction was introduced powered by advent of software like Unity etc. At the top of the technological pyramid, VR systems are focused towards more real- life like environment using state of the art tools like CRYENGINE, UNREAL game engine etc.

Primarily, VR was used for training simulation such as aircraft pilot and driving simulation, equipment training, but now it is being used in treating phobias and improving post-traumatic stress disorder. Besides treating rehabilitated population, VR has now tremendously used for the cognitive training in the field of military and sports (Parsons et al., 2013). In addition, in the field of cognitive neuroscience and psychology, VR platform provides the possibility of controlling stimulus, replicating real life situations, assessing neurobehavioral responses accurately etc. Contributing towards more ecologically valid assessments, VR provides veridical control and rigor of laboratory estimates with a verisimilitude that demonstrates real life situations (Parsons, 2011b).

Moreover, the astronomical increase in computation power and speed contribute towards accurate assessment of systematic presentation of complex stimuli. Consequently, reduced latency between stimuli onset and presentation makes participants to manipulate three-dimensional objects in a virtual environment as of real environment's operations. Upgrading the role of VR from simulator to management by involving it into various fields is now possible with the present technology. For example, different virtual scenarios combined with the standardised neuropsychological test battery can enhance ecological validity and improve diagnosis and treatment planning. These kinds of scenario have been used in the psychiatry disorder (Parsons & Rizzo, 2008), affective disorder (Parsons & Rizzo, 2008), memory (Parsons et al., 2013), attention (Parsons et al., 2007, 2011), executive function (Parsons et al., 2011) and spatial abilities (Akhutina et al., 2003; Moffat, 2009). Moreover, some of the qualities make VR relevant for the hierarchical task that can be delivered and mixed across a range of difficulty levels (Rizzo et al., 2004). In depth, these qualities promote customisation of an individual's treatment plan with the informed gradual progression of challenge.

VIRTUAL ENVIRONMENT (VE) IN PAEDIATRIC REHABILITATION

Developmental disorders impair child's ability to perform routine chores. Abilities are required for exhibiting typical mental and social skills in particular circumstances. For example, neurocognitive impairments may illicit a child to have diminished personality and behavioural functioning such as faulty self-awareness, illogical reasoning and judgement, impaired theory of mind. Rehabilitation allows a child to perform the functionally-oriented task in a more systematic way which enables care-giver to assess and understand child's brain-behaviour deficits. In a clinical perspective, therapeutic practices assist children who are deficit in brain behaviour's ability and improve performance for daily life activities. VR offers a great benefit for clinical applications due to current advances and progressive cost reduction in both software and hardware tools. It provides freedom for the play that can be amusing, challenging and non-threatening which captures the motivation of children for carrying on the activity. Moreover, it permits children to control their actions and to maintain their desired movements for a certain amount of time. As a consequence, neuroplasticity is observed for the affected limb which is the formation of new synapses in the unused brain regions. In addition, VR also focuses on the 'play' factor which is essential for a child in developing motor and social skills. The studies on VR for paediatric rehabilitation are more focused on the control of posture, visual perceptual skills, arm and hand motor skills, social skills, and pain management (Levin, 2011).

Cerebral Palsy (CP)

It is defined as "a group of permanent disorders of the development of movement and posture, causing diminished activity, which is attributed to non-progressive disturbances that occur in the developing foetal or infant brain. The motor disorders are often accompanied by a disturbance of sensation, perception, cognition, communication, behaviour, epilepsy, and by secondary musculoskeletal problems" (Rosenbaum, 2007). The rate of occurrence of CP per 1000 live births ranges 2-2.8 in India (Gladstone, 2010).

The typical management of the child with CP includes a traditional physiotherapy programme that involves positioning, casting, stretching, strengthening, splinting, and the facilitation of movement (Sharan et al., 2012). Intervention with VR might improve conditions of the child with CP because of involved motivation (Harris & Reid, 2005), cerebral reorganisation (Snider et al., 2010), better motor control (Luna-Oliva et al., 2013), and improved cognitive functions (Akhutina et al., 2003; Reid, 2004). In a related study, an effectiveness of VR was examined on the feeling of self-efficacy, upper-extremity control, postural control, and competence through interactive VR games (Reid, 2002). Findings indicated positive impact of VR that allows the sense of mastery and increase the feeling of self-efficacy. Similarly, VR intervention improves the self-image by introducing playful act (Reid, 2004). Also, it provides a positive environment for strengthening preferences for the choices (Harris & Reid, 2005).

In addition to improve social activities, VR plays an active role to improve cognitive ability such as spatial skills. In a research study, promising results were found in the spatial ability by using the battery of virtual environments such as a virtual maze and clown assembly (Akhutina et al., 2003). These types of improvements are also documented in the imaging study where activity in the unused brain areas for children with CP was observed. For example, activity in contralateral primary sensorimotor cortices (SMCs) was detected during affected elbow movements after providing VR therapy which is important for the task of enhanced motor skills (You et al., 2005). The result supports the evidence of neuroplasticity in the brain regions of the affected body parts. Considering a review paper, Chiu et al (2015) investigated the efficacy of VR intervention in children with CP. Authors reported that experimental group who were exposed to VR intervention such as EyeToy: Play, Gesture Xtreme, custom engineered computer game and Nintendo Wii had 30% improvement with compare to control group who were exposed to no intervention. The outcome suggests that VR intervention can supplement traditional therapy especially for children who are more attracted to the exercise programs. In extension to similar findings, VR was used for improving 'reaching kinematics' (Chen, Garcia-Vergara & Howard, 2015; Chen et al., 2014). VR included games to train children for reaching movements like outwards, upwards towards virtual objects that appeared everywhere on the screen. These games allowed movements, the anticipation of movements, and satisfaction on completing the task. The result showed improvement in the movements of the affected limbs. Similarly, in the other related review study, an efficacy of VR intervention was examined on the brain reorganisation/plasticity, motor capacity, visual-perceptual skills, social participation and personal factors (Snider et al., 2010). Findings of papers indicated that VR has potential benefits for children with CP. However, lacking empirical data and evidence produce hurdle for VR to be a part of systematic clinical settings.

In conclusion, VR as an intervention offers notable improvements in the children with CP. For instance, as suggested by Levac et al. (2012), there are 9 potential active ingredients from VR therapy which could help children with CP to improve their motor skills: (1) practice opportunities, (2) task specificity between the VR and real-world movements, (3) Person-specific flexibility for treatment measures, (4) visual and/or auditory feedback, (5) involvement in play situation equivalent to social play, (6) neuroplasticity changes, (7) problem solving through different virtual contexts, (8) motivation since children can select the games they like or compete with peers (Chen et al., 2015), and (9) role of a support person (a parent or therapist) with verbal backing and assistance.

Pain Distraction

Experimental Pain

A considerable number of researches have shown that experimental pain could be reduced by using VR distraction (Malloy & Milling, 2010). In one reported study, cold pressor pain was reduced by using two VR distraction interventions (Dahlquist et al, 2007). These interventions comprised of interactive VR distraction intervention and passive VR distraction intervention. Former used an adjustable head-mounted display helmet with integrated headphones to play the Sony Play-station 2 Finding Nemo "Jellyfish Race" game while latter used the head-mounted display helmet to see and hear pre-recorded video of another person playing the same game. Total three trials were given to the 40 participants, trial 1(no intervention), trial 2 (Interactive VR intervention), and trial 3 (passive VR intervention). Participants in trial 2 showed highest pain tolerance and threshold while in trial 1 felt lowest pain tolerance and threshold. Findings showed effectiveness of interactive VR because of the underlying active cognitive processing which was encouraged by tactile and kinaesthetic feedback to participants. Similarly, interactive VR intervention can also be used for improving pain tolerance, especially in older children (Dahlquist et al., 2009).

Cancer Pain Reduction

Non-pharmacological interventions (such as VR) have captured the attention of researcher for children submitted to painful and distressing procedures. Generally, interventions are given during implanted venous catheter puncture and apply of topic local anaesthetics before the procedure (Gershon et al., 2004).

Port Access/Venous Puncture (Malloy & Milling, 2010)

A port is an appliance which is surgically implanted under the skin through which drugs can be repeatedly injected and blood samples can be taken. Ports are primarily used to treat cancer patients, delivering chemotherapy agents. Application of port access or venous puncture can be very painful. To reduce such pain, non-immersive VR distraction can be used. For example, in a study, authors (Nilsson et al., 2009 demonstrated) that VR games lower the self-reported pain scores during and after the procedures. The result encourages VR as a positive experiences for the children undergoing venous puncture or a subcutaneous venous port access. Similarly, VR distraction offers advantageous leap over no distraction for youngsters (ages 7–19) undergoing port access (Gershon et al., 2003). In a study, three kinds of interventions, no-distraction control condition, non- VR distraction, and VR distraction, were used for relieving the distress experienced by participants. The VR distraction was Virtual Gorilla, an educational tool for children visiting the gorilla habitat at Zoo Atlanta. This program consisted of the responding behaviour of other gorillas in a virtual gorilla habitat which depends on the participant's action as a Gorilla. Result showed differences on the child, parent, and observers' ratings of pain for VR distraction.

A new term 'VR anaesthesia' has also been used in clinical case studies and randomized control trials (Gold et al., 2005). VR anaesthesia diminishes the risk associated with sedation by minimizing exposure to pharmacological therapy. However, this term is still in infancy. Despite VR limitation, it shows satisfaction and innovation for pain reduction. In summary, children felt less pain during VR distraction condition but differences were non-significant. Those differences can be significant if we can combine analog scale (VAS) and physiological measures during intervention program.

Intravenous Placement

An intravenous (IV) catheter is used to introduce medications or fluids directly into the bloodstream (Malloy & Milling, 2010). It can be painful for children ; therefore, it requires VR distraction for alleviating children's distress during IV placement. In one study, children were randomly assigned to either VR distraction or standard medical care control conditions (Gold et al., 2006). In the VR distraction condition, subjects experienced the Street Luge virtual environment in which they raced downhill laying on top of a big skateboard. Subjects wore a head-mounted display helmet and navigated through the virtual environment using a rumble pad that provided tactile feedback and music through headphones. The result showed significant differences between treatment conditions on parents' beliefs about how much the intervention had lowered their child's pain, while the control group had four times larger pain during IV placement.

Burn Injury

For the reduction of chronic pain in children hospitalized due to excessive burns, VR distraction 'SnowWorld' was used (Hoffman et al., 2008). In SnowWorld, patients ''go into'' an icy, cool 3-dimensional virtual environment. The results showcased lower pain ratings during VR distraction including worst pain, unpleasantness of pain and total time spent thinking about the pain. In another study, augmented reality (computer-generated enhancements atop an existing reality) was used to relieve the pain of children undergoing dressing changes for burn injuries (Mott et al., 2008). Participants were randomly assigned to the augmented reality task or standard medical care control condition (cognitive therapy). The augmented reality intervention featured a 7 in. LCD screen and a camera into which the child inserted plastic figurines. This created a 3-dimensional character called "Hospital Harry" that the child was instructed via audiotape to manipulate (Malloy & Milling, 2010). The standard care condition included the use of distraction, positive reinforcement, relaxation, and an age-appropriate video program. The result showed that the augmented reality intervention had shown analgesic effectiveness when the children were having longer dressing changes (more than 30 minutes).

Autism

Autism is characterised by the absence of typical social and communication behaviours and the presence of stereotyped, repetitive behaviours (American Psychiatric Association, 1994). To address impairments in social interaction, one study used virtual cafe (Mitchell et al., 2007). Here, the subjects executed some specific tasks that a normal individual would go about doing in an actual environment i.e. finding a place to sit, ordering, paying etc. The difficulty in the execution of the activities was gradually increased and then the individuals were evaluated on the basis of the verbal description of their execution and resulting behaviour and decision making, hence paving the way for an effective investigation of generalisation of social learning. In a similar study, 'virtual supermarket' was used to conduct numerous exercises about the physical, functional, and symbolic use of objects. It was found that the performance of children increased after the interventions and one child was able to transfer the acquired skills to the real environment (Herrera et al., 2008). In extension to this, VR was also used for teaching and reinforcing key social skills like eye contact, turn-taking, sharing and jointly directed behaviour (Bauminger et al., 2007). Training was given using StoryTable and MarbleWorks. StoryTable interface was integrated with the Diamond-Touch table (Circle Twelve Inc., Framingham, multitouch Mass., USA), a state-of-the-art multitouch display table, enabling many people to interact with objects on the table-top display screen simultaneously through touch. The ratings were given on the social behaviour from StoryTable and behaviours from MarbleWorks. The results showcased marked improvements in positive social behaviours, quality of plays, and relevant narrative utterances after VR intervention. Not only social skills but emotion recognition and manifestation can also be regulated using VR. In such studies, Collaborative Virtual Environments (CVEs) which maintain multiple simultaneous users were used to explore the ability to identify emotions, manifest emotions, and understand the emotion of others (Moore et al, 2005). In the lab of Biomedical Engineering department of Institute of Nuclear Medicine & Allied Sciences (INMAS), some virtual environment scenarios such as the park, metro station, school etc. (see Figure 1) were created to assess emotion recognition in autistic children with contextual storytelling. The emotion was displayed on the virtual avatar after some dialogue delivery, children's task was to identify whether displayed emotion on the face of avatar was appropriate or inappropriate. The children's response helps them to recognise contextual emotion. Children with autism get assistance in particularly well constructed VR-integrated interventions: firstly, children with autism are acute visual learners and are often easily engaged by computers and television (Iovannone et al., 2003), secondly, some well-established treatments, such as applied behavioural analysis are based on principles of reinforcement.

Thus, VR has the potential to provide treatment for Autistic children and to help caretakers and educators to improve social behaviour among these individuals. Future scope of the VR interventions in Autism would comprise of the investigation for understanding skill transfer from VR to real life setting and percentage of improvements in social ability.

Attention Deficit Hyperactivity Disorder (ADHD)

The primary deficits of ADHD include the presence and frequency of inattentive, impulsive and hyperactive behaviours (American Psychiatric Association, 1994). The virtual classroom is the most popular virtual environment for the management of ADHD people (Adams et al., 2009; Rizzo et al., 2000). The Virtual Classroom (VC) utilises a continuous performance task paradigm (CPT) commonly used in the assessment of ADHD. Participants are instructed to view a series of letters presented continuously on a computer screen. They are asked to respond via a mouse click only after they view the letter "X" preceded by the letter "A." Emphasis is placed on speed and accuracy. Individuals with ADHD have generally been shown to make more omission errors (failing to respond to a target) and commission errors (responding to a non-target) on CPT tests. Omission error indicated the lack of attention while commission errors indicate hyperactivity. In the high distraction task, external interference control is also assessed. Adopting similar paradigm, virtual classroom (VC) is created. In VC, the participant is immersed in the

Figure 1. Virtual Environment, a) Metro Station, and b) Park, for treatment of Autistic children

a.

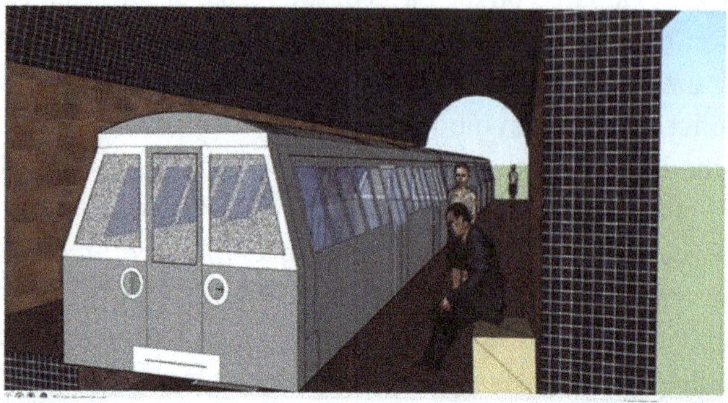

b.

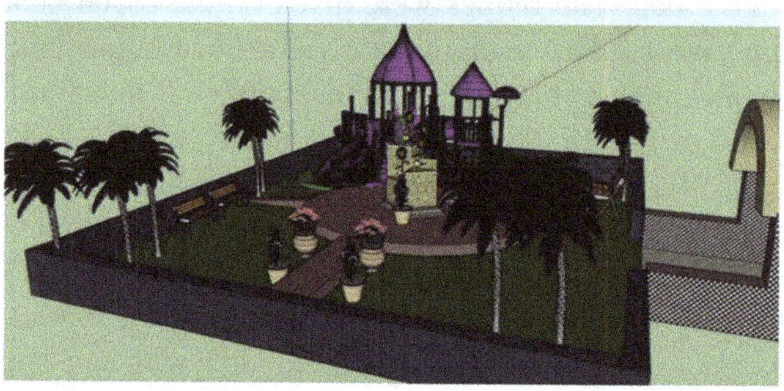

classroom, and seated at a desk near the centre of the classroom with a view of other children, a teacher, and a window, among other things (see Figure 2). After instructions are communicated to participants via computer speakers, the task begins (similarly to CPT). During the task, different auditory and visual distractors are presented in the various areas of the classroom. Audiovisual distractors include a school bus driving by, paper flying, ball rolling, pedestrian movements, children passing notes, a child raising his hand, the teacher answering the classroom door, and the principal entering the room (Parsons, 2015). These distractors are dispersed throughout the left, centre, and middle of the classroom. An important feature of the VC is the ability to mimic the complexity of the real world in a controlled environment. VC can assess attentional abnormalities along with behavioural abnormalities altogether. In one such study, examiners have compared 10 children with ADHD with 10 typically developing children (Adams et al., 2009). They found that children with ADHD were more influenced by distracted stimuli; had more commission and omission errors; showed more overall body movement. Also, VC was found to be significantly correlated with traditional measures and behaviour checklists. The result showed that VC was able to distinguish between ADHD and control groups more than the traditional continuous performance test. Ecologically valid distractors presented in the task led participants with ADHD to have poor performance because they were less competent to cope with the novelty of the situation than those in the control group. Not only on the clinical setting with non-pharmacological assessment, VC seems to be more sensitive to attention deficient than traditional measures combining pharmacological intervention. In one such study, authors investigated the effect of methylphenidate (MPH), a drug used in the treatment of ADHD (Pollack et al., 2010). They found out that MPH reduced omission errors, especially in VC compare with CPT and Test of Variables of Attention (TOVA). Besides medication,

Figure 2. Virtual Classroom displaying letter on blackboard

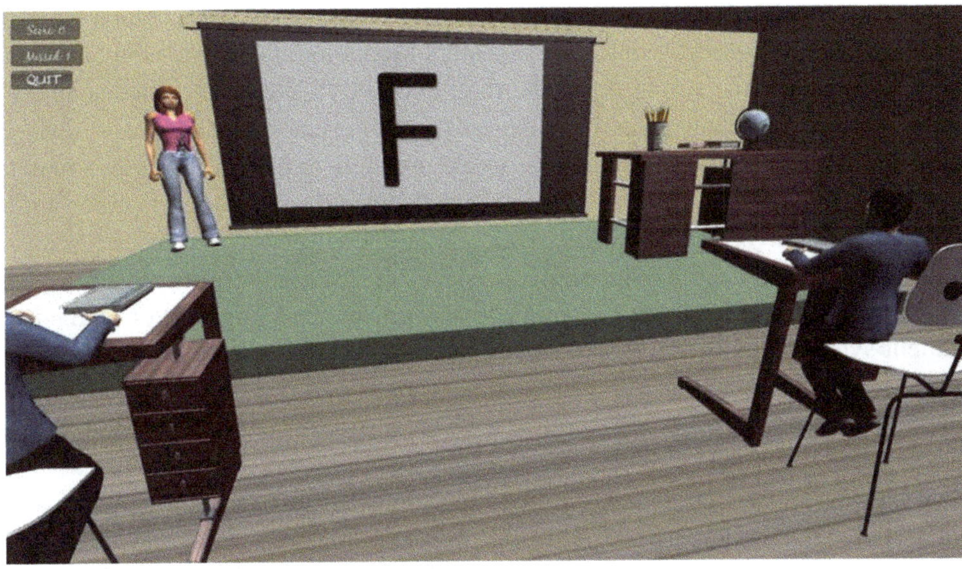

time can also play a big role in the performance of ADHD children. One study identified that for a prolonged time ADHD children's performance was worse than control in VC. This indicates that VC can also become sensitive to the time-bound performance for ADHD management (Bioulac et al., 2012).

In summary, VC has good potential for measuring controlled performance within an ecologically valid environment. In addition, it selects out significant effects under the distraction stimuli which are important to identify the attention deficient children.

VIRTUAL ENVIRONMENT IN ELDER REHABILITATION

The process of ageing is linked with functional deficits in visuospatial abilities, executive functions, episodic memory, attention, and language. In other words, ageing leads to cognitive decline which can be prevented if an appropriate intervention is introduced at the right time. It is important to consider elder population because a better lifestyle and medical facilities have escalated life expectancy which will also increase cognitive impairment in proportion. Cognitive impairment is included in major neurodegenerative disorders such as Dementia, Parkinson, Alzheimer, Executive function loss etc. VR as an intervention can be used in rehabilitation for elder people with the management of cognitive impairments. The VR technology can be widely used to design games which can augment methods of traditional rehabilitation interventions. The VR is available at home which may assist ageing people with and into a disability for training and treatment (Kamieth et al., 2010)." Available at home technology" can provide an opportunity of telerehabilitation for stroke patients (Flores et al., 2008). This technology can improve their lifespan as well as the level of independence. In addition, it enhances patient motivation and appraises recovery progress for improving rehabilitation in proprioception (Cho et al., 2010). Further use of VR involves 'virtual avatar' who can serve as simulated doctors or healthcare workers for establishing communication for bedside soft-skills training (Cabrera-Umpierrez et al., 2006).

In such a study, to improve navigation in elder drivers, an approach of augmented reality was used. Instead, to display information through GPS navigation system which increases cognitive load, navigation information can be projected directly onto the windshield that would remove switching time between looking at the road and the navigation system (Kim & Dey, 2009). This can reduce spatial recognition problems and improve ability to understand context sensitive information. In another study, for the usage of VR interfaces, VR was used to improve access to elder people to navigate complex real scenes (Pittarello & De Faveri, 2006). These interfaces provided assistance for object descriptions and navigation on the basis of user's cognitive deficiencies.

A major brain disease, Dementia, which affects more than 100 million people per year in India, is one of the largest problems in the world. Memory loss is one of the symptoms of Dementia. Memory loss is a prevalent symptom of ageing which can either be delayed or treated using VR technology. In one study, authors provided new methods for the treatment of memory deficits in elderly individuals (Optale et al., 2010). In this, VR memory training (VRMT), auditory stimulation and VR experiences in path-finding were used on the elder subjects. The subjects who were impaired on the Verbal Story Recall Test had six months training on VRMT. The result showed improvement in memory function by increasing focused attention.

In addition, People with dementia face the high rate of forgetting as well as difficulties in storing new information; therefore, it becomes important to address problems of immediate and delayed retention. To train elder population suffering from dementia, one such study used virtual environment 'MULTITASK ' (Schreiber, 1999). In the immediate retention mode, all the targets were provided in the instructions, and participants had to seek them immediately (e.g. "Please find the chair, the cupboard, and the TV"). In the delayed retention mode, the instruction was to memorise the preceding task and to try it again. The preceding task was always a correctly solved immediate task. Therefore, participants worked again on a problem which had already been solved in the delayed task. Effect of training was evaluated using neuropsychological assessment which showed improvement in retention of meaningful visual-figurative and topographic material. Furthermore, subjects were able to transfer learned skills to real-life settings.

The efficient ways to sustain memory functions in elder population, various memory techniques such as retrieval strategies, space retrieval can be incorporated in VR for successful interventions. For example, a study explored the clinical utility of a memory training programme delivered in either a VR or a therapist-led mode for older adults with Mild Cognitive Impairments (MCI) (Man et al., 2012). Result found that subjects who had used VR intervention had better encoding functioning of episodic information while Non-VR group showed significantly better contentment in the subjective appraisal of memory functioning. Memory impairment due to Acquired Brain Injury (ABI) can cause significant disability in the daily life of elders. VR training can help in alleviating memory impairment, but the volume of such studies are less in number. Not only memory impairment but improvements in executive function can easily be accomplished using VR intervention in elder population (Kizony et al., 2012). One such VR intervention, Virtual Action Planning – Supermarket (VAP-S) which was a fully textured, medium-sized supermarket, used on the participants with non-amnesic or multi-domain amnesic (mixed) MCI. Participants entered into the supermarket, a list of items appeared in front of them and the user was asked to shop for those items (see Figure 3). The result showed improvement in the scoring of Multiple Errands Test - Simplified Version (MET-SV) test; henceforth, this study indicates the potential of using the VAP-S as an intervention tool for training Executive Function in people with MCI.

VR has been proven to be a useful and innovative technique for Alzheimer patients in improving cognitive functioning and instrumental activities of daily living (IADL) (Jekel et al., 2015). For example, in one study virtual kitchen was used for the assessment of IADL in Alzheimer patient, which was correlated with the non-immersive virtual coffee task (NI-VCT) and caregiver-reported IADL functioning. VR technique can additionally provide a clue for the onset of Alzheimer disease in the patient of MCI. For instance, virtual reality day-out task (VR-DOT) was used to estimate predictive value in patients with mild cognitive impairment (MCI) (Tarnanas et al., 2014).

In summary, VR technique can be used for assessment, diagnosis, and training in Alzheimer patient for IADL, memory, attention, navigation, and orientation that altogether changing or improving the life of the patient.

VIRTUAL ENVIRONMENT IN MILITARY

For the military psychologist, it becomes challenging to recognise the ability of a military personnel to "return to active duty". This kind of judgments is required for the soldiers who have suffered from post-traumatic stress disorder (PTSD), blast injuries, and Traumatic brain injury (TBI). Current "Return-to-Duty" assessments are based upon guidelines and Automated Neuropsychological Assessment Metrics (ANAM) that have its own limitations such as patient's specific difficulty levels, addressing everyday activities etc.This raised the questions on the decision related to resuming activities. The solution lies in merging adaptive assessment for distinct patient's profile and improving ecological validity of assessment and treatment modules using the progression of technology. The similar solution was adopted by Parsons

Figure 3. Virtual Mall, a) displaying shopping list to remember, b) purchasing items from the memorised list

a.

b.

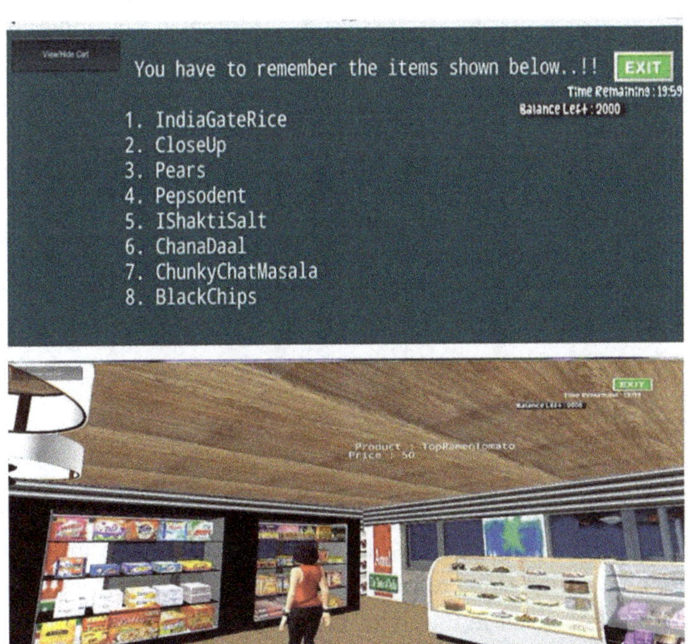

et al. (2008, 2009, 2012; Parsons & Reinebold, 2012; Parsons & Rizzo, 2008) by developing comprehensive, standardised, norm-based virtual reality cognitive performance assessment test (VRCPAT) battery. It utilises the ecologically valid environment to measure neurocognitive components such as attention, memory, reasoning abilities etc. VR environment has a simulation of a city environment, resembling the Iraqi and Afghani city, and participants perform task embedded in the environment with the complete 360-degree view using head-mounted display (HMD). During immersion in the VRCPAT, participants are seated at a desk and have a complete 360-degree view of the city environment. Application of VR-CPAT in context to military has been explained by Parson et al (Parsons & Reinebold, 2012) relative to a user's neurocognitive processing: 1) information load via the intensity and complexity of target stimuli; 2) temporal constraints during varied sustained assessment conditions; 3) distracting activities during the neurocognitive assessments; 4) sensory modality of the information presentation that needs to be attended to; 5) presentation of aversive stimuli for stressed performance evaluations; and 6) the development of a Normative Database whereby neuropsychological performance could be assessed under known conditions supported by normative standards. For example, in the VRCPAT Memory Module, participants toured to 5 zones for identifying 10 targets in a virtual city. Psychometric scores were computed for acquisition phase and retrieval phased, termed as learning score and memory score respectively (Parsons & Rizzo, 2008). In convergent validity measures, authors used Hopkins Verbal Learning Test – Revised (HVLT) and the Brief Visuospatial Memory Test – Revised (BVMT). Discriminant validity measures included Digit Span (Forward and Backward), Digit Symbol Coding, Trail Making Test Part A & Test Part B, Controlled Oral Word Association Test (FAS and Animals), and Stroop Color & Word Test. The result showed that the VRCPAT Memory Module correlated significantly with the HVLT and BVMT while no correlation with the measures of Discriminant validity.

Similarly for VRCPAT attentional module, "HUMVEE Attention Task" scenario was used in which four digit number was displayed on the virtual shield (Parsons et al., 2009). The position of number appearance determined stimulus "complexity" while "safe" (low intensity) and "ambush" (high intensity) settings determined stimulus "intensity". The result indicated dropping in the performance under high complexity and intensity. Aforementioned VRCPAT studies were conducted on the healthy adult. To certify VRCPAT on the military convoy, Virtual Reality Stroop Task (VRST) was used with simulated combat threats. Four conditions, word reading, colour naming, interference, and a complex interference, in a VRST, were presented on the windshield of virtual military Humvee which was automatically driven down a desert road in Iraq. The result showed convergent and discriminant validity of the VRST on the military cohort.

In summary, VR can become the potential tool for cognitive assessment and training for military personnel because it is cost-effective compared to field training, tasks can be reproduced, trials are reviewable and analyzable, and it permits administration over the simulation (Smith & Steel, 2001).

VIRTUAL ENVIRONMENT IN SPORTS

For a sports person, cognitive training is equally important as physical training. Sometimes, peer pressure, victory ratio, anxiety, and other factors lead worst performance in a game. The cause is centred in the mind where cognitive thoughts are processed; therefore, it reduces the capability of an athlete to focus on the relevant information in the game (Oudejans & Nieuwenhuys, 2009). This indicates the importance to inculcate VR intervention with cognitive training to a sports person for a particular sport. VR serves as an efficient platform for developing an athlete specific mental training module which can assist in getting them acclimatised to different situations which they may encounter and hence improve their tactical adroitness, mental acuity and strategy formulation, all in an optimal time frame. In addition, it can aid decision related to 'return to play' after the sports injury. To simulate a virtual environment closely resembling a real environment, large crowds manipulated with either positive boosting or negative hooting could be introduced for generating anxiety. Anxiety generation is induced in the Virtual Environment by audio streaming boosting and hooting voices among simulated crowds henceforth closely resembling a real environment. This enables the coaches/instructors to manipulate the different variables associated with the virtual environment in accordance with the requirements of the player.

In one study, VR goalkeeper system simulated a soccer environment in which participants had to defend penalty kicks (Stinson, 2013). Simultaneously, participants were tracked with physiological measures such as heart rate (HR), heart rate variability (HRV), and were rated on the presence questionnaires and user rankings. The results showed no significant differences in the observed variables i.e. the field of regard (FOR), simulation fidelity (SF), and competitive realism (individual versus pair conditions), but the participants gave some constructive feedbacks during their respective interviews. They suggested more refinement in VR goalkeeper system such as more ecological valid simulation, as the number of provided attempts were not enough to raise their anxiety. However, physiological data showed promising results, the high FOR/high SF conditions were the only conditions to elicit a visible spike in the HRV data. Positive outcome might indicate both FOR and SF were influential in activating anxiety in participants. The result also showcased that the level of anxiety had an inadvertent effect on performance. In addition, it showed significance of using physiological measures along with VR intervention to record the improvement in the performance.

VR AND BRAIN COMPUTER INTERFACE (BCI) IN NEURO-REHABILITATION

The interaction between systems and humans have seemingly increased with the evolution of civilisation. This interaction has gradually led to the design and development of Brain-Computer Interface (BCI), hence enabling the user to directly communicate with the system through brain waves. EMOTIV-EPOC Electroencephalography (EEG) system is arguably the best brain-computer interface system till date; offering an easy real-time assessment of cognitive traits and subsequent feedback to the system (Chandra et al., 2015, 2016, 2017). The primary use of BCI was thought with the biomedical application, but recent progress in the technology of VR prompts both, VR & BCI, to generate miracle for rehabilitated as well as healthy population. For example, patients like amputees and stroke victims with diminished motor-sensory skills can control modern devices such as prosthetic limbs or powered robotic exoskeletons using VR based BCI applications (Contreras-Vidal et al., 2012).

To assess the behaviour of drivers using BCI, VR technology was used to create an environment for testing the drivers (Jingkun et al., 2010). VR includes a combination of audio-visual information with a generic task. The result showed that the VR environment was very effective in the assessment of output with imagined movements. Authors also indicated that it could be very useful if the subjects were taken from the pool of disabled people.

In another study, BCI was used to fly a helicopter in 3D space (Royer et al., 2010). In this task, imagined movement by subject initiated action in the helicopter which was flying action in the virtual environment. This technique is incredibly useful for video game industry, where rather than using any peripheral device subject can take advantage of his/her own brain signals to control virtual objects.

DISCUSSION

It is imperative to embrace progression of technology in the field of neuropsychology; therefore, the significance of virtual reality has been recognised as the potential tool for intervention. Virtual reality offers several advantages over the traditional methods of cognitive assessment and training including improvement in ecological validity i.e. verisimilitude and veridicality, repetitive measures, control of administrators on the variables. VR is successfully implemented in the rehabilitation of children and elder population with various clinical disorder, as well as, for the training of military personnel and sports person. Numerous research demonstrate that VR-based assessment/training drastically improves the accuracy of the prediction generated by traditional test battery. Relatively low-cost and user-friendly application bridges the gap between the technology and the method of neuropsychological assessment. Amalgamation of these kinds are possible by virtual reality which improve the external validity and reliability of the designed test. Although, several limitations exist with the available studies of VR intervention such as lack of properly controlled study, small sample size etc, but it still has a huge impact on the methods of treatment for ameliorating the condition of rehabilitated population. Aiding with subjective scale and interview, VR results can be improved along with the involvement of physiological measurements. In military psychology, it can assist decision-making about resuming activity through assessment of cognitive processing like attention, memory, executive function. However, it is still in the preliminary stage with less number of available data on military cohort, but it offers innovative and interactive method for assessing cognitive processing. Usually, traditional methods lack creativity because of repetitive monotonous activity that can be neutralised by using VR. On the other hand, in sports, VR is used to improve performance of an athlete under stressful situation. VR serves as an efficient platform for developing an athlete specific mental training module which can assist in getting them acclimatised to different situations which they may encounter and hence improve their tactical adroitness, mental acuity and strategy formulation, all in an optimal time frame. Ultimately, sports person will be trained for developing tolerance on anxiety, team pressure, public noise etc. which can be incorporated as a cognitive training just like physical training for building an endurance in the muscle. In future, assessment of cognitive and affective skills could be possible in more ecologically valid situation through VR. In addition, VR can be used to create customised training module which can be individual specific and targeted towards more specific population.

REFERENCES

Adams, R., Finn, P., Moes, E., Flannery, K., & Rizzo, A. S. (2009). Distractibility in attention/deficit/hyperactivity disorder (ADHD): The virtual reality classroom. *Child Neuropsychology*, *15*(2), 120–135. doi:10.1080/09297040802169077 PMID:18608217

Akhutina, T. Y., Foreman, N., Krichevets, A., Matikka, L., Narhi, V., Pylaeva, N., & Vahakuopus, J. (2003). Improving spatial functioning in children with cerebral palsy using computerized and traditional game tasks. *Disability and Rehabilitation*, *25*(24), 1361–1371. doi:10.1080/09638280310001616358 PMID:14660204

American Psychiatric Association. (1994). *Diagnostic and statistical manual of mental disorders (DSM)*. Washington, DC: American Psychiatric Association.

Bauminger, N., Goren-Bar, D., Gal, E., Weiss, P. L., Yifat, R., Kupersmitt, J., . . . Zancanaro, M. (2007, October). Enhancing social communication in high-functioning children with autism through a co-located interface. In *Multimedia Signal Processing, 2007. MMSP 2007. IEEE 9th Workshop on* (pp. 18-21). IEEE. doi:10.1109/MMSP.2007.4412808

Bilder, R. M. (2011). Neuropsychology 3.0: Evidence-based science and practice. *Journal of the International Neuropsychological Society*, *17*(01), 7–13. doi:10.1017/S1355617710001396 PMID:21092355

Bioulac, S., Lallemand, S., Rizzo, A., Philip, P., Fabrigoule, C., & Bouvard, M. P. (2012). Impact of time on task on ADHD patient's performances in a virtual classroom. *European Journal of Paediatric Neurology, 16*(5), 514-521.

Cabrera-Umpierrez, M. F., Ramirez, C. M., Sevillano, A., Arredondo, M. T., & DeSmedt, A. (2006, May). Medical educational e-Platform through virtual reality technologies. In MELECON 2006-2006 IEEE Mediterranean Electrotechnical Conference (pp. 453-456). IEEE. doi:10.1109/MELCON.2006.1653136

Chandra, S., Sharma, G., Mittal, A. P., & Jha, D. (2016). Effect of Sudarshan Kriya (meditation) on gamma, alpha, and theta rhythm during working memory task. *International Journal of Yoga*, *9*(1), 72.

Chandra, S., Sharma, G., Sharma, M., Jha, D., & Mittal, A. P. (2017). Workload regulation by Sudarshan Kriya: an EEG and ECG perspective. *Brain Informatics*, 1-13.

Chandra, S., Verma, K. L., Sharma, G., Mittal, A., & Jha, D. (2015). EEG based cognitive workload classification during NASA MATB-II multitasking. *International Journal of Cognitive Research in Science English Education*, *3*(1), 35–41.

Chaytor, N., & Schmitter-Edgecombe, M. (2003). The ecological validity of neuropsychological tests: A review of the literature on everyday cognitive skills. *Neuropsychology Review*, *13*(4), 181–197. doi:10.1023/B:NERV.0000009483.91468.fb PMID:15000225

Chen, Y., Garcia-Vergara, S., & Howard, A. M. (2015). Effect of a home-based virtual reality intervention for children with cerebral palsy using super pop vr evaluation metrics: A feasibility study. *Rehabilitation Research and Practice*. PMID:26457202

Chen, Y. P., Caldwell, M., Dickerhoof, E., Hall, A., Odakura, B., Morelli, K., & Fanchiang, H. C. (2014). Game analysis, validation, and potential application of EyeToy play and play 2 to upper-extremity rehabilitation. *Rehabilitation Research and Practice*. PMID:25610652

Chiu, H. C., & Kuo, P. W. (2015). Effects of Virtual Reality in Children with Cerebral Palsy: A Systematic Review. *物理治療*, *40*(3), 136-144.

Cho, S. W., Ku, J. H., Kang, Y. J., Lee, K. H., Song, J. Y., Kim, H. J., . . . Kim, S. I. (2010). A Pilot Study for Development of Shoulder Proprioception Training System Using Virtual Reality for Patients with Stroke: The Effect of Manipulated Visual Feedback. In *XII Mediterranean Conference on Medical and Biological Engineering and Computing 2010* (pp. 722-724). Springer Berlin Heidelberg. doi:10.1007/978-3-642-13039-7_182

Contreras-Vidal, J. L., Presacco, A., Agashe, H., & Paek, A. (2012). Restoration of whole body movement: toward a noninvasive brain-machine interface system. *IEEE Pulse, 3*(1), 34-37.

Dahlquist, L. M., McKenna, K. D., Jones, K. K., Dillinger, L., Weiss, K. E., & Ackerman, C. S. (2007). Active and passive distraction using a head-mounted display helmet: Effects on cold pressor pain in children. *Health Psychology, 26*(6), 794–801. doi:10.1037/0278-6133.26.6.794 PMID:18020853

Dahlquist, L. M., Weiss, K. E., Clendaniel, L. D., Law, E. F., Ackerman, C. S., & McKenna, K. D. (2009). Effects of videogame distraction using a virtual reality type head-mounted display helmet on cold pressor pain in children. *Journal of Pediatric Psychology, 34*(5), 574–584. doi:10.1093/jpepsy/jsn023 PMID:18367495

Dodrill, C. B. (1997). Myths of neuropsychology. *The Clinical Neuropsychologist, 11*(1), 1–17. doi:10.1080/13854049708407025 PMID:10806469

Flores, E., Tobon, G., Cavallaro, E., Cavallaro, F. I., Perry, J. C., & Keller, T. (2008, December). Improving patient motivation in game development for motor deficit rehabilitation. In *Proceedings of the 2008 International Conference on Advances in Computer Entertainment Technology* (pp. 381-384). ACM. doi:10.1145/1501750.1501839

Gershon, J., Zimand, E., Lemos, R., Rothbaum, B. O., & Hodges, L. (2003). Use of virtual reality as a distractor for painful procedures in a patient with pediatric cancer: A case study. *Cyberpsychology & Behavior, 6*(6), 657–661. doi:10.1089/109493103322725450 PMID:14756933

Gershon, J., Zimand, E., Pickering, M., Rothbaum, B. O., & Hodges, L. (2004). A pilot and feasibility study of virtual reality as a distraction for children with cancer. *Journal of the American Academy of Child and Adolescent Psychiatry, 43*(10), 1243–1249. doi:10.1097/01.chi.0000135621.23145.05 PMID:15381891

Gladstone, M. (2010). A review of the incidence and prevalence, types and aetiology of childhood cerebral palsy in resource-poor settings. *Annals of Tropical Paediatrics, 30*(3), 181–196. doi:10.1179/146532810X12786388978481 PMID:20828451

Gold, J. I., Kant, A. J., & Kim, S. H. (2005, December). Virtual anesthesia: the use of virtual reality for pain distraction during acute medical interventions. In Seminars in Anesthesia, Perioperative Medicine and Pain (Vol. 24, No. 4, pp. 203-210). WB Saunders. doi:10.1053/j.sane.2005.10.005

Gold, J. I., Kim, S. H., Kant, A. J., Joseph, M. H., & Rizzo, A. S. (2006). Effectiveness of virtual reality for pediatric pain distraction during IV placement. *Cyberpsychology & Behavior, 9*(2), 207–212. doi:10.1089/cpb.2006.9.207 PMID:16640481

Harris, K., & Reid, D. (2005). The influence of virtual reality play on childrens motivation. *Canadian Journal of Occupational Therapy, 72*(1), 21–29. doi:10.1177/000841740507200107 PMID:15727045

Harris, K., & Reid, D. (2005). The influence of virtual reality play on childrens motivation. *Canadian Journal of Occupational Therapy*, *72*(1), 21–29. doi:10.1177/000841740507200107 PMID:15727045

Herrera, G., Alcantud, F., Jordan, R., Blanquer, A., Labajo, G., & De Pablo, C. (2008). Development of symbolic play through the use of virtual reality tools in children with autistic spectrum disorders Two case studies. *Autism*, *12*(2), 143–157. doi:10.1177/1362361307086657 PMID:18308764

Hoffman, H. G., Patterson, D. R., Seibel, E., Soltani, M., Jewett-Leahy, L., & Sharar, S. R. (2008). Virtual reality pain control during burn wound debridement in the hydrotank. *The Clinical Journal of Pain*, *24*(4), 299–304. doi:10.1097/AJP.0b013e318164d2cc PMID:18427228

Iovannone, R., Dunlap, G., Huber, H., & Kincaid, D. (2003). Effective educational practices for students with autism spectrum disorders. *Focus on Autism and Other Developmental Disabilities*, *18*(3), 150–165. doi:10.1177/10883576030180030301

Jekel, K., Damian, M., Wattmo, C., Hausner, L., Bullock, R., Connelly, P. J., & Kramberger, M. G. et al. (2015). Mild cognitive impairment and deficits in instrumental activities of daily living: A systematic review. *Alzheimers Research & Therapy*, *7*(1), 1. doi:10.1186/s13195-015-0099-0 PMID:25815063

Jingkun, L., Guizhi, X., Jianrong, G., Feng, Z., & Xiuyan, F. (2010, May). Analysis of virtual simulation environment for driving behavior based on imaging movements. In *Networking and Digital Society (ICNDS), 2010 2nd International Conference on* (Vol. 1, pp. 246-248). IEEE. doi:10.1109/ICNDS.2010.5479148

Kamieth, F., Arca, A., Villalar, J. L., Arredondo, M. T., Dähne, P., Wichert, R., & Jimenez-Mixco, V. (2010). *Exploring the Potential of Virtual Reality for the Elderly and People with Disabilities*. INTECH Open Access Publisher.

Kim, S., & Dey, A. K. (2009, April). Simulated augmented reality windshield display as a cognitive mapping aid for elder driver navigation. In *Proceedings of the SIGCHI Conference on Human Factors in Computing Systems* (pp. 133-142). ACM. doi:10.1145/1518701.1518724

Kizony, R., Korman, M., Sinoff, G., Klinger, E., Josman, N., Sharky, P. M., & Klinger, E. (2012). Using a virtual supermarket as a tool for training executive functions in people with mild cognitive impairment. *Proceedings of the 9th International Conference on Disability, Virtual Reality and Associated Technologies*, 41-46.

Levac, D., Rivard, L., & Missiuna, C. (2012). Defining the active ingredients of interactive computer play interventions for children with neuromotor impairments: A scoping review. *Research in Developmental Disabilities*, *33*(1), 214–223. doi:10.1016/j.ridd.2011.09.007 PMID:22093667

Levin, M.F. (2011). *Virtual reality: Rehabilitation applications in children with disabilities*. Academic Press.

Luna-Oliva, L., Ortiz-Gutiérrez, R. M., Cano-de la Cuerda, R., Piédrola, R. M., Alguacil-Diego, I. M., Sánchez-Camarero, C., & Martínez Culebras, M. D. C. (2013). Kinect Xbox 360 as a therapeutic modality for children with cerebral palsy in a school environment: A preliminary study. *NeuroRehabilitation*, *33*(4), 513–521. PMID:24018364

Malloy, K. M., & Milling, L. S. (2010). The effectiveness of virtual reality distraction for pain reduction: A systematic review. *Clinical Psychology Review*, *30*(8), 1011–1018. doi:10.1016/j.cpr.2010.07.001 PMID:20691523

Man, D. W., Chung, J. C., & Lee, G. Y. (2012). Evaluation of a virtual reality-based memory training programme for Hong Kong Chinese older adults with questionable dementia: A pilot study. *International Journal of Geriatric Psychiatry*, *27*(5), 513–520. doi:10.1002/gps.2746 PMID:21681818

Meyer, R. E. (1996). Neuropsychopharmacology: Are we ready for a paradigm shift? *Neuropsychopharmacology*, *14*(3), 169–179. doi:10.1016/0893-133X(95)00074-N PMID:8866700

Mitchell, P., Parsons, S., & Leonard, A. (2007). Using virtual environments for teaching social understanding to 6 adolescents with autistic spectrum disorders. *Journal of Autism and Developmental Disorders*, *37*(3), 589–600. doi:10.1007/s10803-006-0189-8 PMID:16900403

Moffat, S. D. (2009). Aging and spatial navigation: What do we know and where do we go? *Neuropsychology Review*, *19*(4), 478–489. doi:10.1007/s11065-009-9120-3 PMID:19936933

Moore, D., Cheng, Y., McGrath, P., & Powell, N. J. (2005). Collaborative virtual environment technology for people with autism. *Focus on Autism and Other Developmental Disabilities*, *20*(4), 231–243. doi:10.1177/10883576050200040501

Mott, J., Bucolo, S., Cuttle, L., Mill, J., Hilder, M., Miller, K., & Kimble, R. M. (2008). The efficacy of an augmented virtual reality system to alleviate pain in children undergoing burns dressing changes: A randomised controlled trial. *Burns*, *34*(6), 803–808. doi:10.1016/j.burns.2007.10.010 PMID:18325675

Nilsson, S., Finnström, B., Kokinsky, E., & Enskär, K. (2009). The use of Virtual Reality for needle-related procedural pain and distress in children and adolescents in a paediatric oncology unit. *European Journal of Oncology Nursing*, *13*(2), 102–109. doi:10.1016/j.ejon.2009.01.003 PMID:19230769

Optale, G., Urgesi, C., Busato, V., Marin, S., Piron, L., Priftis, K., & Bordin, A. et al. (2010). Controlling memory impairment in elderly adults using virtual reality memory training: A randomized controlled pilot study. *Neurorehabilitation and Neural Repair*, *24*(4), 348–357. doi:10.1177/1545968309353328 PMID:19934445

Oudejans, R. R., & Nieuwenhuys, A. (2009). Perceiving and moving in sports and other high-pressure contexts. *Progress in Brain Research*, *174*, 35–48. doi:10.1016/S0079-6123(09)01304-1 PMID:19477328

Parsons, T. D. (2011a). Neuropsychological assessment using virtual environments: enhanced assessment technology for improved ecological validity. In Advanced Computational Intelligence Paradigms in Healthcare 6. Virtual Reality in Psychotherapy, Rehabilitation, and Assessment (pp. 271-289). Springer Berlin Heidelberg. doi:10.1007/978-3-642-17824-5_13

Parsons, T. D. (2011b). Neuropsychological assessment using virtual environments: enhanced assessment technology for improved ecological validity. In *Advanced computational intelligence paradigms in healthcare 6. Virtual reality in psychotherapy, rehabilitation, and assessment* (pp. 271–289). Springer Berlin Heidelberg. doi:10.1007/978-3-642-17824-5_13

Parsons, T. D. (2015). Ecological validity in virtual reality-based neuropsychological assessment. *Information Science and Technology,*, 214-223.

Parsons, T. D., Bowerly, T., Buckwalter, J. G., & Rizzo, A. A. (2007). A controlled clinical comparison of attention performance in children with ADHD in a virtual reality classroom compared to standard neuropsychological methods. *Child Neuropsychology*, *13*(4), 363–381. doi:10.1080/13825580600943473 PMID:17564852

Parsons, T. D., Courtney, C. G., Arizmendi, B. J., & Dawson, M. E. (2011, February). *Virtual Reality Stroop Task for neurocognitive assessment*. MMVR.

Parsons, T. D., Courtney, C. G., Dawson, M. E., Rizzo, A. A., & Arizmendi, B. J. (2013, July). Visuospatial processing and learning effects in virtual reality based mental rotation and navigational tasks. In *International Conference on Engineering Psychology and Cognitive Ergonomics* (pp. 75-83). Springer Berlin Heidelberg. doi:10.1007/978-3-642-39360-0_9

Parsons, T. D., Iyer, A., Cosand, L., Courtney, C., & Rizzo, A. A. (2009). Neurocognitive and psychophysiological analysis of human performance within virtual reality environments. *Studies in Health Technology and Informatics*, *142*, 247–252. PMID:19377160

Parsons, T. D., McPherson, S., & Interrante, V. (2013, March). Enhancing neurocognitive assessment using immersive virtual reality. In *Virtual and Augmented Assistive Technology (VAAT), 2013 1st Workshop on* (pp. 27-34). IEEE. doi:10.1109/VAAT.2013.6786190

Parsons, T. D., & Reinebold, J. L. (2012). Adaptive virtual environments for neuropsychological assessment in serious games. *IEEE Transactions on Consumer Electronics*, *58*(2), 197–204. doi:10.1109/TCE.2012.6227413

Parsons, T. D., & Rizzo, A. A. (2008). Affective outcomes of virtual reality exposure therapy for anxiety and specific phobias: A meta-analysis. *Journal of Behavior Therapy and Experimental Psychiatry*, *39*(3), 250–261. doi:10.1016/j.jbtep.2007.07.007 PMID:17720136

Parsons, T. D., & Rizzo, A. A. (2008). Initial validation of a virtual environment for assessment of memory functioning: Virtual reality cognitive performance assessment test. *Cyberpsychology & Behavior*, *11*(1), 17–25. doi:10.1089/cpb.2007.9934 PMID:18275308

Pittarello, F., & De Faveri, A. (2006, May). Improving access of elderly people to real environments: a semantic based approach. In *Proceedings of the working conference on Advanced visual interfaces* (pp. 364-368). ACM. doi:10.1145/1133265.1133341

Pollak, Y., Shomaly, H. B., Weiss, P. L., Rizzo, A. A., & Gross-Tsur, V. (2010). Methylphenidate effect in children with ADHD can be measured by an ecologically valid continuous performance test embedded in virtual reality. *CNS Spectrums*, *15*(02), 125–130. doi:10.1017/S109285290002736X PMID:20414157

Rabin, L. A., Burton, L. A., & Barr, W. B. (2007). Utilization rates of ecologically oriented instruments among clinical neuropsychologists. *The Clinical Neuropsychologist*, *21*(5), 727–743. doi:10.1080/13854040600888776 PMID:17676540

Reid, D. (2004). The influence of virtual reality on playfulness in children with cerebral palsy: A pilot study. *Occupational Therapy International*, *11*(3), 131–144. doi:10.1002/oti.202 PMID:15297894

Reid, D. T. (2002). Benefits of a virtual play rehabilitation environment for children with cerebral palsy on perceptions of self-efficacy: A pilot study. *Pediatric Rehabilitation*, *5*(3), 141–148. doi:10.1080/1363849021000039344 PMID:12581476

Rizzo, A. A., Buckwalter, J. G., Bowerly, T., Van Der Zaag, C., Humphrey, L., Neumann, U., & Sisemore, D. et al. (2000). The virtual classroom: A virtual reality environment for the assessment and rehabilitation of attention deficits. *Cyberpsychology & Behavior*, *3*(3), 483–499. doi:10.1089/10949310050078940

Rizzo, A. A., Schultheis, M., Kerns, K. A., & Mateer, C. (2004). Analysis of assets for virtual reality applications in neuropsychology. *Neuropsychological Rehabilitation*, *14*(1-2), 207–239. doi:10.1080/09602010343000183

Rosenbaum, P., Paneth, N., Leviton, A., Goldstein, M., Bax, M., Damiano, D., & Jacobsson, B. et al. (2007). A report: The definition and classification of cerebral palsy April 2006. *Developmental Medicine and Child Neurology. Supplement*, *109*(suppl 109), 8–14. PMID:17370477

Royer, A. S., Doud, A. J., Rose, M. L., & He, B. (2010). EEG control of a virtual helicopter in 3-dimensional space using intelligent control strategies. *IEEE Transactions on Neural Systems and Rehabilitation Engineering*, *18*(6), 581–589. doi:10.1109/TNSRE.2010.2077654 PMID:20876032

Schreiber, M. (1999). Potential of an interactive computer-based training in the rehabilitation of dementia: An initial study. *Neuropsychological Rehabilitation*, *9*(2), 155–167. doi:10.1080/713755596

Sharan, D., Ajeesh, P. S., Rameshkumar, R., Mathankumar, M., Paulina, R. J., & Manjula, M. (2012). Virtual reality based therapy for post operative rehabilitation of children with cerebral palsy. *Work (Reading, Mass.)*, *41*(Supplement 1), 3612–3615. PMID:22317271

Smith, J. D., & Steel, M. J. (2001). *The use of virtual simulation for dismounted infantry training*. Cranfield University/RMCS Shrivenham. (Unpublished)

Snider, L., Majnemer, A., & Darsaklis, V. (2010). Virtual reality as a therapeutic modality for children with cerebral palsy. *Developmental Neurorehabilitation*, *13*(2), 120–128. doi:10.3109/17518420903357753 PMID:20222773

Sternberg, R. J. (1997). Intelligence and lifelong learning: Whats new and how can we use it? *The American Psychologist*, *52*(10), 1134–1139. doi:10.1037/0003-066X.52.10.1134 PMID:9329294

Stinson, C. A. (2013). *Virtual Reality for Sport Training* (Doctoral dissertation). Virginia Tech.

Tarnanas, I., Tsolaki, M., Nef, T., Müri, R. M., & Mosimann, U. P. (2014). Can a novel computerized cognitive screening test provide additional information for early detection of Alzheimers disease? *Alzheimers & Dementia*, *10*(6), 790–798. doi:10.1016/j.jalz.2014.01.002 PMID:24656838

You, S. H., Jang, S. H., Kim, Y. H., Kwon, Y. H., Barrow, I., & Hallett, M. (2005). Cortical reorganization induced by virtual reality therapy in a child with hemiparetic cerebral palsy. *Developmental Medicine and Child Neurology*, *47*(09), 628–635. doi:10.1111/j.1469-8749.2005.tb01216.x PMID:16138671

Chapter 12
Development of a Wireless Controlled Iontophoretic Drug Delivery System

Preeti Madhuri Pandey
National Institute of Technology Rourkela, India

Suraj Kumar Nayak
National Institute of Technology Rourkela, India

Biswajeet Champaty
National Institute of Technology Rourkela, India

Indranil Banerjee
National Institute of Technology Rourkela, India

D. N. Tibarewala
Jadavpur University, India

Kunal Pal
National Institute of Technology Rourkela, India

ABSTRACT

The current study describes the development of a wireless controlled iontophoretic drug delivery system. The control system was made using ZigBee communication protocol. The performance analysis of the current injecting circuit was performed to ascertain minimal error combined with high efficiency. Finally, the developed controlled system was used to manipulate the functioning of the two independent iontophoretic drug delivery systems. In gist, a wireless controlled drug delivery system based on ZigBee communication protocol was developed and tested successfully.

DOI: 10.4018/978-1-5225-2829-6.ch012

INTRODUCTION

The term iontophoresis has become a common terminology in the medical fraternity. The process involves delivery of drug molecules (having a physiological activity) for the treatment of a disease by passing an electric current through the human body. For this purpose, the human body is connected with a current injecting electrode and a reference electrode (required for the completing the electrical path). These electrodes are connected to an electrical circuit, which is capable of providing a voltage gradient across the electrodes. This voltage gradient is responsible for pushing the ionic drug molecules into the body. This process was first described by LeDus (1900) (Ciach & Moscicka-Studzinska, 2011; Leduc, 1900). The movement of the charged drug molecules occurs in such a fashion that they move towards the electrode, which is oppositely charged. Hence, care should be taken to place the drug under a suitable electrode. Mistakenly, if the drug molecules are placed under the electrode, which is counter charged, then no delivery of drug will happen. As a matter of fact, the cationic and the neutral drug molecules should always be placed under the positive electrode, whereas, the anionic drug molecules should always be placed on the negative electrode. The delivery of a drug by this method is governed by two phenomena, namely, electromigration and electroosmosis. Electromigration is a mass transfer process, which occurs due to the electrostatic interaction. As per this process, the charged drug molecules are electrostatically repelled by the active electrode (having the same charge) into the body. This process is predominant if the drug molecules are charged species. The process of electroosmosis has predominant effect in tissues, which are negatively charged (e.g. skin and buccal mucosa). As the ionic drug molecules move through the tissues under the electric field, the movement of the cationic molecules will be enhanced, whereas, the movement of the anionic molecules will be retarded. This influences the movement of the solvent molecules and other uncharged molecules. Such transfer is reported to occur by simple momentum transfer (Ciach & Moscicka-Studzinska, 2011). This phenomenon allows delivery of neutral drug molecules. Since the tissues are negatively charged, the delivery efficiency of cationic molecules has been found to be much higher as compared to the anionic drug molecules.

In the last two decades, there has been a considerable advancement in the technologies associated with the microcontroller design. This has allowed in developing current injecting devices at affordable prices. Due to this reason, along with the smooth delivery of drugs into the systemic circulation in a non-invasive manner, the use of these devices has been explored for personal healthcare, which was previously mainly confined to the treatment of the patients in the hospitals. The iontophoretic devices can find the application in the management of the patients in the hospitals. In most of the hospitals, there is a shortage of nursing staff. This issue is valid not only for developing countries but also for developed countries. Due to this reason, many scientists are working on the development of medical devices which are capable of reducing the workload of nursing staff. Herein, we propose to develop a wireless controlled iontophoretic delivery system. The control system will be able to manipulate the operation of the iontophoretic device from a remote location (e.g. nursing station of an intensive care unit (ICU)). The controlled system has been made to control multiple iontophoretic devices.

BACKGROUND

Drugs are administered through various routes like oral, ocular, intravenous, topical and transdermal. Amongst them, the drug administration through topical and transdermal routes is relatively easier and hence, is receiving special attention of the physicians in recent years (Sai Sateesh, Prasanjit, Kunal, & Sirsendu Sekhar, 2015). The topical drug delivery systems provide local administration of the drugs on the skin surface. On the other hand, the transdermal drug delivery systems allow the administration of the drugs into the blood circulation by applying them on the skin surface (Balfour & Heel, 1991; Küchler, et al., 2009). Transdermal drug delivery provides considerable potential for the non-invasive administration of the therapeutic agents (Kalia, Naik, Garrison, & Guy, 2004). The use of skin for drug delivery eliminates the hepatic first-pass effect and the probable chemical degradation in the antagonistic atmosphere of the gastrointestinal tract along with providing a large surface area (Naik, Kalia, & Guy, 2000). However, the transdermal delivery of drugs requires the improvement in the permeability of the drugs through the skin in order to allow the passage of the drug molecules through the stratum corneum (i.e. the outermost layer of the skin comprising of keratinoids) (Kalia, et al., 2004; Küchler, et al., 2009; Potts & Francoeur, 1991). This is because the stratum corneum possesses a multilamellar lipid structure that restricts the number of drug molecules, which can be passively transferred through the skin (Kalia, Merino, & Guy, 1998; Potts & Francoeur, 1991). Only a few drugs with low molecular weight like clonidine, fentanyl, nicotine and oxybutynin have been explored for passive transdermal drug delivery (Kalia, et al., 1998). In the last few decades, many physical and chemical enhancement methods have been proposed to minimize the skin barrier in a reversible manner without causing any skin irritation effect. Amongst them, the methods involving electrical and physical forces are regarded as the energy-driven permeation-enhancement methods (Barry, 2001; Morrow, McCarron, Woolfson, & Donnelly, 2007). Some examples of the energy-driven permeation-enhancement methods are ultrasound, jet injection, electrophoresis, magnetophoresis and iontophoresis (Barry, 2001; Morrow, et al., 2007). The iontophoretic transdermal drug delivery has been reported to provide numerous advantages like improved onset and offset times, desired drug input kinetics (i.e. continuous or pulsatile) and delivery of ionized as well as unionized drugs, which set it apart from other methods (Kalia, et al., 2004). Iontophoresis can be defined as the use of a constant electric current across the skin (by applying an electrical potential) to enable the efficient transdermal delivery of therapeutic agents (Wang, Thakur, Fan, & Michniak, 2005). Due to the use of electric current, iontophoresis is time and again categorized under the class of active drug delivery methods. The applied current induces an alteration in the skin physiology, which in turn, enhances the permeability of the drug molecules across the skin (Dhote, Bhatnagar, Mishra, Mahajan, & Mishra, 2012).

The working mechanism of iontophoresis is based on the general principle of electricity, which states that like charges repel and opposite charges attract each other. Therefore, for the delivery of a positively charged drug, the drug is dissolved in the electrolyte under the anode, the vice versa being true for a negatively charged drug. The anode is placed at the desired place of application and the cathode is placed at a nearby location on the skin surface. When a low voltage (generally < 10 V) is applied, the charged drug molecules are repelled by the anode and travel across the stratum corneum to the cathode (Glikfeld, Cullander, Hinz, & Guy, 1988). In case of a neutral drug, the movement of drug molecules takes place through convection. This becomes possible because of the electro-osmotic and osmotic forces occurring due to the application of electric current (Green, Flanagan, Shroot, & Guy, 1993). The convective solvent motion generated due to the electromigration of ions during iontophoresis drags neutral drug molecules along with it and is regarded as electro-osmosis (R. R. Burnette & Ongpipattanakul, 1987). On the other hand, an osmotic force is generated between the cathode and the anode due to the electrochemical gradient resulting from different transport numbers of cations and anions. This osmotic force induces the flow of water molecules from anode to cathode, which also transport the neutral drug molecules present within the anode with them (Harris, 1967; Sloan & Soltani, 1986; Wang, et al., 2005). A number of studies have been performed to describe the rate of iontophoretic drug delivery due to its complex nature (Srinivasan & Higuchi, 1990; Wang, et al., 2005). The Nernst-Planck equation is a reformulation of Fick's diffusion law and is used describe the movement of a charged chemical substance in a fluid (Maex, 2013; Samson & Marchand, 1999; Sokalski, Lingenfelter, & Lewenstam, 2003; Tedesco, Hamelers, & Biesheuvel, 2016; Tsuru, Urairi, Nakao, & Kimura, 1991). However, Srinivasan *et al.* (1990), Pikal *et al.* (1990) and Singh *et al.* (1993) have reported the modification of Nernst-Planck equation to predict the iontophoretic enhancement ratio (i.e. the ratio of steady state flux in the presence and the absence of electrical potential) because the original equation does not take the convective electro-osmotic flow into account (Pikal, 1990; Pikal & Shah, 1990a, 1990b; Singh & Maibach, 1993; Srinivasan & Higuchi, 1990). The modified equation can be represented as given in Equation 1 below.

$$J_i = -D_i \frac{\partial C_i}{\partial x} - D_i \frac{C_i z_i F}{RF} \frac{\partial E}{\partial x} \pm C_i J_v \quad (1)$$

where D_i = diffusion coefficient of solute

$\frac{\partial C_i}{\partial x}$ = solute concentration gradient

zi = the solute charge

F = Faraday constant

R = gas constant

T = absolute temperature

J_v= velocity of convective flow

It has been revealed from a number of studies that the transport of drug molecules during iontophoresis takes place through the appendageal pores like sweat glands and hair follicles (Chien, 1991; Chien, et al., 1999; Nair, Pillai, Poduri, & Panchagnula, 1999; Pillai, Nair, Poduri, & Panchagnula, 1999). However, the comparison of the outcomes of iontophoretic drug delivery in hairless and normal rats has suggested that the involvement of the sweat glands and ducts is more than that of the hair follicles (R. Burnette, 1989; R. R. Burnette & Bagniefski, 1988; Jue-Chen, Ying, Siddiqui, Wei-min, & John, 1988; Wang, et al., 2005). Cullander *et al.* (1991) had reported the use of a vibrating probe electrode for identification and vectorization of site-specific ion flow that occurred in hairless mouse skin (Cullander & Guy, 1991). The results suggested that certain skin appendages like small hairs carry most of the iontophoretic current. However, the same research group, in 1992, reported that although the transport of drug molecules takes place mainly through pores but the pores not necessarily mean the skin appendages. Paracellular transport also occurs for the delivery of water and uncharged drug molecules and can be a foremost pathway of permeation (Cullander, 1992). Singh *et al.* (1993) have proposed the potential-dependent pore formation as a pathway of iontophoretic drug delivery (Singh & Maibach, 1993).

Iontophoresis can be affected by various factors like p^H, type of electrodes, the strength of co-ions, type of current and its magnitude, the strength of solute in the donor, temperature and the type of the delivery vehicle (Wang, et al., 2005). The p^H of the drug solution influences iontophoresis in two ways. Firstly, it manipulates the p^H of the skin. When the p^H of the skin goes above 4, the carboxylic acid moieties present in the skin get ionized. This can promote the delivery of positively charged drugs if placed under the anode. Secondly, the p^H of the drug solution also influences the ionization of the drug molecules itself. As a result, the weakly basic drug is ionized to a lower extent when p^H is greater than its p^{Ka}. This, in turn, reduces the permeation of the drug molecules through electromigration during iontophoresis and the transport of drug molecules mainly occurs due to electro-osmosis. The type of electrodes employed also influences the iontophoretic drug delivery by causing a change in the p^H value. It generally occurs in the case of platinum or Zn/$ZnCl_2$ electrodes. The Ag/AgCl electrode opposes the changes in the p^H and is regarded the most suitable electrode for iontophoresis in the present scenario (Phipps, Padmanabhan, & Lattin, 1989). The type of electric current applied is another important parameter that affects the pattern of the iontophoretic drug delivery. The application of continuous direct current can cause polarization of the skin leading to skin damage. Therefore, the use of pulsed direct current or alternating current has been recommended to avoid the skin damage (Okabe, Yamaguchi, & Kawai, 1986).

Iontophoretic drug delivery has been successfully used for the treatment of a number of diseases. Hill *et al.* (1981) have reported the use of tap water iontophoresis for the treatment of hyperhydrosis. Karakoc *et al.* (2002) have proposed the working mechanism behind this treatment (Karakoç, Aydemir, Kalkan, & Ünal, 2002). Sakamoto *et al.* (2004) have found the improvement in dermatitis through the iontophoretic delivery of antisense oligonucleotides in NC/Nga mice (Sakamoto, et al., 2004). Over the years, the non-invasive delivery of proteins and peptides (e.g. LHRH, salmon calcitonin, human parathyroid hormone) has emerged as a promising application of iontophoretic drug delivery (Chang, Hofmann, Zhang, Deftos, & Banga, 2003; Medi & Singh, 2003; Raiman, Koljonen, Huikko, Kostiainen, & Hirvonen, 2004).

Although the development of different types of iontophoretic drug delivery devices has been extensively studied in the last few decades for the non-invasive, transdermal administration of a range of drugs, the wireless control of the iontophoretic devices has not been much explored.

MAIN FOCUS OF THE CHAPTER

Over the years, the development of iontophoretic drug delivery devices has received special attention of the researchers. However, not much work has been done on the hands-free wireless control of these devices. The main focus of the current study was to develop a Wireless controlled iontophoretic drug delivery system. Zigbee wireless communication protocol was used for the development of the proposed system.

MATERIALS

Arduino UNO (Arduino, Italy) was used for signal processing. Xbee Series-1 (Digi International, USA) was used for wireless data transmission and reception. Basic electronic components like variable resistors (5 kΩ and 10 kΩ), capacitors (0.1 μF and 1nF), resistors (1 kΩ, 2.7 kΩ, and 3.9 kΩ), push buttons, LEDs (red and green), power supply (± 12V) and double pole double throw (DPDT) relay were collected from a local market. Operational amplifier (UA741CN) from Texas Instruments and waveform generator (ICL8038) from Intersil Corporation were used in the study. Gelatin (HiMedia Private Limited, India) was used for the preparation of the hydrogels. 0.25 ml of glutaraldehyde (Merck specialists Private Limited, India), 0.2 ml of 0.1% N hydrochloric acid (Merck specialists Private Limited, India) and 0.05 ml of ethanol (Honyon International, Inc., Hong Yong Chemical Corporation, China) were mixed to obtain the crosslinking reagent. Salicylic acid (Loba Chemie Private Limited, India) was used as a model drug for iontophoresis study.

METHODS

Generation of Sinusoidal Wave Using IC 8038

A sinusoidal signal of a frequency of 5 kHz and amplitude of 4.40 V was developed using IC8038. The circuit diagram of the signal generator has been shown in Figure 1. The output of the signal generator was fed to a voltage divider to adjust the amplitude.

Development of an Iontophoretic Setup

An iontophoretic setup was developed in-house. It consisted of a buffer circuit at the primary stage, which was supposed to receive input from the signal generator. After that, a wideband band-pass filter (f_L = 408.08 Hz and f_H = 58.946 kHz) was implemented to select the particular frequency. The output of the voltage divider was fed to a buffer so as to prevent the loading of the previous circuit. The output of

Figure 1. Circuit diagram of IC 8038

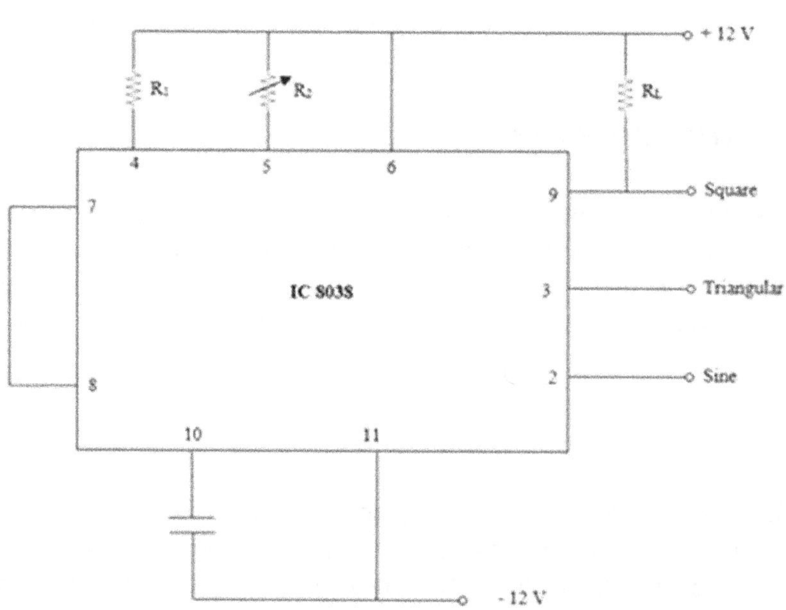

the band-pass filter was used as the input to a constant current source, which was developed as per the previous literature. The circuit diagram of the complete iontophoretic setup has been shown in Figure 2.

The drug release study was done using the iontophoretic drug delivery setup. A hydrogel was developed using carboxymethyl chitosan (CMC) and gelatine. The hydrogel was loaded with salicylic acid (model drug). The composition of the hydrogel has been tabulated in Table 1.

Wireless Control System

A ZigBee-based control system was developed. The control system consisted of two switches. The initial pressing of a switch generated a HIGH output signal at the digital output channel (Channel 1) of the Arduino UNO. The output was transmitted through ZigBee transmitter unit. The ZigBee receiver units received the wirelessly communicated signal. The received signal was transferred to Arduino UNO, which was used to control a relay. The relay was used as a switching device for controlling the output of the signal generator, whose circuit was slightly modified (Figure 3). When the switch was pressed for the second time, the output from the Arduino UNO (transmitter section) was LOW.

In this study, two switches were used so as to control two iontophoretic devices. The block diagram of the developed devices has been shown in Figure 4.

Testing of the Wireless Controlled Iontophoretic Devices

The working of the iontophoretic drug delivery system was tested using the developed representative hydrogel. The ability of the developed control system was tested by manipulating the switching states of the switches and correspondingly monitoring the output of the voltage across the iontophoretic cell.

Figure 2. Circuit diagram of the complete iontophoretic setup

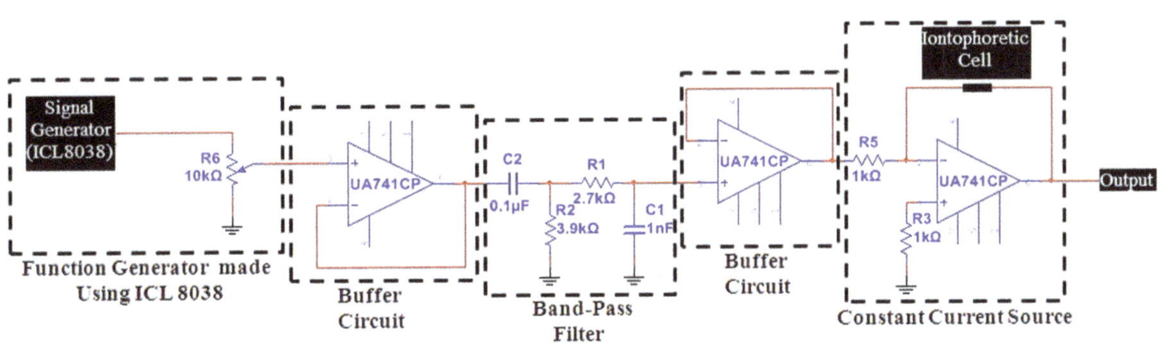

Table 1. Composition of Hydrogels

Formulations	Gelatin solution (20%) (g)	Carboxymethyl chitosan (2%)(g)	Crosslinker (ml)	Salicylic acid (1%) (g)
GC	10	10	1	-
GCS	10	10	1	0.2

Figure 3. Modified circuit of signal generator

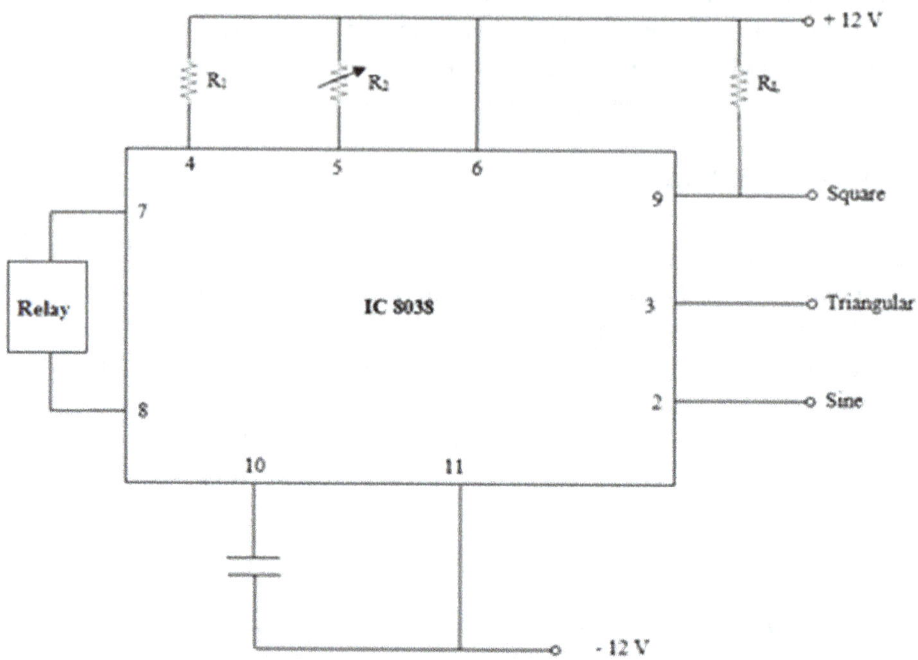

Figure 4. Block Diagram of the developed device

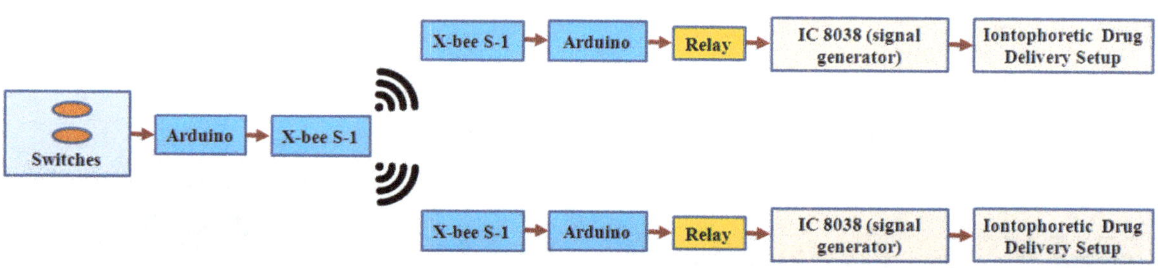

RESULTS AND DISCUSSION

Generation of Sinusoidal Wave Using IC 8038

A signal generator, generating a sinusoidal wave of 4.40 V_{pp} amplitude and 5 kHz frequency was developed using IC8038. The circuit was developed as per the circuit diagram, given in Figure 1.Visual analysis of the output signal confirmed the generation of a sinusoidal signal. The sinusoidal output from the signal generator and its corresponding Fourier transform have been shown in Figure 5.

The sinusoidal output showed an offset of 1.00 V added to the sinusoidal waveform of 4.40 V_{pp}. The output of the signal generator was fed to the voltage divider. The output of the voltage divider was 1.2 V_{pp} with an offset voltage of 1.00 V (Figure 6).

Figure 5. (a) Output of signal generator and (b) its corresponding FFT

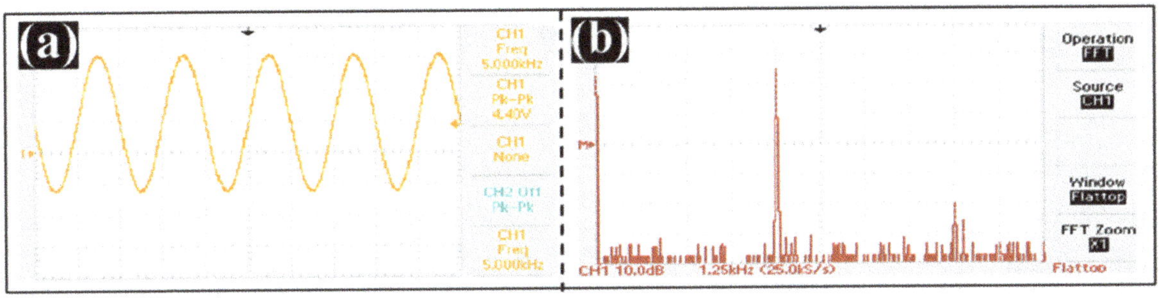

Figure 6. Input from IC8038 and its corresponding output of voltage divider showing 1.2 V_{pp} with offset of 1.00 V

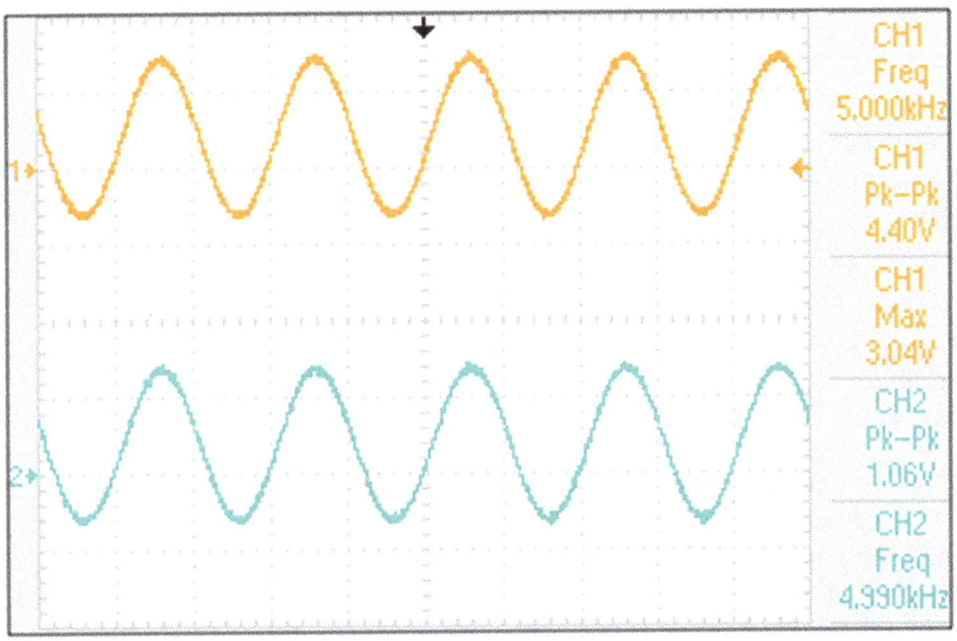

Development of an Iontophoretic Setup

The circuit for the iontophoretic setup was developed as per the circuit diagram, shown in Figure 2. The efficiency of the buffer circuit was tested by giving sinusoidal signals of varied amplitudes at its input and correspondingly measuring the output of the buffer circuit. The input and the output waveforms have been shown in Figure 7.

The measurements have been tabulated in Table 2. The theoretical output is the expected output considering the ideal nature of the op-amp, which is equal to the input signal. The percentage error in the output signal corresponding to the theoretical output was calculated. It was found that the percentage error of the output of the buffer circuit was within 5% in all cases.

Figure 7. Input and output waveforms of the buffer circuit

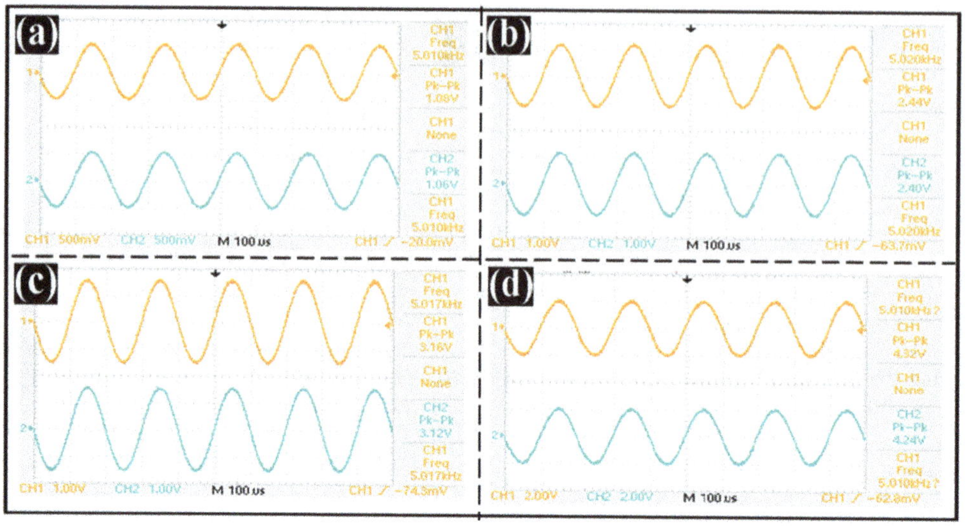

Table 2. Measurement of buffer circuit (1st Stage)

Vin (Vpp)	Practical Vout (Vpp)	Theoretical Vout (Vpp)	% Error
	1.04	1.08	3.7
2.44	2.40	2.44	1.6
3.16	3.12	3.16	1.2
4.32	4.24	4.32	1.8

In the second stage of the iontophoretic circuit, a band-pass filter was implemented. The band-pass filter was introduced in the circuit to eliminate the offset voltage obtained at the output of the signal generator and band limit the signal so as to analyze the signals in a computer/ laptop if needed. The amplitude response of the filter has been plotted in Figure 8 (a). The circuit was designed so as to have an f_L of 408.08 Hz and f_H of 58.946 kHz. The theoretical bandwidth (f_H - f_L) of the filter was 58.538 kHz. The calculated center frequency was 4.904 kHz. The practical cut-off frequencies (f'_L and f'_H) were determined from the amplitude plot at -3 dB gain. The practical cut-off frequencies f'_L and f'_H was 414.425 Hz and 62.35 kHz, respectively. Hence, the practical bandwidth of the filter was 61.9 kHz. The center frequency of the filter was found to be 5.08 kHz. The 'Q' factor was calculated using the f'_L and f'_H values. The calculated 'Q' factor was 0.0815 Hz. From the calculated 'Q' factor, it can be ascertained that the developed filter is a wideband filter (since 'Q' value was less than 10).

The output of the band-pass filter served as the input for a second buffer circuit. The analysis of the buffer circuit was done and it was found to be similar to that of the buffer circuit previously analyzed. The analysis parameter of this buffer circuit has been tabulated in Table 3. The percentage error in the output of the buffer circuit was lower than 5%.

The output of the buffer circuit was fed into a constant current source working in the inverting mode. The efficiency of the constant current source circuit was estimated by changing the load resistance (in place of the iontophoretic cell) and measuring the current passing through the load resistance. The re-

Figure 8. (a) Frequency response, (b) (c) and (d) input signal details, input waveform and output waveform of band-pass filter, respectively

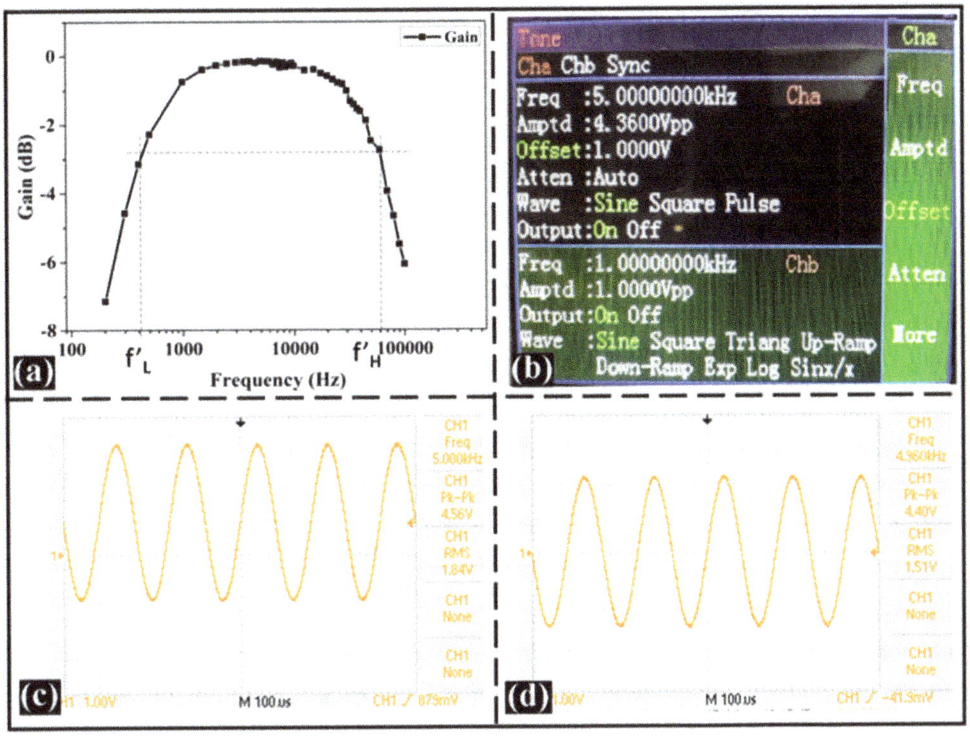

Table 3. Measurement of buffer circuit (3rd Stage)

Vin (Vpp)	Practical Vout (Vpp)	Theoretical Vout (Vpp)	% Error
1.08	1.10	1.08	1.8
2.16	2.12	2.16	1.8
3.16	3.12	3.16	1.2
4.32	4.24	4.32	1.8

sults suggested that even though the load resistance was changed, there was no significant change in the current flowing through the load resistance (Table 4 and Figure 4.4).

The amplitude of the current can be governed by varying the resistance 'R5'. It can be seen from the input and the output signals that there was a near 180° phase shift across the load resistance, which can be attributed to the property of an inverting amplifier.

The iontophoretic delivery system was tested using an in-vitro test. For this purpose, CMC-gelatin hydrogel was used as the matrix for salicylic acid drug release. It was found that the release of the drug under electrical stimulation was slightly higher than the passive drug release (Figure 10). Though the release of the drug under electrical field was higher, there was not much difference in the cumulative percentage drug release. This can be explained by the hydrophilic nature of the drug.

Table 4. Stability of constant current source

Load Resistance (kΩ)	V_{rms}(V)	I_{rms}(mA)
0.560	0.226	0.40
1	0.381	0.381
1.5	0.579	0.386
1.8	0.692	0.385
2.7	1.025	0.379
3.3	1.240	0.376
3.9	1.449	0.372
4.7	1.746	0.372
5.6	2.100	0.375
6.8	2.510	0.369
8.2	3.054	0.373
10	3.712	0.371
13	4.808	0.370
14.7	5.480	0.373

Figure 9. (a) Input (5 kHz, 1 V_{pp}), (b) output profile by using various load resistances, (c) and (d) input and output waveforms across constant current source with a load resistance of 560 Ω and 1 kΩ, respectively

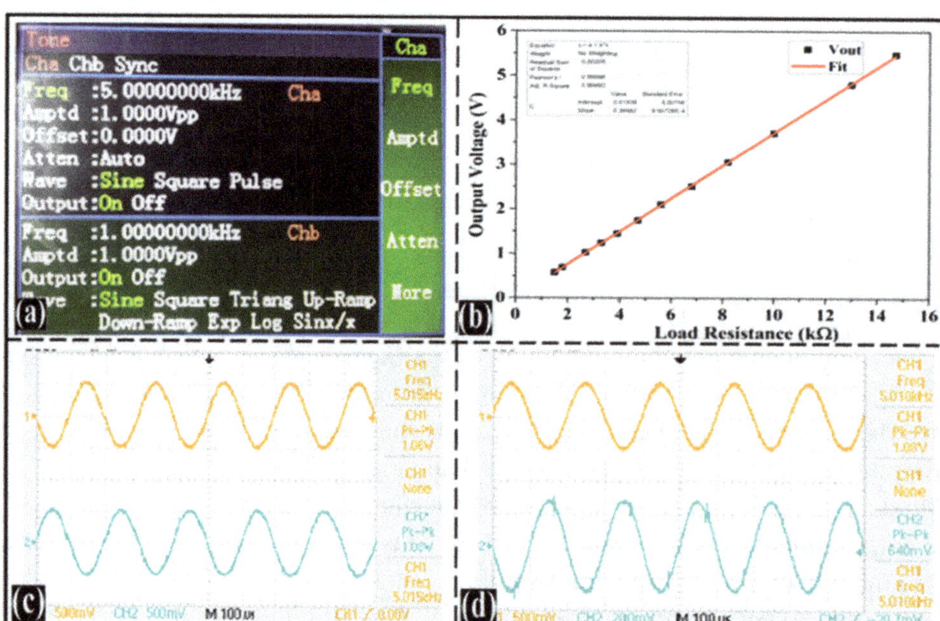

Figure 10. (a) Passive and (b) Active (iontophoresis) drug release profile of GCS hydrogel

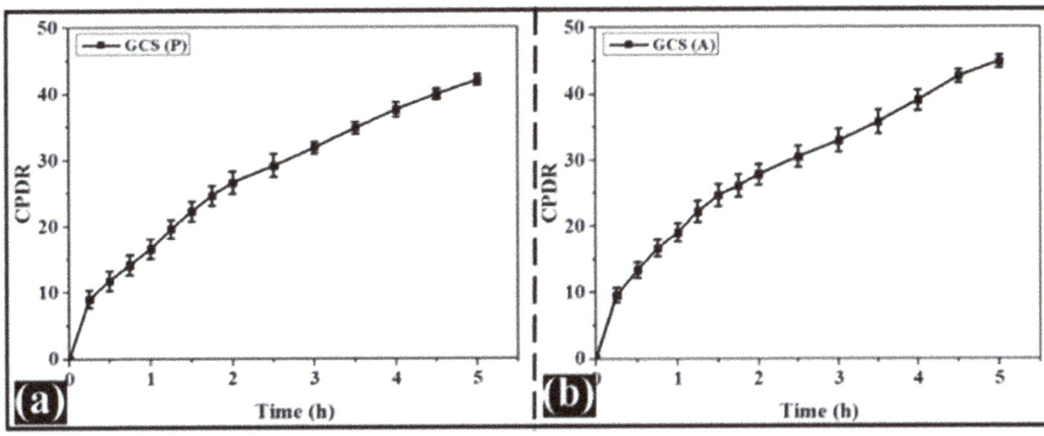

Wireless Control System

A wireless control system was developed so as to control two or more iontophoretic devices simultaneously. In this study, a hand-held switching device was made (Figure 11). This switching device consisted of two switches. The switches were used to send HIGH and LOW commands to the iontophoretic drug delivery setup via ZigBee wireless communication protocol.

The algorithm to describe the functioning of the transmitter unit has been shown in Figure 12. The algorithm for the operation of the receiver units has been shown in Figure 13.

Testing of the Wireless Controlled Iontophoretic Devices

The functioning of the device using the developed wireless control system was tested. The output across the load resistance when the switches were put on HIGH and LOW modes has been shown in Figure 14. A visual observation of the output signal suggested that the developed device was functioning properly and could be used for developing Wireless Controlled drug delivery systems.

Figure 11. (a) Switching device, (b) operation of switching device using Arduino

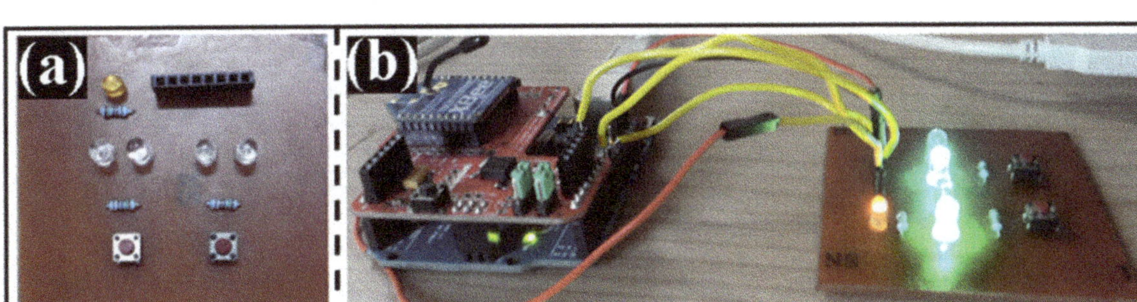

Figure 12. Algorithm of operation of the transmitter unit

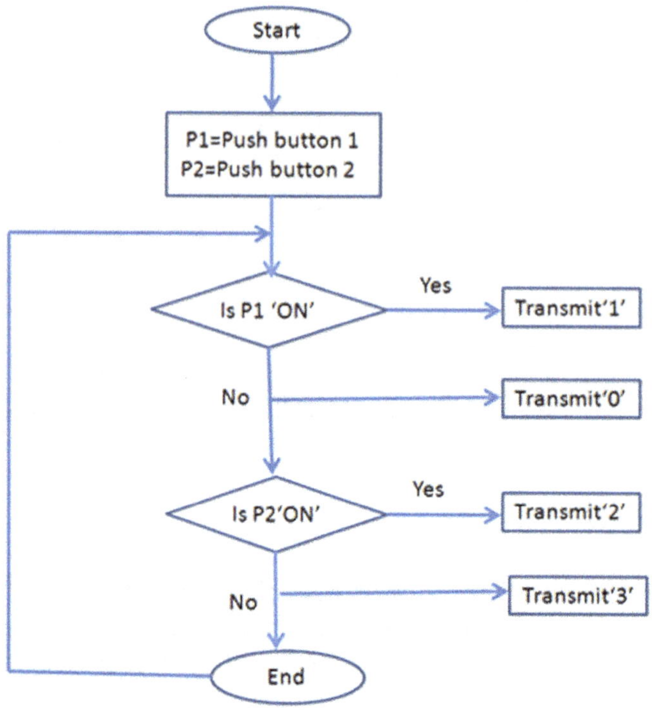

Figure 13. Algorithm of operation in the receiver units

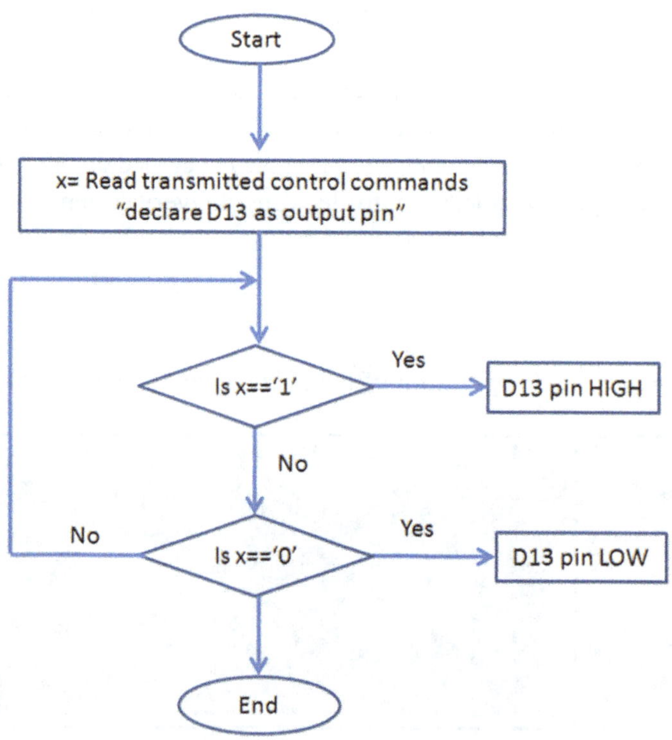

Figure 14. Wireless Controlled iontophoretic drug delivery setup: (a) when both switches are OFF, (b), (c) One of the switches is ON, and (d) Both the switches are ON

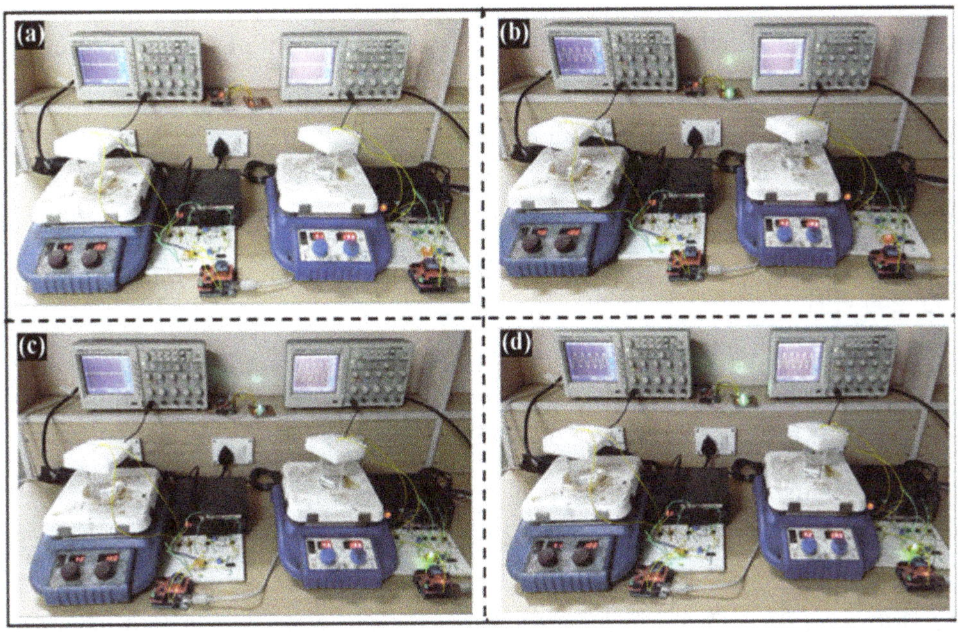

FUTURE RESEARCH DIRECTIONS

The current study was focussed on the development of a Wireless Controlled iontophoretic drug delivery device using ZigBee wireless communication protocol. The iontophoresis process was performed continuous sinusoidal current. Future studies can be performed the development of a Wireless Controlled iontophoretic drug delivery device using other wireless communication technologies like Bluetooth, radio frequency (RF) modules and Wi-Fi. The use of continuous current can be replaced with a pulsed current to obtain a different iontophoretic drug delivery profile.

CONCLUSION

In recent years, iontophoretic drug delivery has received much importance in the medical fraternity. This can be explained by the fact that iontophoretic drug delivery allows delivery of the drugs into the systemic circulation in a non-invasive manner. Due to this reason, such devices can be used effectively with minimal training to the patient. In this study, we have developed a Wireless Controlled iontophoretic drug delivery device, which can be used for ICU patient management. The control system can be kept at the central nursing station, which can allow the nursing staff to deliver the drugs to the ICU patients from their working seat. The proposed device is expected to minimize the working load of the nursing staff.

REFERENCES

Balfour, J., & Heel, R. (1991). 90365515 Transdermal estradiol. A review of its pharmacodynamic and pharmacokinetic properties, and therapeutic efficacy in the treatment of menopausal complaints. *Maturitas, 13*(3), 254–255. doi:10.1016/0378-5122(91)90204-4

Barry, B. W. (2001). Novel mechanisms and devices to enable successful transdermal drug delivery. *European Journal of Pharmaceutical Sciences, 14*(2), 101–114. doi:10.1016/S0928-0987(01)00167-1 PMID:11500256

Burnette, R. (1989). Iontophoresis. *Transdermal Drug Delivery: Developmental Issues and Research Initiatives, 35*, 247–292.

Burnette, R. R., & Bagniefski, T. M. (1988). Influence of constant current iontophoresis on the impedance and passive Na+ permeability of excised nude mouse skin. *Journal of Pharmaceutical Sciences, 77*(6), 492–497. doi:10.1002/jps.2600770606 PMID:3171927

Burnette, R. R., & Ongpipattanakul, B. (1987). Characterization of the permselective properties of excised human skin during iontophoresis. *Journal of Pharmaceutical Sciences, 76*(10), 765–773. doi:10.1002/jps.2600761003 PMID:3123641

Chang, S.-L., Hofmann, G. A., Zhang, L., Deftos, L. J., & Banga, A. K. (2003). Stability of a transdermal salmon calcitonin formulation. *Drug Delivery, 10*(1), 41–45. doi:10.1080/713840326 PMID:12554363

Chien, Y. W. (1991). *Transdermal route of peptide and protein drug delivery Peptide and Protein Drug Delivery* (pp. 667–689). Marcel Dekker New York.

Chien, Y. W., Li, J. K.-J., Liu, J.-C., Shi, W.-M., Siddiqui, O., & Sun, Y. (1999). *Iontotherapeutic device and process and iontotherapeutic unit dose*. Google Patents.

Ciach, T., & Moscicka-Studzinska, A. (2011). Buccal iontophoresis: An opportunity for drug delivery and metabolite monitoring. *Drug Discovery Today, 16*(7-8), 361–366. doi:10.1016/j.drudis.2011.01.012 PMID:21300173

Cullander, C. (1992). What are the pathways of iontophoretic current flow through mammalian skin? *Advanced Drug Delivery Reviews, 9*(2-3), 119–135. doi:10.1016/0169-409X(92)90021-H

Cullander, C., & Guy, R. H. (1991). Sites of iontophoretic current flow into the skin: Identification and characterization with the vibrating probe electrode. *The Journal of Investigative Dermatology, 97*(1), 55–64. doi:10.1111/1523-1747.ep12478060 PMID:2056194

Dhote, V., Bhatnagar, P., Mishra, P. K., Mahajan, S. C., & Mishra, D. K. (2012). Iontophoresis: A potential emergence of a transdermal drug delivery system. *Scientia Pharmaceutica, 80*(1), 1–28. doi:10.3797/scipharm.1108-20 PMID:22396901

Glikfeld, P., Cullander, C., Hinz, R. S., & Guy, R. H. (1988). A new system for in vitro studies of iontophoresis. *Pharmaceutical Research, 5*(7), 443–446. doi:10.1023/A:1015944619348 PMID:3247315

Green, P. G., Flanagan, M., Shroot, B., & Guy, R. H. (1993). Iontophoretic drug delivery. *Drugs and the Pharmaceutical Sciences, 59*, 311-333.

Harris, R. (1967). *Iontophoresis* (Vol. 15). Baltimore, MD: Waverly Press.

Jue-Chen, L., Ying, S., Siddiqui, O., Wei-min, S., & John, L. (1988). Blood glucose control in diabetic rats by transdermal iontophoretic delivery of insulin. *International Journal of Pharmaceutics*, *44*(1-3), 197–204. doi:10.1016/0378-5173(88)90116-0

Kalia, Y. N., Merino, V., & Guy, R. H. (1998). Transdermal drug delivery: Clinical aspects. *Dermatologic Clinics*, *16*(2), 289–299. doi:10.1016/S0733-8635(05)70011-5 PMID:9589202

Kalia, Y. N., Naik, A., Garrison, J., & Guy, R. H. (2004). Iontophoretic drug delivery. *Advanced Drug Delivery Reviews*, *56*(5), 619–658. doi:10.1016/j.addr.2003.10.026 PMID:15019750

Karakoç, Y., Aydemir, E. H., Kalkan, M. T., & Ünal, G. (2002). Safe control of palmoplantar hyperhidrosis with direct electrical current. *International Journal of Dermatology*, *41*(9), 602–605. doi:10.1046/j.1365-4362.2002.01473.x PMID:12358834

Küchler, S., Abdel-Mottaleb, M., Lamprecht, A., Radowski, M. R., Haag, R., & Schäfer-Korting, M. (2009). Influence of nanocarrier type and size on skin delivery of hydrophilic agents. *International Journal of Pharmaceutics*, *377*(1), 169–172. doi:10.1016/j.ijpharm.2009.04.046 PMID:19439166

Leduc, S. (1900). Introduction of medicinal substances into the depth of tissues by electric current. *Ann. Electrobiol*, *3*, 545–560.

Maex, R. (2013). Nernst-Planck Equation. In D. Jaeger & R. Jung (Eds.), *Encyclopedia of Computational Neuroscience* (pp. 1–7). New York, NY: Springer New York.

Medi, B. M., & Singh, J. (2003). Electronically facilitated transdermal delivery of human parathyroid hormone (1–34). *International Journal of Pharmaceutics*, *263*(1), 25–33. doi:10.1016/S0378-5173(03)00337-5 PMID:12954177

Morrow, D., McCarron, P., Woolfson, A., & Donnelly, R. (2007). Innovative strategies for enhancing topical and transdermal drug delivery. *The Open Drug Delivery Journal*, *1*, 36-59.

Naik, A., Kalia, Y. N., & Guy, R. H. (2000). Transdermal drug delivery: Overcoming the skins barrier function. *Pharmaceutical Science & Technology Today*, *3*(9), 318–326. doi:10.1016/S1461-5347(00)00295-9 PMID:10996573

Nair, V., Pillai, O., Poduri, R., & Panchagnula, R. (1999). Transdermal iontophoresis. Part I: Basic principles and considerations. *Methods and Findings in Experimental and Clinical Pharmacology*, *21*(2), 139–151. doi:10.1358/mf.1999.21.2.529241 PMID:10327395

Okabe, K., Yamaguchi, H., & Kawai, Y. (1986). New iontophoretic transdermal administration of the beta-blocker metoprolol. *Journal of Controlled Release*, *4*(2), 79–85. doi:10.1016/0168-3659(86)90043-X

Phipps, J., Padmanabhan, R., & Lattin, G. (1989). Iontophoretic delivery model inorganic and drug ions. *Journal of Pharmaceutical Sciences*, *78*(5), 365–369. doi:10.1002/jps.2600780505 PMID:2746475

Pikal, M. J. (1990). Transport mechanisms in iontophoresis. I. A theoretical model for the effect of electroosmotic flow on flux enhancement in transdermal iontophoresis. *Pharmaceutical Research*, *7*(2), 118–126. doi:10.1023/A:1015816532532 PMID:2308891

Pikal, M. J., & Shah, S. (1990a). Transport mechanisms in iontophoresis. II. Electroosmotic flow and transference number measurements for hairless mouse skin. *Pharmaceutical Research*, *7*(3), 213–221. doi:10.1023/A:1015857608850 PMID:2339092

Pikal, M. J., & Shah, S. (1990b). Transport mechanisms in iontophoresis. III. An experimental study of the contributions of electroosmotic flow and permeability change in transport of low and high molecular weight solutes. *Pharmaceutical Research*, *7*(3), 222–229. doi:10.1023/A:1015809725688 PMID:2339093

Pillai, O., Nair, V., Poduri, R., & Panchagnula, R. (1999). Transdermal iontophoresis. Part II: Peptide and protein delivery. *Methods and Findings in Experimental and Clinical Pharmacology*, *21*(3), 229–240. doi:10.1358/mf.1999.21.3.534833 PMID:10389126

Potts, R. O., & Francoeur, M. L. (1991). The influence of stratum corneum morphology on water permeability. *The Journal of Investigative Dermatology*, *96*(4), 495–499. doi:10.1111/1523-1747.ep12470197 PMID:2007788

Raiman, J., Koljonen, M., Huikko, K., Kostiainen, R., & Hirvonen, J. (2004). Delivery and stability of LHRH and Nafarelin in human skin: The effect of constant/pulsed iontophoresis. *European Journal of Pharmaceutical Sciences*, *21*(2), 371–377. doi:10.1016/j.ejps.2003.11.003 PMID:14757511

Sai Sateesh, S., Prasanjit, P., Kunal, P., & Sirsendu Sekhar, R. (2015). *Drug Delivery: Iontophoretic. In Encyclopedia of Biomedical Polymers and Polymeric Biomaterials* (pp. 2726–2740). CRC Press.

Sakamoto, T., Miyazaki, E., Aramaki, Y., Arima, H., Takahashi, M., Kato, Y., & Tsuchiya, S. et al. (2004). Improvement of dermatitis by iontophoretically delivered antisense oligonucleotides for interleukin-10 in NC/Nga mice. *Gene Therapy*, *11*(3), 317–324. doi:10.1038/sj.gt.3302171 PMID:14737092

Samson, E., & Marchand, J. (1999). Numerical solution of the extended Nernst–Planck model. *Journal of Colloid and Interface Science*, *215*(1), 1–8. doi:10.1006/jcis.1999.6145 PMID:10362465

Singh, P., & Maibach, H. I. (1993). Iontophoresis in drug delivery: Basic principles and applications. *Critical Reviews in Therapeutic Drug Carrier Systems*, *11*(2-3), 161–213. PMID:7600587

Sloan, J. B., & Soltani, K. (1986). Iontophoresis in dermatology: A review. *Journal of the American Academy of Dermatology*, *15*(4), 671–684. doi:10.1016/S0190-9622(86)70223-5 PMID:3534013

Sokalski, T., Lingenfelter, P., & Lewenstam, A. (2003). Numerical solution of the coupled Nernst-Planck and Poisson equations for liquid junction and ion selective membrane potentials. *The Journal of Physical Chemistry B*, *107*(11), 2443–2452. doi:10.1021/jp026406a

Srinivasan, V., & Higuchi, W. (1990). A model for iontophoresis incroporating the effect of convective solvent flow. *International Journal of Pharmaceutics*, *60*(2), 133–138. doi:10.1016/0378-5173(90)90298-I

Tedesco, M., Hamelers, H., & Biesheuvel, P. (2016). Nernst-Planck transport theory for (reverse) electrodialysis: I. Effect of co-ion transport through the membranes. *Journal of Membrane Science*, *510*, 370–381. doi:10.1016/j.memsci.2016.03.012

Tsuru, T., Urairi, M., Nakao, S.-i., & Kimura, S. (1991). Reverse osmosis of single and mixed electrolytes with charged membranes: Experiment and analysis. *Journal of Chemical Engineering of Japan*, *24*(4), 518–524. doi:10.1252/jcej.24.518

Wang, Y., Thakur, R., Fan, Q., & Michniak, B. (2005). Transdermal iontophoresis: Combination strategies to improve transdermal iontophoretic drug delivery. *European Journal of Pharmaceutics and Biopharmaceutics*, *60*(2), 179–191. doi:10.1016/j.ejpb.2004.12.008 PMID:15939232

ADDITIONAL READING

Amichai, B., Nitzan, B., Mosckovitz, R., & Shemer, A. (2010). Iontophoretic delivery of terbinafine in onychomycosis: A preliminary study. *The British Journal of Dermatology*, *162*(1), 46–50. doi:10.1111/j.1365-2133.2009.09414.x PMID:19785609

Banga, A. K., & Chien, Y. W. (1993). Hydrogel-based lontotherapeutic delivery devices for transdermal delivery of peptide/protein drugs. *Pharmaceutical Research*, *10*(5), 697–702. doi:10.1023/A:1018955631835 PMID:8321834

Barry, B. (2002). Drug delivery routes in skin: A novel approach. *Advanced Drug Delivery Reviews*, *54*, S31–S40. doi:10.1016/S0169-409X(02)00113-8 PMID:12460714

Barry, B. W. (2001). Novel mechanisms and devices to enable successful transdermal drug delivery. *European Journal of Pharmaceutical Sciences*, *14*(2), 101–114. doi:10.1016/S0928-0987(01)00167-1 PMID:11500256

Benson, H. A. (2005). Transdermal drug delivery: Penetration enhancement techniques. *Current Drug Delivery*, *2*(1), 23–33. doi:10.2174/1567201052772915 PMID:16305405

Brounéus, F., Karami, K., Beronius, P., & Sundelöf, L.-O. (2001). Diffusive transport properties of some local anesthetics applicable for iontophoretic formulation of the drugs. *International Journal of Pharmaceutics*, *218*(1), 57–62. doi:10.1016/S0378-5173(01)00612-3 PMID:11337149

Calatayud-Pascual, M., Balaguer-Fernandez, C., Serna-Jiménez, C., Del Rio-Sancho, S., Femenia-Font, A., Merino, V., & López-Castellano, A. (2011). Effect of iontophoresis on in vitro transdermal absorption of almotriptan. *International Journal of Pharmaceutics*, *416*(1), 189–194. doi:10.1016/j.ijpharm.2011.06.039 PMID:21736929

Cázares-Delgadillo, J., Balaguer-Fernandez, C., Calatayud-Pascual, A., Ganem-Rondero, A., Quintanar-Guerrero, D., López-Castellano, A., & Kalia, Y. N. et al. (2010). Transdermal iontophoresis of dexamethasone sodium phosphate in vitro and in vivo: Effect of experimental parameters and skin type on drug stability and transport kinetics. *European Journal of Pharmaceutics and Biopharmaceutics*, *75*(2), 173–178. doi:10.1016/j.ejpb.2010.03.011 PMID:20332024

Cázares-Delgadillo, J., Ganem-Rondero, A., Quintanar-Guerrero, D., López-Castellano, A. C., Merino, V., & Kalia, Y. N. (2010). Using transdermal iontophoresis to increase granisetron delivery across skin in vitro and in vivo: Effect of experimental conditions and a comparison with other enhancement strategies. *European Journal of Pharmaceutical Sciences*, *39*(5), 387–393. doi:10.1016/j.ejps.2010.01.008 PMID:20096354

Chansai, P., Sirivat, A., Niamlang, S., Chotpattananont, D., & Viravaidya-Pasuwat, K. (2009). Controlled transdermal iontophoresis of sulfosalicylic acid from polypyrrole/poly (acrylic acid) hydrogel. *International Journal of Pharmaceutics*, *381*(1), 25–33. doi:10.1016/j.ijpharm.2009.07.019 PMID:19643172

Curdy, C., Kalia, Y. N., & Guy, R. H. (2001). Non-invasive assessment of the effects of iontophoresis on human skin in-vivo. *The Journal of Pharmacy and Pharmacology*, *53*(6), 769–777. doi:10.1211/0022357011776117 PMID:11428652

Curdy, C., Kalia, Y. N., Naik, A., & Guy, R. H. (2001). Piroxicam delivery into human stratum corneum in vivo: Iontophoresis versus passive diffusion. *Journal of Controlled Release*, *76*(1), 73–79. doi:10.1016/S0168-3659(01)00418-7 PMID:11532314

del Rio-Sancho, S., Serna-Jiménez, C., Calatayud-Pascual, M., Balaguer-Fernández, C., Femenía-Font, A., Merino, V., & López-Castellano, A. (2012). Transdermal absorption of memantine–Effect of chemical enhancers, iontophoresis, and role of enhancer lipophilicity. *European Journal of Pharmaceutics and Biopharmaceutics*, *82*(1), 164–170. doi:10.1016/j.ejpb.2012.06.005 PMID:22732268

Eljarrat-Binstock, E., & Domb, A. J. (2006). Iontophoresis: A non-invasive ocular drug delivery. *Journal of Controlled Release*, *110*(3), 479–489. doi:10.1016/j.jconrel.2005.09.049 PMID:16343678

Eljarrat-Binstock, E., Domb, A. J., Orucov, F., Dagan, A., Frucht-Pery, J., & Peer, J. (2008). In vitro and in vivo evaluation of carboplatin delivery to the eye using hydrogel-iontophoresis. *Current Eye Research*, *33*(3), 269–275. doi:10.1080/02713680701871140 PMID:18350438

Eljarrat–Binstock, E., Domb, A. J., Orucov, F., Frucht–Pery, J., & Peer, J. (2007). Methotrexate delivery to the eye using transscleral hydrogel iontophoresis. *Current Eye Research*, *32*(7-8), 639–646. doi:10.1080/02713680701528674 PMID:17852187

Eljarrat-Binstock, E., Raiskup, F., Frucht-Pery, J., & Domb, A. J. (2004). Hydrogel probe for iontophoresis drug delivery to the eye. *Journal of Biomaterials Science. Polymer Edition*, *15*(4), 397–413. doi:10.1163/156856204323005271 PMID:15212325

Eljarrat-Binstock, E., Raiskup, F., Stepensky, D., Domb, A. J., & Frucht-Pery, J. (2004). Delivery of gentamicin to the rabbit eye by drug-loaded hydrogel iontophoresis. *Investigative Ophthalmology & Visual Science*, *45*(8), 2543–2548. doi:10.1167/iovs.03-1294 PMID:15277475

Fang, J.-Y., Hsu, L.-R., Huang, Y.-B., & Tsai, Y.-H. (1999). Evaluation of transdermal iontophoresis of enoxacin from polymer formulations: In vitro skin permeation and in vivo microdialysis using Wistar rat as an animal model. *International Journal of Pharmaceutics*, *180*(2), 137–149. doi:10.1016/S0378-5173(98)00287-7 PMID:10370184

Fang, J. Y., Sung, K., Wang, J. J., Chu, C. C., & Chen, K. T. (2002). The effects of iontophoresis and electroporation on transdermal delivery of buprenorphine from solutions and hydrogels. *The Journal of Pharmacy and Pharmacology*, *54*(10), 1329–1337. doi:10.1211/002235702760345392 PMID:12396293

Finnin, B. C., & Morgan, T. M. (1999). Transdermal penetration enhancers: Applications, limitations, and potential. *Journal of Pharmaceutical Sciences*, *88*(10), 955–958. doi:10.1021/js990154g PMID:10514338

Frucht-Pery, J., Goren, D., Solomon, A., Siganos, C. S., Mechoulam, H., Solomon, A., & Shapiro, M. et al. (1999). The distribution of gentamicin in the rabbit cornea following iontophoresis to the central cornea. *Journal of Ocular Pharmacology and Therapeutics*, *15*(3), 251–256. doi:10.1089/jop.1999.15.251 PMID:10385134

Frucht-Pery, J., Mechoulam, H., Siganos, C. S., Ever-Hadani, P., Shapiro, M., & Domb, A. (2004). Iontophoresis–gentamicin delivery into the rabbit cornea, using a hydrogel delivery probe. *Experimental Eye Research*, *78*(3), 745–749. doi:10.1016/S0014-4835(03)00215-X PMID:15106954

Green, P., Shroot, B., Bernard, F., Pilgrim, W. R., & Guy, R. H. (1992). In vitro and in vivo iontophoresis of a tripeptide across nude rat skin. *Journal of Controlled Release*, *20*(3), 209–217. doi:10.1016/0168-3659(92)90123-9

Green, P. G. (1996). Iontophoretic delivery of peptide drugs. *Journal of Controlled Release*, *41*(1), 33–48. doi:10.1016/0168-3659(96)01354-5

Guy, R. H. (1998). Iontophoresis—recent developments. *The Journal of Pharmacy and Pharmacology*, *50*(4), 371–374. doi:10.1111/j.2042-7158.1998.tb06875.x PMID:9625480

Haida, H., Ando, S., Ogami, S., Wakita, R., Kohase, H., & Saito, N. et al.. (2012). In vitro evaluation of calcium alginate gels as matrix for iontophoresis electrodes. *Journal of Medical and Dental Sciences*, *59*(1), 9–16. PMID:23896960

Kalaria, D. R., Patel, P., Patravale, V., & Kalia, Y. N. (2012). Comparison of the cutaneous iontophoretic delivery of rasagiline and selegiline across porcine and human skin in vitro. *International Journal of Pharmaceutics*, *438*(1), 202–208. doi:10.1016/j.ijpharm.2012.08.037 PMID:22954444

Kanikkannan, N. (2002). Iontophoresis-based transdermal delivery systems. *BioDrugs*, *16*(5), 339–347. doi:10.2165/00063030-200216050-00003 PMID:12408738

Kanjilal, B., Dasgupta, R., & Banthia, A. K. (2011). Iontophoretic study on Salicylic acid and Disprin loaded polymer hydrogels. *International Journal of Plastics Technology*, *15*(1), 19–29. doi:10.1007/s12588-011-9003-3

Kigasawa, K., Kajimoto, K., Watanabe, M., Kanamura, K., Saito, A., & Kogure, K. (2009). In vivo transdermal delivery of diclofenac by ion-exchange iontophoresis with geraniol. *Biological & Pharmaceutical Bulletin*, *32*(4), 684–687. doi:10.1248/bpb.32.684 PMID:19336905

Knoblauch, P., & Moll, F. (1993). In vitro pulsatile and continuous transdermal delivery of buserelin by iontophoresis. *Journal of Controlled Release*, *26*(3), 203–212. doi:10.1016/0168-3659(93)90187-A

Malakar, J., Sen, S. O., Nayak, A. K., & Sen, K. K. (2012). Formulation, optimization and evaluation of transferosomal gel for transdermal insulin delivery. *Saudi Pharmaceutical Journal*, *20*(4), 355–363. doi:10.1016/j.jsps.2012.02.001 PMID:23960810

Nair, V., & Panchagnula, R. (2003). Poloxamer gel as vehicle for transdermal iontophoretic delivery of arginine vasopressin: Evaluation of in vivo performance in rats. *Pharmacological Research*, *47*(6), 555–562. doi:10.1016/S1043-6618(03)00043-4 PMID:12742011

Nemanic, M. K., & Elias, P. M. (1980). In situ precipitation: A novel cytochemical technique for visualization of permeability pathways in mammalian stratum corneum. *The Journal of Histochemistry and Cytochemistry*, *28*(6), 573–578. doi:10.1177/28.6.7190175 PMID:7190175

Panchagnula, R., Pillai, O., Nair, V. B., & Ramarao, P. (2000). Transdermal iontophoresis revisited. *Current Opinion in Chemical Biology*, *4*(4), 468–473. doi:10.1016/S1367-5931(00)00111-3 PMID:10959777

Pescina, S., Ferrari, G., Govoni, P., Macaluso, C., Padula, C., Santi, P., & Nicoli, S. (2010). In-vitro permeation of bevacizumab through human sclera: Effect of iontophoresis application. *The Journal of Pharmacy and Pharmacology*, *62*(9), 1189–1194. doi:10.1111/j.2042-7158.2010.01153.x PMID:20796199

Petersen, J. (2008). Water electrolysis to facilitate drug delivery by iontophoresis: Google Patents.

Pliquett, U. F., Zewert, T. E., Chen, T., Langer, R., & Weaver, J. C. (1996). Imaging of fluorescent molecule and small ion transport through human stratum corneum during high voltage pulsing: Localized transport regions are involved. *Biophysical Chemistry*, *58*(1), 185–204. doi:10.1016/0301-4622(95)00098-4 PMID:8679918

Prasad, R., Anand, S., Khar, R. K., Dinda, A. K., & Koul, V. (2009). Studies on in vitro and in vivo transdermal flux enhancement of methotrexate by a combinational approach in comparison to oral delivery. *Drug Development and Industrial Pharmacy*, *35*(11), 1281–1292. doi:10.3109/03639040902882322 PMID:19832628

Prausnitz, M. R. (1997). Reversible skin permeabilization for transdermal delivery of macromolecules. *Critical Reviews™ in Therapeutic Drug Carrier Systems, 14*(4).

Prausnitz, M. R. (1999). A practical assessment of transdermal drug delivery by skin electroporation. *Advanced Drug Delivery Reviews*, *35*(1), 61–76. doi:10.1016/S0169-409X(98)00063-5 PMID:10837689

Ramanathan, S., & Block, L. H. (2001). The use of chitosan gels as matrices for electrically-modulated drug delivery. *Journal of Controlled Release*, *70*(1), 109–123. doi:10.1016/S0168-3659(00)00333-3 PMID:11166412

Roberts, M. (1997). Targeted drug delivery to the skin and deeper tissues: Role of physiology, solute structure and disease. *Clinical and Experimental Pharmacology & Physiology*, *24*(11), 874–879. doi:10.1111/j.1440-1681.1997.tb02708.x PMID:9363373

Sakamoto, T., Miyazaki, E., Aramaki, Y., Arima, H., Takahashi, M., Kato, Y., & Tsuchiya, S. et al. (2004). Improvement of dermatitis by iontophoretically delivered antisense oligonucleotides for interleukin-10 in NC/Nga mice. *Gene Therapy*, *11*(3), 317–324. doi:10.1038/sj.gt.3302171 PMID:14737092

Scott, E. R., Laplaza, A. I., White, H. S., & Phipps, J. B. (1993). Transport of ionic species in skin: Contribution of pores to the overall skin conductance. *Pharmaceutical Research*, *10*(12), 1699–1709. doi:10.1023/A:1018909811672 PMID:8302754

Shukla, C., Friden, P., Juluru, R., & Stagni, G. (2009). In vivo quantification of acyclovir exposure in the dermis following iontophoresis of semisolid formulations. *Journal of Pharmaceutical Sciences*, *98*(3), 917–925. doi:10.1002/jps.21474 PMID:18623192

Sieg, A., Guy, R. H., & Delgado-Charro, M. B. (2004). Noninvasive glucose monitoring by reverse iontophoresis in vivo: Application of the internal standard concept. *Clinical Chemistry*, *50*(8), 1383–1390. doi:10.1373/clinchem.2004.032862 PMID:15155544

Singh, I., & Sri, P. (2010). Percutaneous penetration enhancement in transdermal drug delivery. *Asian Journal of Pharmaceutics*, *4*(2), 92. doi:10.4103/0973-8398.68459

Sloan, J. B., & Soltani, K. (1986). Iontophoresis in dermatology: A review. *Journal of the American Academy of Dermatology*, *15*(4), 671–684. doi:10.1016/S0190-9622(86)70223-5 PMID:3534013

Tomoda, K., Terashima, H., Suzuki, K., Inagi, T., Terada, H., & Makino, K. (2012). Enhanced transdermal delivery of indomethacin using combination of PLGA nanoparticles and iontophoresis in vivo. *Colloids and Surfaces. B, Biointerfaces*, *92*, 50–54. doi:10.1016/j.colsurfb.2011.11.016 PMID:22154100

Touitou, E. (2002). Drug delivery across the skin. *Expert Opinion on Biological Therapy*, *2*(7), 723–733. doi:10.1517/14712598.2.7.723 PMID:12387671

Vaghani, S, S., Gurjar, M., Singh, S., Sureja, S., Koradia, S., P Jivani, N., et al. (. (2010). Effect of iontophoresis and permeation enhancers on the permeation of an acyclovir gel. *Current Drug Delivery*, *7*(4), 329–333. doi:10.2174/156720110793360603 PMID:20695844

KEY WORDS AND DEFINITIONS

Band-Pass Filter: A band-pass filter is an electronic circuit, which permits the passage of signals through it having frequency between two defined values. The defined frequency values are called as the lower and the higher cut-off frequencies.

Dermatitis: Dermatitis is a disease that causes the inflammation of the skin. It is also known as eczema.

Hyperhydrosis: Hyperhydrosis is a clinical condition that causes excessive sweating in the upper and lower limbs.

Iontophoresis: Iontophoresis is one of the methods of transdermal delivery of drugs by applying a small electric current across the skin surface.

Operational Amplifier: An operational amplifier is an integrated circuit amplifier possessing high gain and high input impedance. It is named so because it can be used to perform various arithmetic operations on signals.

Relay: A Relay is an electrical apparatus used to open or close an electrical circuit.

ZigBee: ZigBee is a wireless communication protocol useful for creating a simple, low-cost wireless personal area network.

Compilation of References

Abdullah, M. H., Abdullah, J. M., & Abdullah, M. Z. (2012). Seizure detection by means of hidden Markov model and stationary wavelet transform of electroencephalograph signals. *International Conference on Biomedical and Health Informatics*, 62-65. doi:10.1109/BHI.2012.6211506

Abo-Zahhad, M., Al-Ajlouni, A. F., Ahmed, S. M., & Schilling, R. J. (2013). A new algorithm for the compression of ECG signals based on mother wavelet parameterization and best-threshold levels selection. *Digital Signal Processing*, *23*(3), 1002–1011. doi:10.1016/j.dsp.2012.11.005

Acharya, U. R., Faust, O., Kadri, N. A., Suri, J. S., & Yu, W. (2013). Automated identification of normal and diabetes heart rate signals using nonlinear measures. *Computers in Biology and Medicine*, *43*(10), 1523–1529. doi:10.1016/j.compbiomed.2013.05.024 PMID:24034744

Adams, R., Finn, P., Moes, E., Flannery, K., & Rizzo, A. S. (2009). Distractibility in attention/deficit/hyperactivity disorder (ADHD): The virtual reality classroom. *Child Neuropsychology*, *15*(2), 120–135. doi:10.1080/09297040802169077 PMID:18608217

Adeli, H., Ghosh-Dastidar, S., & Dadmehr, N. (2008). A spatio-temporal wavelet-chaos methodology for EEG-based diagnosis of Alzheimers disease. *Neuroscience Letters*, *444*(2), 190–194. doi:10.1016/j.neulet.2008.08.008 PMID:18706477

Adeli, H., Zhou, Z., & Dadmehr, N. (2003). Analysis of EEG records in an epileptic patient using wavelet transform. *Journal of Neuroscience Methods*, *123*(1), 69–87. doi:10.1016/S0165-0270(02)00340-0 PMID:12581851

Aguado, D., Montoya, T., Borras, L., Seco, A., & Ferrer, J. (2008). Using SOM and PCA for analysing and interpreting data from a P-removal SBR. *Engineering Applications of Artificial Intelligence*, *21*(6), 919–930. doi:10.1016/j.engappai.2007.08.001

Ahmadlou, M., & Adeli, H. (2014). Electroencephalograms in diagnosis of autism. In V. B. Patel, V. R. Preedy, & C. R. Martin (Eds.), *Comprehensive Guide to Autism* (pp. 327–343). doi:10.1007/978-1-4614-4788-7_204

Ahmadlou, M., Adeli, H., & Adeli, A. (2010). Fractality and a wavelet-chaos-neural network methodology for EEG-based diagnosis of autistic spectrum disorder. *Journal of Clinical Neurophysiology*, *27*(5), 328–333. doi:10.1097/WNP.0b013e3181f40dc8 PMID:20844443

Ah-Pine, J., Bressan, M., Clinchant, S., Csurka, G., Hoppenot, Y., & Renders, J. (2009). Crossing Textual and Visual content in different application scenarios. *Multimedia Tools and Applications*, *42*(1), 31–56. doi:10.1007/s11042-008-0246-8

Ahrabian, A., Rehman, N. U., & Mandic, D. (2013). Bivariate empirical mode decomposition for unbalanced real-world signals. *IEEE Signal Processing Letters*, *20*(3), 245–248. doi:10.1109/LSP.2013.2242062

Aisen, M., Broderick, L., Winer-Muram, H., Brodley, C., Kak, A., Pavlopoulou, C., & Marchori, A. et al. (2003). Automated Storage and Retrieval of thin-section CT images to assist diagnosis:System description and Preliminary Assessment. *Radiology*, *228*(1), 265–270. doi:10.1148/radiol.2281020126 PMID:12832587

Akgül, C., Rubin, D., Napel, S., Beaulieu, C., Greenspan, H., & Acar, B. (2011). Content-based image retrieval in radiology: Current status and future directions. *Journal of Digital Imaging*, *24*(2), 208–222. doi:10.1007/s10278-010-9290-9 PMID:20376525

Akhutina, T. Y., Foreman, N., Krichevets, A., Matikka, L., Narhi, V., Pylaeva, N., & Vahakuopus, J. (2003). Improving spatial functioning in children with cerebral palsy using computerized and traditional game tasks. *Disability and Rehabilitation*, *25*(24), 1361–1371. doi:10.1080/09638280310001616358 PMID:14660204

Akram, M. U., Tariq, A., Khan, S. A., & Javed, M. Y. (2014). Automated detection of exudates and macula for grading of diabetic macular edema. *Computer Methods and Programs in Biomedicine*, *114*(2), 141–152. doi:10.1016/j.cmpb.2014.01.010 PMID:24548898

Al-Diri, B., Hunter, A., & Steel, D. (2009). An active contour model for segmenting and measuring retinal vessels. *IEEE Transactions on Medical Imaging*, *28*(9), 1488–1497. doi:10.1109/TMI.2009.2017941 PMID:19336294

Alexander, M. E., Baumgartner, R., Summers, A. R., Windischberger, C., Klarhoefer, M., Moser, E., & Somorjai, R. L. (2000). A wavelet-based method for improving signal-to-noise ratio and contrast in MR images. *Magnetic Resonance Imaging*, *18*(2), 169–180. doi:10.1016/S0730-725X(99)00128-9 PMID:10722977

Allen, V. A., & Belina, J. (1992, October). ECG data compression using the discrete cosine transform (DCT). In Computers in Cardiology 1992, Proceedings of (pp. 687-690). IEEE.

Altaf, M. U. B., Gautama, T., Tanaka, T., & Mandic, D. P. (2007). Rotation invariant complex empirical mode decomposition. In *IEEE International Conference on Acoustics, Speech and Signal Processing*, (pp. III–1009–III–1012). Honolulu, HI: IEEE.

American Psychiatric Association. (1994). *Diagnostic and statistical manual of mental disorders (DSM)*. Washington, DC: American Psychiatric Association.

Amiya Halder et al. (2011). *Edge Detection: A Statistical Approach*. IEEE.

Amoud, H., Snoussi, H., Hewson, D., & Duchêne, J. (2008). Univariate and bivariate empirical mode decomposition for postural stability analysis. *EURASIP Journal on Advances in Signal Processing*, *657391*, 1–11.

Anand, C. S., & Sahambi, J. S. (2010). Wavelet domain non-linear filtering for MRI denoising. *Magnetic Resonance Imaging*, *28*(6), 842–861. doi:10.1016/j.mri.2010.03.013 PMID:20418039

Andreão, R. V., Dorizzi, B., & Boudy, J. (2006). ECG signal analysis through hidden Markov models. *IEEE Transactions on Bio-Medical Engineering*, *53*(8), 1541–1549. doi:10.1109/TBME.2006.877103 PMID:16916088

Andrzejak, R. G., Schindler, K., & Rummel, C. (2012). Nonrandomness, nonlinear dependence, and nonstationarity of electroencephalographic recordings from epilepsy patients. *Physical Review E*, *86*(4).

Andrzejak, R. G., Schindler, K., & Rummel, C. (2012). Nonrandomness, nonlinear dependence, and nonstationarity of electroencephalographic recordings from epilepsy patients. *Physical Review E: Statistical, Nonlinear, and Soft Matter Physics*, *86*(046206), 1–17. PMID:23214662

Angulo, J., & Flandrin, G. (2003). Microscopic image analysis using mathematical morphology: application to hematological cytology. In A. Mendez-Vilas (Ed.), Science, Technology and Education of Microscopy: An overview (pp. 304–312). Academic Press.

Antal, B., & Hajdu, A. (2012). An ensemble-based system for microaneurysm detection and diabetic retinopathy grading. *IEEE Transactions on Bio-Medical Engineering*, *59*(6), 1720–1726. doi:10.1109/TBME.2012.2193126 PMID:22481810

Antani, S., Lee, D., Long, L., & Thoma, G. (2004). Evaluation of shape similarity measurement methods for spine X-ray images. *Journal of Visual Communication and Image Representation*, *15*(3), 285–302. doi:10.1016/j.jvcir.2004.04.005

Arbel, T., Morandi, X., Comeau, R., & Collins, D.L. (2004). Automatic non-linear mri-ultrasound registration for the correction of intraoperative brain deformations. *Comput Aided Surg, 9*(4), 123–136.

Aronson, A. (2006). Metamap: Mapping text to the UMLS metathesaurus. Bethesda, MD: NLM, NIH, DHHS.

Article 18: council of Europian Union. (2015). *Draft data protection regulation.* Retrieved from http.data.consiliun.europa.eu/doc/documents/ST-9565-2015-INIT/en/pdf

Asadi, M., Vahedi, A., & Amindavar, H. (2006) Leukemia Cell Recognition with Zernike Moments of Holographic Images. *Proceedings of the 7th Nordic Signal Processing Symposium*, 214-217. doi:10.1109/NORSIG.2006.275226

Asha, T., Natarajan, S., & Murthy, K. N. B. (2010, July). Notice of Retraction Diagnosis of tuberculosis using ensemble methods. *3rd IEEE International Conference on Computer Science and Information Technology (ICCSIT)*, 8, 409-412.

Atrey, P., Hossain, M., El Saddik, A., & Kankanhalli, M. (2010). Multimodal fusion for multimedia analysis: A survey. *Multimedia Systems*, *16*(6), 345–379. doi:10.1007/s00530-010-0182-0

Aurich, V., & Weule, J. (*1995*). Nonlinear Gaussian Filters Performing Edge preserving Diffusion. *Mutererkennung 17, DAGM-Symposium*, 538-545.

Avants, B., Epstein, C., Grossman, M., & Gee, J. (2008). Symmetric diffeomorphic image registration with cross-correlation: Evaluating automated labeling of elderly and neurodegenerative brain. *Medical Image Analysis*, *12*(1), 26–41. doi:10.1016/j.media.2007.06.004 PMID:17659998

Avni, U., Greenspan, H., Konen, E., Sharon, M., & Goldberger, J. (2011). X-ray categorization and retrieval on the organ and pathology level, using patch- based visual words. *IEEE Transactions on Medical Imaging*, *30*(3), 733–746. doi:10.1109/TMI.2010.2095026 PMID:21118769

Ayas, S., & Ekinci, M. (2014). Random forest-based tuberculosis bacteria classification in images of ZN-stained sputum smear samples. *Signal, Image and Video Processing, 8*(1), 49–61.

Azar, A. T., & El-Said, S. A. (2014). Performance analysis of support vector machines classifiers in breast cancer mammography recognition. *Neural Computing & Applications*, *24*(5), 1163–1177. doi:10.1007/s00521-012-1324-4

Bach, J., Fuller, C., Gupta, A., Hampapur, A., Horowitz, B., Humphrey, R., & Shu, C. (1996, March). Virage image search engine: An open framework for image management. In Electronic Imaging: Science & Technology (pp. 76-87). International Society for Optics and Photonics.

Badawy, R. A. B., Curatolo, J. M., Newton, M., Berkovic, S. F., & Macdonell, R. A. L. (2007). Changes in cortical excitability differentiate generalized and focal epilepsy. *Annals of Neurology*, *61*(4), 324–331. doi:10.1002/ana.21087 PMID:17358004

Baldassano, S., Wulsin, D., Ung, H., Blevins, T., Brown, M. G., Fox, E., & Litt, B. (2016). A novel seizure detection algorithm informed by hidden Markov model event states. *Journal of Neural Engineering, 13*(3).

Balfour, J., & Heel, R. (1991). 90365515 Transdermal estradiol. A review of its pharmacodynamic and pharmacokinetic properties, and therapeutic efficacy in the treatment of menopausal complaints. *Maturitas*, *13*(3), 254–255. doi:10.1016/0378-5122(91)90204-4

Barro, S., Fernandez-Delgado, M., Vila-Sobrino, J. A., Regueiro, C. V., & Sanchez, E. (1998). Classifying multichannel ECG patterns with an adaptive neural network. *IEEE Engineering in Medicine and Biology Magazine*, *17*(1), 45–55. doi:10.1109/51.646221 PMID:9460620

Barry, B. W. (2001). Novel mechanisms and devices to enable successful transdermal drug delivery. *European Journal of Pharmaceutical Sciences*, *14*(2), 101–114. doi:10.1016/S0928-0987(01)00167-1 PMID:11500256

Bauminger, N., Goren-Bar, D., Gal, E., Weiss, P. L., Yifat, R., Kupersmitt, J., . . . Zancanaro, M. (2007, October). Enhancing social communication in high-functioning children with autism through a co-located interface. In *Multimedia Signal Processing, 2007. MMSP 2007. IEEE 9th Workshop on* (pp. 18-21). IEEE. doi:10.1109/MMSP.2007.4412808

Bay, H., Ess, A., Tuytelaars, T., & Van Gool, L. (2008). Speeded-up robust features (SURF). *Computer Vision and Image Understanding*, *110*(3), 346–359. doi:10.1016/j.cviu.2007.09.014

Beil, M., Irinopoulou, T., Vassy, J., & Wolf, G. (1995). A dual approach to structural texture analysis in microscopic cell images. *Computer Methods and Programs in Biomedicine*, *48*(3), 211–219. doi:10.1016/0169-2607(96)81866-9 PMID:8925647

Beltagy, E., Mohamed, A., & Mohamed, K. (2010). Role of intraoperative ultrasound in resection of pediatric brain tumors. *Childs Nerv Syst, 26*, 1189–1193.

Benavent, J., Benavent, X., de Ves, E., Granados, R., & García-Serrano, A. (2010). Experiences at ImageCLEF 2010 using CBIR and TBIR Mixing Information Approaches. CLEF (Notebook Papers/LABs/Workshops).

Ben-Jacob, E., Doron, I., Gazit, T., Rephaeli, E., Sagher, O., & Towle, V. L. (2007). Mapping and assessment of epileptogenic foci using frequency-entropy templates. *Physical Review E: Statistical, Nonlinear, and Soft Matter Physics*, *76*(051903), 1–8. PMID:18233683

Berber, T., & Alpkoc¸ak, A. (2009). DEU at ImageCLEFmed 2009: Evaluating re–ranking and integrated retrieval model. Working Notes of CLEF 2009.

Bers, D. M. (2002). Cardiac excitation–contraction coupling. *Nature, 415*(6868), 198-205.

Besancon, R., & Millet, C. (2005). Merging results from different media: Lic2m experiments at ImageCLEF 2005. *Cross Language Evaluation Forum 2005 Workshop*.

Besl, P. J., & McKay, N. D. (1992, February). A Method for Registration of 3-D Shapes. *IEEE Transactions on Pattern Analysis and Machine Intelligence*, *14*(2), 239–256. doi:10.1109/34.121791

Bhattacharjee, R., & Saini, L. M. (2015) Robust Technique for the Detection of Acute Lymphoblastic Leukemia. *IEEE Power, Communication and Information Technology Conference*, 657-662. doi:10.1109/PCITC.2015.7438079

Bhattacharyya, A., Pachori, R. B., & Acharya, U. R. (2017). Tunable-Q wavelet transform based multivariate sub-band fuzzy entropy with application to focal EEG signal analysis. *Entropy*, *19*(3).

Bhattacharyya, A., Sharma, M., Pachori, R. B., Sircar, P., & Acharya, U. R. (2016). A novel approach for automated detection of focal EEG signals using empirical wavelet transform. *Neural Computing & Applications*, 1–11.

Bhaumik, S., & Biswas, T. (2012). India makes tuberculosis a notifiable disease. *Canadian Medical Association Journal*, *184*(10), E519–E520. doi:10.1503/cmaj.109-4213 PMID:22641684

Bikhet, S., Darwish, A., Tolba, H., & Shaheen, S. (2000) Segmentation and classification of white blood cells. *IEEE International Conference on Acoustics, Speech, and Signal Processing,* 2259-2261. doi:10.1109/ICASSP.2000.859289

Bilder, R. M. (2011). Neuropsychology 3.0: Evidence-based science and practice. *Journal of the International Neuropsychological Society*, *17*(01), 7–13. doi:10.1017/S1355617710001396 PMID:21092355

Bilgin, A., Marcellin, M. W., & Altbach, M. I. (2003). Compression of electrocardiogram signals using JPEG2000. *IEEE Transactions on Consumer Electronics*, *49*(4), 833–840. doi:10.1109/TCE.2003.1261162

Bioulac, S., Lallemand, S., Rizzo, A., Philip, P., Fabrigoule, C., & Bouvard, M. P. (2012). Impact of time on task on ADHD patient's performances in a virtual classroom. *European Journal of Paediatric Neurology, 16*(5), 514-521.

Boneau, C. A. (1960). The effects of violations of assumptions underlying the t test. *Psychological Bulletin*, *57*(1), 49–64. doi:10.1037/h0041412 PMID:13802482

Bosyk, G. M., Portesi, M., & Plastino, A. (2012). Collision entropy and optimal uncertainty. *Physical Review A, 85*(1).

Bovik, W. Z., Bovic, A.C., Sheikh, H.R., & Simoncelli, E.P. (2004). Image Quality Assessment: From Error Visibility to Structural Similarity. *IEEE Transactions on Image Processing, 13*(4), 600-612.

Breslauer, D. N., Maamari, R. N., Switz, N. A., Lam, W. A., & Fletcher, D. A. (2009). Mobile Phone Based Clinical Microscopy for Global Health Applications. *PLoS ONE*, *4*(7), e6320. doi:10.1371/journal.pone.0006320 PMID:19623251

Brown, L. G. (1992). A Survey of Image Registration Techniques. *ACM Computing Surveys, 24*(4).

Browning, D. J. (2010). Screening for diabetic retinopathy. In *Diabetic Retinopathy* (pp. 369–385). Springer New York. doi:10.1007/978-0-387-85900-2_14

Brutsaert, D. L. (2003). Cardiac endothelial-myocardial signalling: its role in cardiac growth, contractile performance, and rhythmicity. *Physiological Reviews, 83*(1), 59-115.

Buades, . (2005). A Non Local Algorithm For Image Denoising. *IEEE International Conference on Computer Vision and Pattern Recognition*, 2, s60-65. doi:10.1109/CVPR.2005.38

Burnette, R. (1989). Iontophoresis. *Transdermal Drug Delivery: Developmental Issues and Research Initiatives, 35*, 247–292.

Burnette, R. R., & Bagniefski, T. M. (1988). Influence of constant current iontophoresis on the impedance and passive Na+ permeability of excised nude mouse skin. *Journal of Pharmaceutical Sciences*, *77*(6), 492–497. doi:10.1002/jps.2600770606 PMID:3171927

Burnette, R. R., & Ongpipattanakul, B. (1987). Characterization of the permselective properties of excised human skin during iontophoresis. *Journal of Pharmaceutical Sciences*, *76*(10), 765–773. doi:10.1002/jps.2600761003 PMID:3123641

Cabrera-Umpierrez, M. F., Ramirez, C. M., Sevillano, A., Arredondo, M. T., & DeSmedt, A. (2006, May). Medical educational e-Platform through virtual reality technologies. In MELECON 2006-2006 IEEE Mediterranean Electrotechnical Conference (pp. 453-456). IEEE. doi:10.1109/MELCON.2006.1653136

Caicedo, J., Cruz, A., & Gonzalez, F. (2009). Histopathology image classification using bag of features and kernel functions. In *Artificial Intelligence in Medicine* (pp. 126–135). Berlin: Springer. doi:10.1007/978-3-642-02976-9_17

Cancer Research UK. (n.d.). *Worldwide cancer statistics*. Retrieved from http://www.cancerresearchuk.org

Caritá, E., Seraphim, E., Honda, M., & Azevedo-Marques, P. (2008). Implementation and evaluation of a medical image management system with content-based retrieval support. *Radiologia Brasileira*, *41*(5), 331–336.

Carpineto, C., & Romano, G. (2012). A survey of automatic query expansion in information retrieval. *ACM Computing Surveys*, *44*(1), 1–23. doi:10.1145/2071389.2071390

Carter, T., Tanner, C., Beechey-Newman, N., Barratt, D., & Hawkes, D. (2008). MR navigated breast surgery: method and initial clinical experience. *Proc. Int. Conf. Med. Image Comput. Comput.-Assist. Intervent.*, 356–363. doi:10.1007/978-3-540-85990-1_43

Chandra, S., Sharma, G., Mittal, A. P., & Jha, D. (2016). Effect of Sudarshan Kriya (meditation) on gamma, alpha, and theta rhythm during working memory task. *International Journal of Yoga*, *9*(1), 72.

Chandra, S., Sharma, G., Sharma, M., Jha, D., & Mittal, A. P. (2017). Workload regulation by Sudarshan Kriya: an EEG and ECG perspective. *Brain Informatics*, 1-13.

Chandra, S., Verma, K. L., Sharma, G., Mittal, A., & Jha, D. (2015). EEG based cognitive workload classification during NASA MATB-II multitasking. *International Journal of Cognitive Research in Science English Education*, *3*(1), 35–41.

Chandy, D., Johnson, J., & Selvan, S. (2013). Texture feature extraction using gray level statistical matrix for content-based mammogram retrieval. *Multimedia Tools and Applications*, 1–14.

Chang, J., Arbelaez, P., Switz, N., Reber, C., Tapley, A., Davis, J. L., & Malik, J. et al. (2012). Automated tuberculosis diagnosis using fluorescence images from a mobile microscope. *Medical Image Computing and Computer-Assisted Intervention.*, *15*(3), 345–352. PMID:23286149

Chang, S.-L., Hofmann, G. A., Zhang, L., Deftos, L. J., & Banga, A. K. (2003). Stability of a transdermal salmon calcitonin formulation. *Drug Delivery*, *10*(1), 41–45. doi:10.1080/713840326 PMID:12554363

Chanwimaluang, T., Fan, G., & Fransen, S. R. (2006). Hybrid retinal image registration. *IEEE Transactions on Information Technology in Biomedicine*, *10*(1), 129–142. doi:10.1109/TITB.2005.856859 PMID:16445258

Chapman, W., Bridewell, W., Hanbury, P., Cooper, G., & Buchanan, B. (2001). A simple algorithm for identifying negated findings and diseases in discharge summaries. *Journal of Biomedical Informatics*, *34*(5), 301–310. doi:10.1006/jbin.2001.1029 PMID:12123149

Chaytor, N., & Schmitter-Edgecombe, M. (2003). The ecological validity of neuropsychological tests: A review of the literature on everyday cognitive skills. *Neuropsychology Review*, *13*(4), 181–197. doi:10.1023/B:NERV.0000009483.91468.fb PMID:15000225

Cheitlin, M. D., Armstrong, W. F., & Aurigemma, G. P. (2003). ACC/AHA/ASE 2003 Guideline update for the clinical application of echocardiography: Summary article. A report of the American College of Cardiology/American Heart Association Task Force on Practice Guidelines (ACC/AHA/ASE Committee to Update the 1997 Guidelines for the Clinical Application of Echocardiography). *Journal of the American Society of Echocardiography*, *16*, 1091. PMID:14566308

Chel, H., Nandi, D., & Bora, P. K. (2015). Image registration in presence of multiplicative noise by Particle Swarm Optimization. *2015 Third International Conference on Image Information Processing (ICIIP)*, 135-140. doi:10.1109/ICIIP.2015.7414754

Chen, G. (2006). *International Conf. on Acoustic, Speech and Signal processing*. IEEE Xplore Digital Library.

Chen, D., Wan, S., & Bao, F. S. (2015) Epileptic focus localization using EEG based on discrete wavelet transform through full-level decomposition. *IEEE International Workshop on Machine Learning for Signal Processing*, 1–6. doi:10.1109/MLSP.2015.7324317

Cheng, P., Chien, B., Ke, H., & Yang, W. (2005). NCTU-DBLAB@ImageCLEFmed 2005: Automatic annotation task. Working Notes of CLEF 2005.

Chen, J., Tian, J., Lee, N., Zheng, J., Smith, R. T., & Laine, A. F. (2010). A partial intensity invariant feature descriptor for multimodal retinal image registration. *IEEE Transactions on Bio-Medical Engineering*, *57*(7), 1707–1718. doi:10.1109/TBME.2010.2042169 PMID:20176538

Chen, S. T., Guo, Y. J., Huang, H. N., Kung, W. M., Tseng, K. K., & Tu, S. Y. (2014). Hiding Patients Confidential Datainthe ECG Signal viaa Transform-Domain Quantization Scheme. *Journal of Medical Systems*, *38*(6), 54. doi:10.1007/s10916-014-0054-9 PMID:24832688

Chen, Y. P., Caldwell, M., Dickerhoof, E., Hall, A., Odakura, B., Morelli, K., & Fanchiang, H. C. (2014). Game analysis, validation, and potential application of EyeToy play and play 2 to upper-extremity rehabilitation. *Rehabilitation Research and Practice*. PMID:25610652

Chen, Y., Garcia-Vergara, S., & Howard, A. M. (2015). Effect of a home-based virtual reality intervention for children with cerebral palsy using super pop vr evaluation metrics: A feasibility study. *Rehabilitation Research and Practice*. PMID:26457202

Chevallet, J., Lim, J., Radhouani, S., & France, C. (2005). *Using ontology dimensions and negative expansion to solve precise queries in clef medical task*. Vienna, Austria: CLEF Workhop, Working Notes Medical Image Track.

Chien, Y. W., Li, J. K.-J., Liu, J.-C., Shi, W.-M., Siddiqui, O., & Sun, Y. (1999). *Iontotherapeutic device and process and iontotherapeutic unit dose*. Google Patents.

Chien, Y. W. (1991). *Transdermal route of peptide and protein drug delivery Peptide and Protein Drug Delivery* (pp. 667–689). Marcel Dekker New York.

Chiu, H. C., & Kuo, P. W. (2015). Effects of Virtual Reality in Children with Cerebral Palsy: A Systematic Review. 物理治療, *40*(3), 136-144.

Cho, S. W., Ku, J. H., Kang, Y. J., Lee, K. H., Song, J. Y., Kim, H. J., . . . Kim, S. I. (2010). A Pilot Study for Development of Shoulder Proprioception Training System Using Virtual Reality for Patients with Stroke: The Effect of Manipulated Visual Feedback. In *XII Mediterranean Conference on Medical and Biological Engineering and Computing 2010* (pp. 722-724). Springer Berlin Heidelberg. doi:10.1007/978-3-642-13039-7_182

Cho, H., Hadjiiski, L., Sahiner, B., Chan, H., Helvie, M., Paramagul, C., & Nees, A. (2011). Similarity evaluation in a content-based image retrieval (CBIR) CADx system for characterization of breast masses on ultrasound images. *Medical Physics*, *38*(4), 1820–1831. doi:10.1118/1.3560877 PMID:21626916

Christensen, G. E., & Johnson, H. J. (2001, July). Consistent image registration. *IEEE Transactions on Medical Imaging*, *20*(7), 568–582. doi:10.1109/42.932742 PMID:11465464

Chu, S., & Cesnik, B. (2001). Knowledge representation and retrieval using conceptual graphs and free text document self-organisation techniques. *International Journal of Medical Informatics*, *62*(2-3), 121–133. doi:10.1016/S1386-5056(01)00156-3 PMID:11470615

Ciach, T., & Moscicka-Studzinska, A. (2011). Buccal iontophoresis: An opportunity for drug delivery and metabolite monitoring. *Drug Discovery Today*, *16*(7-8), 361–366. doi:10.1016/j.drudis.2011.01.012 PMID:21300173

Clinchant, S., Renders, J., & Csurka, G. (2007). XRCE's Participation to ImageCLEFphoto 2007. *Working Notes of the CLEFWorkshop*.

Clinchant, S., Ah-Pine, J., & Csurka, G. (2011, April). Semantic combination of textual and visual information in multimedia retrieval. In *Proceedings of the 1st ACM International Conference on Multimedia Retrieval* (p. 44). ACM. doi:10.1145/1991996.1992040

Coast, D. A., Stern, R. M., Cano, G. G., & Briller, S. A. (1990). An approach to cardiac arrhythmia analysis using hidden Markov models. *IEEE Transactions on Bio-Medical Engineering*, *37*(9), 826–836. doi:10.1109/10.58593 PMID:2227969

Coburger, J., Scheuerle, A., Thal, D. R., Engelke, J., Hlavac, M., Wirtz, C. R., & Konig, R. (2015). Linear array ultrasound in low-grade glioma surgery: Histology-based assessment of accuracy in comparison to conventional intraoperative ultrasound and intraoperative MRI. *Acta Neurochirurgica*, *157*(2), 195–206. doi:10.1007/s00701-014-2314-3 PMID:25559430

Cohn, A., Miller, P., Fisher, P., Mutalik, P., & Swett, H. (1990). Knowledge-based radiologic image retrieval using axes of clinical relevance. *Computers and Biomedical Research, an International Journal*, *23*(3), 199–221. doi:10.1016/0010-4809(90)90017-7 PMID:2350958

Collins, D.L., & Evans, A.C. (1997). Animal: Validation and applications of nonlinear registration-based segmentation. *Int Journal of Pattern Recognition, 11*, 1271–1294.

Comeau, R. M., Fenster, A., & Peters, T. M. (1998). Intraoperative US in Interactive Image guided Neurosurgery. *Radiographics*, *18*(4), 1019–1027.

Contreras-Vidal, J. L., Presacco, A., Agashe, H., & Paek, A. (2012). Restoration of whole body movement: toward a noninvasive brain-machine interface system. *IEEE Pulse, 3*(1), 34-37.

Cortes, C., & Vapnik, V. (1995). Support Vector Networks. *Machine Learning*, *20*(3), 273–297. doi:10.1007/BF00994018

Costa, M. G., Costa Filho, C. F., Sena, J. F., Salem, J., & de Lima, M. O. (2008, August). Automatic identification of mycobacterium tuberculosis with conventional light microscopy. *30th Annual International Conference of the IEEE Engineering in Medicine and Biology Society*, 382-385. doi:10.1109/IEMBS.2008.4649170

Coupe, P., Yger, P., & Barillot, C. (2006). Fast non local means denoising for MR images. *Proceedings at the 9th International Conference on Medical Image Computing and Computer assisted Intervention (MICCAI)*, 33–40. doi:10.1007/11866763_5

Crnčević-Urek, M., Stipić-Marković, A., Kardum-Skelin, I., Stipić, J., Crnek-Kunstelj, V., & Urek, R. (2002). Induced Sputum: A Method for Cytologic Analysis of Bronchial Specimens. *Acta Clinica Croatica*, *41*(2), 89–93.

Csurka, G., Ah-Pine, J., & Clinchant, S. (2014). *Unsupervised Visual and Textual Information Fusion in Multimedia Retrieval-A Graph-based Point of View.* arXiv preprint arXiv:1401.6891

Cullander, C. (1992). What are the pathways of iontophoretic current flow through mammalian skin? *Advanced Drug Delivery Reviews*, *9*(2-3), 119–135. doi:10.1016/0169-409X(92)90021-H

Cullander, C., & Guy, R. H. (1991). Sites of iontophoretic current flow into the skin: Identification and characterization with the vibrating probe electrode. *The Journal of Investigative Dermatology*, *97*(1), 55–64. doi:10.1111/1523-1747.ep12478060 PMID:2056194

Dahlquist, L. M., McKenna, K. D., Jones, K. K., Dillinger, L., Weiss, K. E., & Ackerman, C. S. (2007). Active and passive distraction using a head-mounted display helmet: Effects on cold pressor pain in children. *Health Psychology*, *26*(6), 794–801. doi:10.1037/0278-6133.26.6.794 PMID:18020853

Dahlquist, L. M., Weiss, K. E., Clendaniel, L. D., Law, E. F., Ackerman, C. S., & McKenna, K. D. (2009). Effects of videogame distraction using a virtual reality type head-mounted display helmet on cold pressor pain in children. *Journal of Pediatric Psychology*, *34*(5), 574–584. doi:10.1093/jpepsy/jsn023 PMID:18367495

Dang, P., Kalra, M., Schultz, T., Graham, S., & Dreyer, K. (2009). Informatics in radiology: Render: An online searchable radiology study repository. *Radiographics*, *29*(5), 1233–1246. doi:10.1148/rg.295085036 PMID:19564253

Das A B & Bhuiyan M I H (2016), Discrimination and classification of focal and non-focal EEG signals using entropy-based features in the EMD-DWT domain, Biomedical Signal Proceesing and control, 29, 11-21.

Das, A. B., & Bhuiyan, M. I. H. (2016). Discrimination and classification of focal and non-focal EEG signals using entropy-based features in the EMD-DWT domain. *Biomedical Signal Processing and Control, 29*, 11–21. doi:10.1016/j.bspc.2016.05.004

Dash, D. P., & Kolekar, M. H. (2017), EEG based Epileptic Seizure Detection using Empirical Mode Decomposition and Hidden Markov Model, Int conf Symhealth, Pune.

Dathe, A., Tarquis, A. M., & Perrier, E. (2006). Multifractal analysis of the pore-and solid-phases in binary two-dimensional images of natural porous structures. *Geoderma, 134*(3), 318–326. doi:10.1016/j.geoderma.2006.03.024

Datta, R., Joshi, D., Li, J., & Wang, J. (2008). Image retrieval: Ideas, Influences, and trends of the new age. *ACM Computing Surveys, 40*(2), 1–60. doi:10.1145/1348246.1348248

De Chazal, P., O Dwyer, M., & Reilly, R. B. (2004). Automatic classification of heartbeats using ECG morphology and heartbeat interval features. *IEEE Transactions on Bio-Medical Engineering, 51*(7), 1196–1206. doi:10.1109/TBME.2004.827359 PMID:15248536

De Chazel, P., & Reilly, R. B. (2000). A comparison of the ECG classification performance of different feature sets. *Computers in Cardiology, 2000*, 327–330.

de Herrera, A., Kalpathy–Cramer, J., Demner-Fushman, D., Antani, S., & Müller, H. (2013). Overview of the ImageCLEF 2013 medical tasks. *Working Notes of CLEF.*

Deepak, K. S., & Sivaswamy, J. (2012). Automatic assessment of macular edema from color retinal images. *IEEE Transactions on Medical Imaging, 31*(3), 766–776. doi:10.1109/TMI.2011.2178856 PMID:22167598

Demner-Fushman, D., Chapman, W., & McDonald, C. (2009). What can natural language processing do for clinical decision support? *Journal of Biomedical Informatics, 42*(5), 760–772. doi:10.1016/j.jbi.2009.08.007 PMID:19683066

Deng, Y., & Manjunath, B. (2001). Unsupervised segmentation of color-texture regions in images and video. *IEEE Transactions on Pattern Analysis and Machine Intelligence, 23*(8), 800–810. doi:10.1109/34.946985

Depeursinge, A., & Müller, H. (2010). Fusion techniques for combining textual and visual information retrieval. In *ImageCLEF* (pp. 95–114). Berlin: Springer. doi:10.1007/978-3-642-15181-1_6

Depeursinge, A., Racoceanu, D., Iavindrasana, J., Cohen, G., Platon, A., Poletti, P., & Müller, H. (2010). Fusing visual and clinical information for lung tissue classification in HRCT data. *Artificial Intelligence in Medicine.* doi:10.1016/j.artmed.2010.04.006

Depeursinge, A., Vargas, A., Gaillard, F., Platon, A., Geissbuhler, A., Poletti, P., & Müller, H. (2011). Case-based lung image categorization and retrieval for interstitial lung diseases: Clinical workflows. *International Journal of Computer Assisted Radiology and Surgery, 7*(1), 97–110. doi:10.1007/s11548-011-0618-9 PMID:21629982

Deselaers, T., Gass, T., Weyand, T., & Ney, H. (2007). FIRE in ImageCLEF 2007. Working Notes of CLEF 2007.

Deselaers, T., Weyand, T., & Ney, H. (2006). Image retrieval and annotation using maximum entropy. Working Notes of CLEF 2006.

Deselaers, T., Weyand, T., Keysers, D., Macherey, W., & Ney, H. (2005). FIRE in ImageCLEF 2005: Combining content–based image retrieval with textual information retrieval. *Working Notes of the CLEF Workshop.*

Deshmukh, A., & Panditrao, A. (2014). Automated leukemia detection using contour signature in blood microscopic images. *International Journal of Research in Computer and Communication Technology*, 304-308.

Dhote, V., Bhatnagar, P., Mishra, P. K., Mahajan, S. C., & Mishra, D. K. (2012). Iontophoresis: A potential emergence of a transdermal drug delivery system. *Scientia Pharmaceutica*, *80*(1), 1–28. doi:10.3797/scipharm.1108-20 PMID:22396901

Dodrill, C. B. (1997). Myths of neuropsychology. *The Clinical Neuropsychologist*, *11*(1), 1–17. doi:10.1080/13854049708407025 PMID:10806469

Dollinger, M., Ko, A., & Rosenbaum, E. (2008). *Everyone's guide to cancer therapy*. Riverside: Andrew's McMeel Publishing.

Dorini, L., Minetto, R., & Leite, N. (2007) White blood cell segmentation using morphological operators and scale-space analysis. *XX Brazilian Symposium on Computer Graphics and Image Processing*, 294-304. doi:10.1109/SIBGRAPI.2007.33

Dwivedi, A. R., Bari, H., Nath, S., Bajaj, V., Sharma, D., & Kumar, A. (2016). Analysis of focal and non-focal EEG signals using bivariate empirical mode decomposition. *IEEE Students' Conference on Electrical, Electronics and Computer Science*, 1–3. doi:10.1109/SCEECS.2016.7509318

Dyck, P. J., Kratz, K. M., Karnes, J. L., Litchy, W. J., Klein, R., Pach, J. M., & Melton, L. (1993). The prevalence by staged severity of various types of diabetic neuropathy, retinopathy, and nephropathy in a population-based cohort The Rochester Diabetic Neuropathy Study. *Neurology*, *43*(4), 817–817. doi:10.1212/WNL.43.4.817 PMID:8469345

Eakins, J. P. (2002). Towards intelligent image retrieval. *Pattern Recognition*, *35*(1), 3–14. doi:10.1016/S0031-3203(01)00038-3

Early Treatment Diabetic Retinopathy Study Research Group. (1991). Grading diabetic retinopathy from stereoscopic color fundus photographs—an extension of the modified Airlie House classification: ETDRS report number 10. *Ophthalmology*, *98*(5), 786–806. doi:10.1016/S0161-6420(13)38012-9 PMID:2062513

Efros & Leung. (1999). Texture synthesis by non-parametric sampling. *International Conference on Computer Vision*, 2(9), 1033–1038.

Eisemann, E., & Durand, F. (2002). Flash Photography Enhancement via Intrinsic Relighting. *ACM Transactions on Graphics*, *23*(3), 673–678. doi:10.1145/1015706.1015778

Elad, M. (2002, October). On the Bilateral Filter and Ways To Improve It. *IEEE Transactions on Image Processing*, *11*(10), 1141–1151. doi:10.1109/TIP.2002.801126 PMID:18249686

El-Kwae, E., Xu, H., & Kabuka, M. (2000). Content-based retrieval in picture archiving and communication systems. *Journal of Digital Imaging*, *13*(2), 70–81. doi:10.1007/BF03168371 PMID:10843252

Elmaoğlu, M., & Çelik, A. (2012). *MR Physics, Patient Positioning, and Protocols*. Springer.

Elveren, E., & Yumuşak, N. (2011). Tuberculosis disease diagnosis using artificial neural network trained with genetic algorithm. *Journal of Medical Systems*, *35*(3), 329–332. doi:10.1007/s10916-009-9369-3 PMID:20703557

El-Zahra, El-Gamal, Elmogy, & Atwan. (2016). Current trends in medical image registration and fusion. *Egyptian Informatics Journal*, *17*, 99–124.

Emerson, M. V., Pieramici, D. J., Stoessel, K. M., Berreen, J. P., & Gariano, R. F. (2001). Incidence and rate of disappearance of retinal hemorrhage in newborns. *Ophthalmology*, *108*(1), 36–39. doi:10.1016/S0161-6420(00)00474-7 PMID:11150261

Endo, M., Aramaki, T., Asakura, K., Moriguchi, M., Akimaru, M., Osawa, A., & Yamaguchi, K. (2012). Content-based image- retrieval system in chest computed tomography for a solitary pulmonary nodule: Method and preliminary experiments. *International Journal of Computer Assisted Radiology and Surgery*, *7*(2), 331–338. doi:10.1007/s11548-011-0668-z PMID:22258753

Escalante, H., González, J., Hernández, C., López, A., Montes, M., Morales, E., & Villasenor, L. (2008, September). TIA-INAOE's Participation at ImageCLEF 2008. *Working Notes of the CLEF 2008 Workshop.*

Fakeri-Tabrizi, A., Amini, M., Tollari, S., & Gallinari, P. (2008). *UPMC/LIP6 at ImageCLEF's WikipediaMM: An image–annotation model for an image search–engine. Working Notes of CLEF.*

Farnia, P., Ahmadian, A., Khoshnevisan, A., Jaberzadeh, A. H., Serej, N. D., & Kazerooni, A. F. (2011). *An efficient Point Based Registration of Intra-operative Ultrasound images with MR images for computation of brain shift: A Phantom Study.* 33rd Annual International Conference of the IEEE EMBS Boston, MA.

Feng, P., Pan, Y., Wei, B., Jin, W., & Mi, D. (2007). Enhancing retinal image by the Contourlet transform. *Pattern Recognition Letters*, *28*(4), 516–522. doi:10.1016/j.patrec.2006.09.007

Ferecatu, M., & Sahbi, H. (2008, September). TELECOM ParisTech at ImageClefphoto 2008: Bi-modal text and image retrieval with diversity enhancement. Working Notes for the CLEF 2008 Workshop.

Fetterhoff, D., Kraft, R. A., Sandler, R. A., Opris, I., Sexton, C. A., Marmarelis, V. Z., & Deadwyler, S. A. et al. (2015). Distinguishing cognitive state with multifractal complexity of hippocampal interspike interval sequences. *Frontiers in Systems Neuroscience*, *9*, 130. doi:10.3389/fnsys.2015.00130 PMID:26441562

Filho, C. F. F. C., Levy, P. C., Xavier, C. de M., Fujimoto, L. B. M., & Costa, M. G. F. (2015). Automatic identification of tuberculosis mycobacterium. *Research on Biomedical Engineering*, *31*(1), 33–43. doi:10.1590/2446-4740.0524

Fischer, B., Welter, P., Günther, R., & Deserno, T. (2012). Web-based bone age assessment by content-based image retrieval for case-based reasoning. *International Journal of Computer Assisted Radiology and Surgery*, *7*(3), 389–399. doi:10.1007/s11548-011-0627-8 PMID:21671096

Fleming, A. D., Goatman, K. A., Philip, S., Williams, G. J., Prescott, G. J., Scotland, G. S., & Olson, J. A. (2009). The role of haemorrhage and exudate detection in automated grading of diabetic retinopathy. *The British Journal of Ophthalmology*. PMID:19661069

Flickner, M., Sawhney, H., Niblack, W., Ashley, J., Huang, Q., Dom, B., & Yanker, P. (1995). Query by image and video content: The QBIC system. *Computer*, *28*(9), 23–32. doi:10.1109/2.410146

Florea, F., Rogozan, A., Cornea, V., Bensrhair, A., & Darmoni, S. (2006, September). MedIC/CISMeF at ImageCLEF 2006: Image annotation and retrieval tasks. *Working Notes of the 2006 CLEF Workshop.*

Flores, E., Tobon, G., Cavallaro, E., Cavallaro, F. I., Perry, J. C., & Keller, T. (2008, December). Improving patient motivation in game development for motor deficit rehabilitation. In *Proceedings of the 2008 International Conference on Advances in Computer Entertainment Technology* (pp. 381-384). ACM. doi:10.1145/1501750.1501839

Forero, M. G., Cristóbal, G., & Desco, M. (2006). Automatic identification of Mycobacterium tuberculosis by Gaussian mixture models. *Journal of Microscopy*, *223*(2), 120–132. doi:10.1111/j.1365-2818.2006.01610.x PMID:16911072

Forsberg, D. (2013). *Robust Image Registration for Improved Clinical Efficiency Using Local Structure Analysis and Model-Based Processing*. Linköping Studies in Science and Technology. Dissertations, No. 1514.

Friedman, C., & Elhadad, N. (2014). Natural language processing in health care and biomedicine. In Biomedical. Informatics: Computer Applications in Health Care and Biomedicine. Springer London. doi:10.1007/978-1-4471-4474-8_8

Friedman, C. (2005). Semantic text parsing for patient records. *Medical Informatics*, *8*, 423–448.

Gabor, A. J., Leach, R. R., & Dowla, F. U. (1996). Automated seizure detection using a self-organizing neural network. *Electroencephalography and Clinical Neurophysiology, 99*(3), 257-266.

Gerig, G., Kubler, O., Kikinis, R., & Jolesz, F. A. (1992). Nonlinear anisotropic filtering of MRI data. *IEEE Transactions on Medical Imaging*, *11*(2), 221–232. doi:10.1109/42.141646 PMID:18218376

Gershon, J., Zimand, E., Lemos, R., Rothbaum, B. O., & Hodges, L. (2003). Use of virtual reality as a distractor for painful procedures in a patient with pediatric cancer: A case study. *Cyberpsychology & Behavior*, *6*(6), 657–661. doi:10.1089/109493103322725450 PMID:14756933

Gershon, J., Zimand, E., Pickering, M., Rothbaum, B. O., & Hodges, L. (2004). A pilot and feasibility study of virtual reality as a distraction for children with cancer. *Journal of the American Academy of Child and Adolescent Psychiatry*, *43*(10), 1243–1249. doi:10.1097/01.chi.0000135621.23145.05 PMID:15381891

Gerstmair, A., Daumke, P., Simon, K., Langer, M., & Kotter, E. (2012). Intelligent image retrieval based on radiology reports. *European Radiology*, *22*(12), 2750–2758. doi:10.1007/s00330-012-2608-x PMID:22865274

Ghosh-Dastidar, S., Adeli, H., & Dadmehr, N. (2008). Principal component analysis-enhanced cosine radial basis function neural network for robust epilepsy and seizure detection. *IEEE Transactions on Bio-Medical Engineering*, *55*(2), 512–518. doi:10.1109/TBME.2007.905490 PMID:18269986

Ghosh, P., Antani, S., Rodney, L., & Thoma, G. (2011). Review of medical Image retrieval systems and future. *Computer Based Medical Systems*, *24*, 1–6. doi:10.1109/CBMS.2011.5999142

Giancardo, L., Meriaudeau, F., Karnowski, T. P., Li, Y., Garg, S., Tobin, K. W. Jr, & Chaum, E. (2012). Exudate-based diabetic macular edema detection in fundus images using publicly available datasets. *Medical Image Analysis*, *16*(1), 216–226. doi:10.1016/j.media.2011.07.004 PMID:21865074

Gladstone, M. (2010). A review of the incidence and prevalence, types and aetiology of childhood cerebral palsy in resource-poor settings. *Annals of Tropical Paediatrics*, *30*(3), 181–196. doi:10.1179/146532810X12786388978481 PMID:20828451

Glikfeld, P., Cullander, C., Hinz, R. S., & Guy, R. H. (1988). A new system for in vitro studies of iontophoresis. *Pharmaceutical Research*, *5*(7), 443–446. doi:10.1023/A:1015944619348 PMID:3247315

Global Tuberculosis Control. (2011). WHO Report.

Gobeill, J., Müller, H., & Ruch, P. (2006). *Query and document translation by automatic text categorization: A simple approach to establish a strong textual baseline for ImageCLEFmed 2006. ImageCLEF Working Notes.*

Gold, J. I., Kant, A. J., & Kim, S. H. (2005, December). Virtual anesthesia: the use of virtual reality for pain distraction during acute medical interventions. In Seminars in Anesthesia, Perioperative Medicine and Pain (Vol. 24, No. 4, pp. 203-210). WB Saunders. doi:10.1053/j.sane.2005.10.005

Gold, J. I., Kim, S. H., Kant, A. J., Joseph, M. H., & Rizzo, A. S. (2006). Effectiveness of virtual reality for pediatric pain distraction during IV placement. *Cyberpsychology & Behavior*, *9*(2), 207–212. doi:10.1089/cpb.2006.9.207 PMID:16640481

Goyal, A., Roy, M., Gupta, P., Dutta, M. K., Singh, S. & Garg, V. (2015). Automatic Detection of Mycobacterium tuberculosis in Stained Sputum and Urine Smear Images. *Archives of Clinical Microbiology, 6*(3-5), 1-4.

Green, P. G., Flanagan, M., Shroot, B., & Guy, R. H. (1993). Iontophoretic drug delivery. *Drugs and the Pharmaceutical Sciences, 59*, 311-333.

Gronningsaeter, A., Unsgaerd, G., Ommedal, S., & Angelsen, B. A. J. (1996). Ultrasound-guided neurosurgery: A feasibility study in the 3-30 MHz frequency range. *British Journal of Neurosurgery, 10*(2), 161-168.

Gudbjartsson & Partz. (2008). *The Rician Distribution of Noisy MRI data.* HHS Public Access Manuscript, PMC.

Gutiérrez, J., Alcántara, R., & Medina, V. (2001). Analysis and localization of epileptic events using wavelet packets. *Medical Engineering & Physics, 23*(9), 623–631. doi:10.1016/S1350-4533(01)00096-0 PMID:11755807

Halim, N., Mashor, M., Nasir, A. S. A., Mokhtar, N. R., & Rosline, H. (2011) Nucleus segmentation technique for acute Leukemia. *IEEE 7th International Colloquium on Signal Processing and its Applications*, 192-197. doi:10.1109/CSPA.2011.5759871

Hall, M. A. (1999). *Correlation-based Feature Selection for Machine Learning* (Ph.D. thesis). The University of Waikato, Hamilton, New Zealand.

Hall, M., Frank, E., Holmes, G., Pfahringer, B., Reutemann, P., & Witten, I. H. (2009). The WEKA Data Mining Software: An Update. *SIGKDD Explor. Newsl., 11*(1), 10–18. doi:10.1145/1656274.1656278

Hamarneh, G., & Hradsky, J. (2007). Bilateral filtering of diffusion tensor magnetic resonance images. *IEEE Transactions on Image Processing, 16*(10), 1723–1730. doi:10.1109/TIP.2007.904964 PMID:17926929

Hammoud, Ligon, Elsouki, Shi, Schomer, & Sawaya. (1996). Use of intraoperative ultrasound for localizing tumors and determining the extent of resection: A comparative study with magnetic resonance imaging. *Journal of Neurosurgery, 84*, 737–741.

Haralick, R., Shanmugam, K., & Dinstein, I. (1973). Textural features for image classification. *IEEE Transactions on Systems, Man, and Cybernetics, 3*(6), 610–621. doi:10.1109/TSMC.1973.4309314

Harrar, K., & Khider, M. (2014). Texture analysis using multifractal spectrum. *International Journal of Modeling and Optimization, 4*(4), 336–341. doi:10.7763/IJMO.2014.V4.396

Harris, K., & Reid, D. (2005). The influence of virtual reality play on childrens motivation. *Canadian Journal of Occupational Therapy, 72*(1), 21–29. doi:10.1177/000841740507200107 PMID:15727045

Harris, R. (1967). *Iontophoresis* (Vol. 15). Baltimore, MD: Waverly Press.

Hassan, K., Bukhari, K., Zafar, A., Malik, M., & Akhtar, M. (1992). Acute leukemia in children. French-American-British (FAB) classification and its relation to clinical features. *JPMA. The Journal of the Pakistan Medical Association, 42*, 29–31. PMID:1573762

Haworth, C., Hepplestone, A., Jones, P. M., Campbell, R., & Evans, M. P. D. (1981). Routine Bone Marrow Examination in the Management of Acute Lymphoblastic Leukemia of childhood. *Journal of Clinical Pathology, 34*(5), 483–485. doi:10.1136/jcp.34.5.483 PMID:6941970

Hazlyna, H. N., Mashor, M., Mokhtar, N., Salihah, A. A., Hassan, R., Raof, R., & Osman, M. (2010). Comparison of acute leukemia Image segmentation using HSI and RGB color space. *10th International Conference on Information Sciences Signal Processing and their Applications*, 749-752. doi:10.1109/ISSPA.2010.5605410

Hemsley, A., & Mukundan, R. (2009, December). Multifractal measures for tissue image classification and retrieval. *11th IEEE International Symposium on Multimedia, 2009. ISM'09*, 618-623. doi:10.1109/ISM.2009.94

Hermitage Museum. (2003). *QBIC colour and layout searches.* Retrieved from http://www.hermitagemuseum.org/fcgi-bin/db2www/qbicSearch.mac/qbic?selLang=English

Herrera, G., Alcantud, F., Jordan, R., Blanquer, A., Labajo, G., & De Pablo, C. (2008). Development of symbolic play through the use of virtual reality tools in children with autistic spectrum disorders Two case studies. *Autism, 12*(2), 143–157. doi:10.1177/1362361307086657 PMID:18308764

Hersh, M. A. (2008). Perception, the eye and assistive technology issues. In *Assistive Technology for Visually Impaired and Blind People* (pp. 51–101). Springer London. doi:10.1007/978-1-84628-867-8_2

Hersh, W., & Hickam, D. (1995). Information retrieval in medicine: The SAPHIRE experience. *JASIS, 46*(10), 743–747. doi:10.1002/(SICI)1097-4571(199512)46:10<743::AID-ASI5>3.0.CO;2-C PMID:8591469

Hiremath, P., Bannigidad, P., & Geeta, S. (2010). Automated Identification and Classification of White Blood Cells (Leukocytes) in Digital Microscopic Images. *IJCA,* 59-63.

Hoffman, H. G., Patterson, D. R., Seibel, E., Soltani, M., Jewett-Leahy, L., & Sharar, S. R. (2008). Virtual reality pain control during burn wound debridement in the hydrotank. *The Clinical Journal of Pain, 24*(4), 299–304. doi:10.1097/AJP.0b013e318164d2cc PMID:18427228

Horsch, K., Giger, M., Vyborny, C., Lan, L., Mendelson, E., & Hendrick, R. (2006). Classification of breast lesions with multimodality computer-aided diagnosis: Observer study results on an independent clinical data set 1. *Radiology, 240*(2), 357–368. doi:10.1148/radiol.2401050208 PMID:16864666

Ho, T., Hull, J., & Srihari, S. (1994). Decision combination in multiple classifier systems. *IEEE Transactions on Pattern Analysis and Machine Intelligence, 16*(1), 66–75. doi:10.1109/34.273716

Houston, A., Chen, H., Schatz, B., Hubbard, S., Sewell, R., & Ng, T. (2000). Exploring the use of concept spaces to improve medical information retrieval. *Decision Support Systems, 30*(2), 171–186. doi:10.1016/S0167-9236(00)00097-X

Hsu, C. W., & Lin, C. J. (2002). A comparison of methods for multiclass support vector machines. *IEEE Transactions on Neural Networks, 13*(2), 415–425. doi:10.1109/72.991427 PMID:18244442

Hu, X. (2004). The Past, Present And Future Of Magnetic Resonance Imaging. Frontiers in Biomedical Engineering, 283-294. DOI doi:10.1007/978-1-4419-8967-3_18

Huang, N. E., Shen, Z., Long, S. R., Wu, M. C., Shih, H. H., Zheng, Q., . . . Liu, H. H. (1998). The empirical mode decomposition and the Hilbert spectrum for nonlinear and non-stationary time series analysis. *Proceedings of the Royal Society of London. Series A: Mathematical, Physical and Engineering Sciences, 454*(1971), 903–995. doi:10.1098/rspa.1998.0193

Huang, H., Nielsen, J., Nelson, M., & Liu, L. (2005). Image-matching as a medical diagnostic support tool (DST) for brain diseases in children. *Computerized Medical Imaging and Graphics, 29*(2), 195–202. doi:10.1016/j.compmedimag.2004.09.008 PMID:15755537

Huang, K., Velliste, M., & Murphy, R. F. (2003, June). Feature reduction for improved recognition of subcellular location patterns in fluorescence microscope images. In *Biomedical Optics 2003* (pp. 307–318). International Society for Optics and Photonics.

Humphrey, S., Rogers, W., Kilicoglu, H., Demner-Fushman, D., & Rindflesch, T. (2006). Word sense disambiguation by selecting the best semantic type based on Journal Descriptor Indexing: Preliminary experiment. *Journal of the American Society for Information Science and Technology, 57*(1), 96–113. doi:10.1002/asi.20257 PMID:19890434

Hussain, M., Khan, S., Muhammad, G., Berbar, M., & Bebis, G. (2012, July). Mass detection in digital mammograms using gabor filter bank. *IET Conference on Image Processing (IPR 2012)*, 1-5. doi:10.1049/cp.2012.0465

Hu, Y. H., Palreddy, S., & Tompkins, W. J. (1997). A patient-adaptable ECG beat classifier using a mixture of experts approach. *IEEE Transactions on Bio-Medical Engineering*, *44*(9), 891–900. doi:10.1109/10.623058 PMID:9282481

Hu, Y. H., Tompkins, W. J., Urrusti, J. L., & Afonso, V. X. (1992). Applications of artificial neural networks for ECG signal detection and classification. *Journal of Electrocardiology*, *26*, 66–73. PMID:8189150

Hwang, K., Lee, H., & Choi, D. (2012). Medical image retrieval: Past and present. *Healthcare Informatics Research*, *18*(1), 3–9. doi:10.4258/hir.2012.18.1.3 PMID:22509468

IMAIOS. (n.d.). *Medical websites and e learning for medical professionals*. Retrieved from www.imaios.com

Ince, T., Kiranyaz, S., & Gabbouj, M. (2009). A generic and robust system for automated patient-specific classification of ECG signals. *IEEE Transactions on Bio-Medical Engineering*, *56*(5), 1415–1426. doi:10.1109/TBME.2009.2013934 PMID:19203885

Iniewski, K. (2009). *Medical Imaging Principles, Detectors & Electronics*. John Wiley & Sons, Inc.

Inkpen, D., Stogaitis, M., DeGuire, F., & Alzghool, M. (2009). Clustering for photo retrieval at Image CLEF 2008. In *Evaluating Systems for Multilingual and Multimodal Information Access* (pp. 685–690). Berlin: Springer. doi:10.1007/978-3-642-04447-2_86

International Diabetes Federation (IDF). (2015). Facts & figures. Retrieved from https://www.idf.org/about-diabetes/what-is-diabetes?language=en

Iovannone, R., Dunlap, G., Huber, H., & Kincaid, D. (2003). Effective educational practices for students with autism spectrum disorders. *Focus on Autism and Other Developmental Disabilities*, *18*(3), 150–165. doi:10.1177/10883576030180030301

Iqbal, A., Valous, N. A., Sun, D. W., & Allen, P. (2011). Parsimonious classification of binary lacunarity data computed from food surface images using kernel principal component analysis and artificial neural networks. *Meat Science*, *87*(2), 107–114. doi:10.1016/j.meatsci.2010.08.014 PMID:21062668

Jain, A., & Vailaya, A. (1996). Image retrieval using color and shape. *Pattern Recognition*, *29*(8), 1233–1244. doi:10.1016/0031-3203(95)00160-3

James, T. N. (2002). Structure and function of the sinus node, AV node and his bundle of the human heart: Part I—structure. *Progress in Cardiovascular Diseases, 45*(3), 235-267.

Jégou, H., Douze, M., & Schmid, C. (2010). Improving bag-of-features for large scale image search. *International Journal of Computer Vision*, *87*(3), 316–336. doi:10.1007/s11263-009-0285-2

Jekel, K., Damian, M., Wattmo, C., Hausner, L., Bullock, R., Connelly, P. J., & Kramberger, M. G. et al. (2015). Mild cognitive impairment and deficits in instrumental activities of daily living: A systematic review. *Alzheimers Research & Therapy*, *7*(1), 1. doi:10.1186/s13195-015-0099-0 PMID:25815063

Jenkins, C. R., Thien, F. C. K., Wheatley, J. R., & Reddel, H. K. (2005). Traditional and patient-centred outcomes with three classes of asthma medication. *The European Respiratory Journal*, *26*(1), 36–44. doi:10.1183/09031936.05.00144704 PMID:15994387

Jeon, J., Lavrenko, V., & Manmatha, R. (2003, July). Automatic image annotation and retrieval using cross-media relevance models. In *Proceedings of the 26th annual international ACM SIGIR conference on Research and development in informaion retrieval* (pp. 119-126). ACM. doi:10.1145/860435.860459

Jha, C. K., & Kolekar, M. H. (2016, January). Efficient ECG data compression and transmission algorithm for telemedicine. *International Conference on Communication Systems and Networks*, (pp. 1-6). IEEE. doi:10.1109/COMSNETS.2016.7439988

Jiang, W., & Kong, S. G. (2007). Block-based neural networks for personalized ECG signal classification. *IEEE Transactions on Neural Networks*, *18*(6), 1750–1761. doi:10.1109/TNN.2007.900239 PMID:18051190

Jingkun, L., Guizhi, X., Jianrong, G., Feng, Z., & Xiuyan, F. (2010, May). Analysis of virtual simulation environment for driving behavior based on imaging movements. In *Networking and Digital Society (ICNDS), 2010 2nd International Conference on* (Vol. 1, pp. 246-248). IEEE. doi:10.1109/ICNDS.2010.5479148

Ji, S., Wu, Z., Hartov, A., Roberts, D. W., & Paulsen, K. D. (2008). Mutual-information-based image to patient re-registration using intraoperative ultrasound in image-guided neurosurgery. *Medical Physics*, *35*(10), 4612–4624. doi:10.1118/1.2977728 PMID:18975707

Jolliffe, I. (2002). *Principal component analysis*. John Wiley & Sons, Ltd.

Jones, G., Groves, D., Khasin, A., Lam-Adesina, A., Mellebeek, B., & Way, A. (2005). Dublin City University at CLEF 2004: Experiments with the ImageCLEF St. Andrew's Collection. In *Multilingual Information Access for Text, Speech and Images* (pp. 653–663). Berlin: Springer. doi:10.1007/11519645_64

Joshi, M. A., & Joshi, K. R. (2015). Quantitative analysis of MR image quality is extremely critical for correct interpretation of the clinical data in the image. CRC Press.

Juan, L., & Gwun, O. (2009). A comparison of sift, PCA-sift and surf. *Int. J. Image Process.*, *3*(5), 143–152.

Jue-Chen, L., Ying, S., Siddiqui, O., Wei-min, S., & John, L. (1988). Blood glucose control in diabetic rats by transdermal iontophoretic delivery of insulin. *International Journal of Pharmaceutics*, *44*(1-3), 197–204. doi:10.1016/0378-5173(88)90116-0

Kaivukangas, J., Salni, Y. L., Lakuilala, J., & Oikarinen, J. (1993). Ultrasound -Controlled Neronavigator-guided brain Surgery. *Journal of Neurosurgery*, *79*, 36-42.

Kalia, Y. N., Merino, V., & Guy, R. H. (1998). Transdermal drug delivery: Clinical aspects. *Dermatologic Clinics*, *16*(2), 289–299. doi:10.1016/S0733-8635(05)70011-5 PMID:9589202

Kalia, Y. N., Naik, A., Garrison, J., & Guy, R. H. (2004). Iontophoretic drug delivery. *Advanced Drug Delivery Reviews*, *56*(5), 619–658. doi:10.1016/j.addr.2003.10.026 PMID:15019750

Kamieth, F., Arca, A., Villalar, J. L., Arredondo, M. T., Dähne, P., Wichert, R., & Jimenez-Mixco, V. (2010). *Exploring the Potential of Virtual Reality for the Elderly and People with Disabilities*. INTECH Open Access Publisher.

Kampouraki, A., Manis, G., & Nikou, C. (2009). Heartbeat time series classification with support vector machines. *IEEE Transactions on Information Technology in Biomedicine*, *13*(4), 512–518. doi:10.1109/TITB.2008.2003323 PMID:19273030

Kanaris, I., Kanaris, K., Houvardas, I., & Stamatatos, E. (2007). Words versus character n-grams for anti-spam filtering. *International Journal of Artificial Intelligence Tools*, *16*(06), 1047–1067. doi:10.1142/S0218213007003692

Karacali, B. (2007). Information theoretic deformable registration using local image information. *IJCV,Vol, 72*(3), 219–237. doi:10.1007/s11263-006-8704-0

Karakoç, Y., Aydemir, E. H., Kalkan, M. T., & Ünal, G. (2002). Safe control of palmoplantar hyperhidrosis with direct electrical current. *International Journal of Dermatology, 41*(9), 602–605. doi:10.1046/j.1365-4362.2002.01473.x PMID:12358834

Karvelis, P. S., Fotiadis, D. I., Georgiou, I., & Sakaloglou, P. (2009, September). Enhancement of the classification of multichannel chromosome images using support vector machines. *Annual International Conference of the IEEE Engineering in Medicine and Biology Society*, 3601-3604. doi:10.1109/IEMBS.2009.5333757

Kaupp, U. B., & Seifert, R. (2001). Molecular diversity of pacemaker ion channels. *Annual Review of Physiology, 63*(1), 235-257.

Kelly, P., Cannon, T., & Hush, D. (1995). Query by image example: the CANDID approach. *SPIE 2420 Storage and Retrieval for Image and Video Databases III*, 238-248. doi:.10.1117/12.205289

Keysers, D., Dahmen, J., Ney, H., Wein, B. B., & Lehmann, T. M. (2003). Statistical framework for model-based image retrieval in medical applications. *Journal of Electronic Imaging, 12*(1), 59–68. doi:10.1117/1.1525790

Khandoker, A. H., Lai, D. T. H., Begg, R. K., & Palaniswami, M. (2007). Wavelet-based feature extraction for support vector machines for screening balance impairments in the elderly. *IEEE Transactions on Neural Systems and Rehabilitation Engineering, 15*(4), 587–597. doi:10.1109/TNSRE.2007.906961 PMID:18198717

Khutlang, R., Krishnan, S., Whitelaw, A., & Douglas, T. S. (2010). Automated detection of tuberculosis in Ziehl-Neelsen-stained sputum smears using two one-class classifiers. *Journal of Microscopy, 237*(1), 96–102. doi:10.1111/j.1365-2818.2009.03308.x PMID:20055923

Kim, B. S., Yoo, S. K., & Lee, M. H. (2006). Wavelet-based low-delay ECG compression algorithm for continuous ECG transmission. *IEEE Transactions on Information Technology in Biomedicine, 10*(1), 77–83. doi:10.1109/TITB.2005.856854 PMID:16445252

Kim, J., & Fessler, J. A. (2004, November). Intensity-based image registration using robust correlation coefficients. *IEEE Transactions on Medical Imaging, 23*(11), 1430–1444. doi:10.1109/TMI.2004.835313 PMID:15554130

Kim, S., & Dey, A. K. (2009, April). Simulated augmented reality windshield display as a cognitive mapping aid for elder driver navigation. In *Proceedings of the SIGCHI Conference on Human Factors in Computing Systems* (pp. 133-142). ACM. doi:10.1145/1518701.1518724

Kizony, R., Korman, M., Sinoff, G., Klinger, E., Josman, N., Sharky, P. M., & Klinger, E. (2012). Using a virtual supermarket as a tool for training executive functions in people with mild cognitive impairment. *Proceedings of the 9th International Conference on Disability, Virtual Reality and Associated Technologies*, 41-46.

Kludas, J., Bruno, E., & Marchand-Maillet, S. (2008). Information fusion in multimedia information retrieval. In *Adaptive Multimedial Retrieval: Retrieval, User, and Semantics* (pp. 147–159). Berlin: Springer. doi:10.1007/978-3-540-79860-6_12

Knechel, N. A. (2009). Tuberculosis: Pathophysiology, clinical features, and diagnosis. *Critical Care Nurse, 29*(2), 34–43. doi:10.4037/ccn2009968 PMID:19339446

Kohavi, R. (1995). A study of cross-validation and bootstrap for accuracy estimation and model selection. *Proceedings of the 14th International Joint Conference on Artificial Intelligence.*

Koivukangas, J., & Kelly, P.J. (1986). Application of ultrasound imaging to stereotactic brain tumor surgery. *Annals of Clinical Research Supplement*, (47), 25-32.

Kolb, H., Fernandez, E., & Nelson, R. (1995). *Facts and Figures Concerning the Human Retina--Webvision*. The Organization of the Retina and Visual System.

Kolekar, M. H., & Dash, D. P. (2015). A nonlinear feature based epileptic seizure detection using least square support vector machine classifier. TENCON 2015 - 2015 IEEE Region 10 Conference, 1–6. doi:10.1109/TENCON.2015.7373164

Kolekar, M. H., & Dash, D. P. (2015, November). A nonlinear feature based epileptic seizure detection using least square support vector machine classifier. *TENCON 2015- Region 10 Conference* (pp. 1-6). IEEE.

Kolekar, M. H., & Dash, D. P. 2015, November. A nonlinear feature based epileptic seizure detection using least square support vector machine classifier. In TENCON 2015-2015 IEEE Region 10 Conference (pp. 1-6). IEEE.

Kolekar, M. H., & Sengupta, S. (2015). Bayesian network-based customized highlight generation for broadcast soccer videos. *IEEE Transactions on Broadcasting, 61*(2), 195-209.

Kolekar, M. H., & Sengupta, S. 2004, December. Hidden markov model based video indexing with discrete cosine transform as a likelihood function. In India Annual Conference, 2004. Proceedings of the IEEE INDICON 2004. First (pp. 157-159). IEEE.

Kolekar, M. H. (2011). Bayesian Belief Network Based Broadcast Sports Video Indexing. *Int. Springer Journal of Multimedia Tools and Applications, 54*, 27–54.

Kolekar, M. H., Dash, D. P., & Patil, P. N. (2017). Support Vector Machine Based Extraction of Crime Information in Human Brain Using ERP Image. *International Conference on Computer Vision and Image Processing* (pp. 163-174). Springer. doi:10.1007/978-981-10-2107-7_15

Kolekar, M. H., & Sengupta, S. (2004 Dec), Hidden Markov Model based Video Indexing with Discrete Cosine Transform as a Likelihood Function, *IEEE INDICON Conference*, India.

Kolekar, M. H., & Sengupta, S. (2004). Hidden Markov Model Based Structuring of Cricket Video Sequences Using Motion and Color Features. *Indian Conference on Computer Vision, Graphics and Image Processing*, 632-637.

Kolekar, M. H., & Sengupta, S. (2005). *Semantic Indexing of News Video Sequences: A Multimodal Hierarchical Approach Based on Hidden Markov Model, IEEE Int. Region 10 Conference*. Melbourne, Australia: TENCON.

Kolekar, M. H., & Sengupta, S. (2015). Bayesian Network-Based Customized Highlight Generation for Broadcast Soccer Videos. *IEEE Transactions on Broadcasting, 61*(2), 195–209.

Kolekar, M. H., Talbar, S. N., & Sontakke, T. R. (2000). Texture Segmentation using Fractal Signature. *IETE Journal of Research, India, 46*(5), 319–323.

Küchler, S., Abdel-Mottaleb, M., Lamprecht, A., Radowski, M. R., Haag, R., & Schäfer-Korting, M. (2009). Influence of nanocarrier type and size on skin delivery of hydrophilic agents. *International Journal of Pharmaceutics, 377*(1), 169–172. doi:10.1016/j.ijpharm.2009.04.046 PMID:19439166

Kuklinski, W. S. (1983). Fast Walsh transform data-compression algorithm: ECG applications. *Medical & Biological Engineering & Computing, 21*(4), 465–472. doi:10.1007/BF02442635 PMID:6888014

Kulasuriya, K. H., & Perera, M. (2011) Focal epileptic seizure forecasting in EEG signals using wavelet transform and artificial neural networks. *IEEE International Conference on Control System, Computing and Engineering*, 296–301. doi:10.1109/ICCSCE.2011.6190540

Kulkarni, P., Stranieri, A., Kulkarni, S., Ugon, J., & Mittal, M. (2014b, April). Visual character n-grams for classification and retrieval of radiological images. *International Journal of Multimedia and its Applications, 6*(2), 35-49

Kulkarni, P., Stranieri, A., Kulkarni, S., Ugon, J., & Mittal, M. (2014a, February). Hybrid technique based on n-gram and neural networks for classification of mammographic images. *Second International Conference on Signal, Image Processing and Pattern Recognition*, 297–306. doi:10.5121/csit.2014.4225

Kulkarni, S., & Verma, B. (2003, September). Fuzzy logic based texture queries for CBIR. *Proceedings of Fifth International Conference on Computational Intelligence and Multimedia Applications*, 223-228. doi:10.1109/ICCIMA.2003.1238129

Kumar, A., & Kolekar, M. H. (2014), Machine Learning Approach for Epileptic Seizure Detection Using Wavelet Analysis of EEG Signals, *Int. Conf. on Medical Imaging, M-health and Emerging Communication Systems.*

Kumar, A., & Kolekar, M. H. (2014). Machine learning approach for epileptic seizure detection using wavelet analysis of eeg signals. *International Conference on Medical Imaging, m-Health and Emerging Communication Systems*, 412–416. doi:10.1109/MedCom.2014.7006043

Kumar, R., Kumar, A., & Pandey, R. K. (2013). Beta wavelet based ECG signal compression using lossless encoding with modified thresholding. *Computers & Electrical Engineering*, *39*(1), 130–140. doi:10.1016/j.compeleceng.2012.04.008

Kumar, T. S., Kanhangad, V., & Pachori, R. B. (2014). Classification of seizure and seizure-free EEG signals using multi-level local patterns. *Proceedings of 19th International Conference on Digital Signal Processing*, 646–650. doi:10.1109/ICDSP.2014.6900745

Kurtz, C., Beaulieu, C., Napel, S., & Rubin, D. (2014). A hierarchical knowledge-based approach for retrieving similar medical images described with semantic annotations. *Journal of Biomedical Informatics*, *49*, 227–244. doi:10.1016/j.jbi.2014.02.018 PMID:24632078

Labati, R., Piuri, V., & Scotti, F. (2011). All-IDB: The acute lymphoblastic leukemia image database for image processing. *18th IEEE International Conference on Image Processing*, 2045-2048. doi:10.1109/ICIP.2011.6115881

Lagerholm, M., Peterson, C., Braccini, G., Edenbrandt, L., & Sornmo, L. (2000). Clustering ECG complexes using Hermite functions and self-organizing maps. *IEEE Transactions on Bio-Medical Engineering*, *47*(7), 838–848. doi:10.1109/10.846677 PMID:10916254

Landini, G. (2011). Fractals in microscopy. *Journal of Microscopy*, *241*(1), 1–8. doi:10.1111/j.1365-2818.2010.03454.x PMID:21118245

Langlotz, C. P. (2006). RadLex: A new method for indexing online educational materials1. *Radiographics*, *26*(6), 1595–1597. doi:10.1148/rg.266065168 PMID:17102038

Lavrenko, V., Manmatha, R., & Jeon, J. (2003). A model for learning the semantics of pictures. Advances in Neural Information Processing Systems.

Leduc, S. (1900). Introduction of medicinal substances into the depth of tissues by electric current. *Ann. Electrobiol*, *3*, 545–560.

Lee, J. H. (1997, July). Analyses of multiple evidence combination. *ACM SIGIR Forum, 31*, 267-276. doi:10.1145/258525.258587

Lee, S., & Lee, M. (2008, August). A real-time ECG data compression algorithm for a digital holter system. In *2008 30th Annual International Conference of the IEEE Engineering in Medicine and Biology Society* (pp. 4736-4739). IEEE. doi:10.1109/IEMBS.2008.4650271

Lee, H., & Buckley, K. M. (1999). ECG data compression using cut and align beats approach and 2-D transforms. *IEEE Transactions on Bio-Medical Engineering*, *46*(5), 556–564. doi:10.1109/10.759056 PMID:10230134

Lee, J. (1995, July). Combining multiple evidence from different properties of weighting schemes. In *Proceedings of the 18th annual international ACM SIGIR conference on Research and development in information retrieval* (pp. 180-188). ACM. doi:10.1145/215206.215358

Lee, S., Kim, J., & Lee, M. (2011). A real-time ECG data compression and transmission algorithm for an e-health device. *IEEE Transactions on Bio-Medical Engineering*, *58*(9), 2448–2455. doi:10.1109/TBME.2011.2156794 PMID:21606020

Lehnertz, K., & Elger, C. E. (1995). Spatio-temporal dynamics of the primary epileptogenic area in temporal lobe epilepsy characterized by neuronal complexity loss. *Electroencephalography and Clinical Neurophysiology*, *95*(2), 108–117. doi:10.1016/0013-4694(95)00071-6 PMID:7649002

Lenseigne, B., Brodin, P., Jeon, H. K., Christophe, T., & Genovesio, A. (2007, April). Support vector machines for automatic detection of tuberculosis bacteria in confocal microscopy images. *4th IEEE International Symposium on Biomedical Imaging: From Nano to Macro*, 85-88. doi:10.1109/ISBI.2007.356794

Levac, D., Rivard, L., & Missiuna, C. (2012). Defining the active ingredients of interactive computer play interventions for children with neuromotor impairments: A scoping review. *Research in Developmental Disabilities*, *33*(1), 214–223. doi:10.1016/j.ridd.2011.09.007 PMID:22093667

Levin, M.F. (2011). *Virtual reality: Rehabilitation applications in children with disabilities*. Academic Press.

Lewis, J. J., Chihota, V. N., van der Meulen, M., Fourie, P. B., Fielding, K. L., Grant, A. D., & Churchyard, G. J. et al. (2012). Proof-Of-Concept Evaluation of an Automated Sputum Smear Microscopy System for Tuberculosis Diagnosis. *PLoS ONE*, *7*(11), e50173. doi:10.1371/journal.pone.0050173 PMID:23209666

Li, J., & Wang, J. Z. (2006). *ALIPR: Automatic photo tagging and visual image search*. Retrieved from http://www. alipr. com

Lilly, J. M., & Gascard, J.-C. (2006). Wavelet ridge diagnosis of time-varying elliptical signals with application to an oceanic eddy. *Nonlinear Processes in Geophysics*, *13*(5), 467–483. doi:10.5194/npg-13-467-2006

Lilly, J. M., & Olhede, S. C. (2010). Bivariate instantaneous frequency and bandwidth. *IEEE Transactions on Signal Processing*, *58*(2), 591–603. doi:10.1109/TSP.2009.2031729

Lim, J. H., & Chevallet, J. P. (2005). Vismed: a visual vocabulary approach for medical image indexing and retrieval. In Information Retrieval Technology (pp. 84-96). Springer Berlin Heidelberg. doi:10.1007/11562382_7

Lim, H., Mashor, M., & Hassan, R. (2012). White blood cell segmentation for acute leukemia bone marrow images. *International Conference on Biomedical Engineering*, 357-361. doi:10.1109/ICoBE.2012.6179038

Lin, S., & Hong, Y. (2012). Differential count of white blood cell in noisy normal blood smear. *7th IEEE Conference on Industrial Electronics and Applications*, 1784-1789.

Lionello, G., Sirieix, C., & Baleanin, M. (2014). An effective procedure to create a speckle pattern on biological soft tissue for digital image correlation measurements. *Journal of the Mechanical Behavior of Biomedical Materials*, *39*, 1–8.

Li, Q., Li, F., Shiraishi, J., Katsuragawa, S., Sone, S., & Doi, K. (2003). Investigation of new psychophysical measures for evaluation of similar images on thoracic computed tomography for distinction between benign and malignant nodules. *Medical Physics*, *30*(10), 2584–2593. doi:10.1118/1.1605351 PMID:14596294

Li, Q., & Wu, Y. (2006). Identifying important concepts from medical documents. *Journal of Biomedical Informatics*, *39*(6), 668–679. doi:10.1016/j.jbi.2006.02.001 PMID:16545986

Li, S., Zhou, W., Yuan, Q., Geng, S., & Cai, D. (2013). Feature extraction and recognition of ictal EEG using EMD and SVM. *Computers in Biology and Medicine*, *43*(7), 807–816. doi:10.1016/j.compbiomed.2013.04.002 PMID:23746721

Liu, C. T., Tai, P. L., Chen, A. Y. J., Peng, C. H., Lee, T., & Wang, J. S. (2001, August). A content-based ct lung image retrieval system for assisting differential diagnosis images collection. *2001 IEEE International Conference on Multimedia and Expo (ICME'01).*

Liu, Y., Zhang, D., Lu, G., & Ma, W. Y. (2007). A survey of content-based image retrieval with high-level semantics. *Pattern Recognition*, *40*(1), 262–282. doi:10.1016/j.patcog.2006.04.045

Long, F., Zhang, H., & Feng, D. D. (2003). Fundamentals of content-based image retrieval. In *Multimedia Information Retrieval and Management* (pp. 1–26). Berlin: Springer. doi:10.1007/978-3-662-05300-3_1

Lopes, R., & Betrouni, N. (2009). Fractal and multifractal analysis: A review. *Medical Image Analysis*, *13*(4), 634–649. doi:10.1016/j.media.2009.05.003 PMID:19535282

Lotte, F., Congedo, M., Lécuyer, A., Lamarche, F., & Arnaldi, B. (2007). A review of classification algorithms for EEG-based brain–computer interfaces. *Journal of Neural Engineering*, *4*(2), R1–R13. doi:10.1088/1741-2560/4/2/R01 PMID:17409472

Lowell, J., Hunter, A., Steel, D., Basu, A., Ryder, R., & Kennedy, R. L. (2004). Measurement of retinal vessel widths from fundus images based on 2-D modeling. *IEEE Transactions on Medical Imaging*, *23*(10), 1196–1204. doi:10.1109/TMI.2004.830524 PMID:15493688

Lu, X., Peng, X., Liu, P., Deng, Y., Feng, B., & Liao, B. (2012). A novel feature selection method based on CFS in cancer detection. *IEEE 6th International Conference on Systems Biology*, 226-231.

Luna-Oliva, L., Ortiz-Gutiérrez, R. M., Cano-de la Cuerda, R., Piédrola, R. M., Alguacil-Diego, I. M., Sánchez-Camarero, C., & Martínez Culebras, M. D. C. (2013). Kinect Xbox 360 as a therapeutic modality for children with cerebral palsy in a school environment: A preliminary study. *NeuroRehabilitation*, *33*(4), 513–521. PMID:24018364

Lu, Z., Kim, D. Y., & Pearlman, W. A. (2000). Wavelet compression of ECG signals by the set partitioning in hierarchical trees algorithm. *IEEE Transactions on Bio-Medical Engineering*, *47*(7), 849–856. doi:10.1109/10.846678 PMID:10916255

Madhloom, H., Kareem, S., & Arifin, H. (2012). A Robust Feature Extraction and Selection Method for the Recognition of Lymphocytes versus Acute Lymphoblastic Leukemia. *International Conference on Advanced Computer Science Applications and Technologies*, 330-335. doi:10.1109/ACSAT.2012.62

Maes, F., Collignon, A., Vandermeulen, D., Marchal, G., & Suetens, P. (1997). Multimodality image registration by maximization of mutual information. *IEEE Transactions on Medical Imaging*, *16*(2), 187–198. doi:10.1109/42.563664 PMID:9101328

Maex, R. (2013). Nernst-Planck Equation. In D. Jaeger & R. Jung (Eds.), *Encyclopedia of Computational Neuroscience* (pp. 1–7). New York, NY: Springer New York.

Magalh˜aes, J., Overell, S., & Rüger, S. (2007). Exploring image, text and geographic evidences. *ImageCLEF 2007.*

Maillot, N., Chevallet, J., Valea, V., & Lim, J. (2006). *IPAL inter-media pseudo-relevance feedback approach to imageclef 2006 photo retrieval. CLEF Working Notes.*

Maintz, J. B. A., & Viergever, M. A. (1998). A survey of medical image registration. *Medical Image Analysis*, *2*(1), 1–36. doi:10.1016/S1361-8415(01)80026-8 PMID:10638851

Malhi, A., & Gao, R. X. (2004). PCA-based feature selection scheme for machine defect classification. *IEEE Transactions on Instrumentation and Measurement*, *53*(6), 1517–1525. doi:10.1109/TIM.2004.834070

Malloy, K. M., & Milling, L. S. (2010). The effectiveness of virtual reality distraction for pain reduction: A systematic review. *Clinical Psychology Review*, *30*(8), 1011–1018. doi:10.1016/j.cpr.2010.07.001 PMID:20691523

Man, D. W., Chung, J. C., & Lee, G. Y. (2012). Evaluation of a virtual reality-based memory training programme for Hong Kong Chinese older adults with questionable dementia: A pilot study. *International Journal of Geriatric Psychiatry*, *27*(5), 513–520. doi:10.1002/gps.2746 PMID:21681818

Mandelbrot, B. B. (1967). How long is the coast of Britain. *Science*, *156*(3775), 636–638. doi:10.1126/science.156.3775.636 PMID:17837158

Mandic, D. P., Rehman, N. U., Wu, Z., & Huang, N. E. (2013). Empirical mode decomposition–based time–frequency analysis of multivariate signals: The power of adaptive data analysis. *IEEE Signal Processing Magazine*, *30*(6), 74–86. doi:10.1109/MSP.2013.2267931

Manikandan, S. (2011). Measures of dispersion. *Journal of Pharmacology and Pharmacotherapeutics*, *2*(4), 315–316. doi:10.4103/0976-500X.85931 PMID:22025871

Manjon, Robles, & Thacker. (2007). Multispectral MRI de-noising using non-local means. *Med. Image Understand. Anal. (MIUA)*, 41–46.

Manjón, J. V., Carbonell-Caballero, J., Lull, J. J., García-Martí, G., Martí-Bonmatí, L., & Robles, M. (2008). MRI denoising using non-local means. *Medical Image Analysis*, *12*(4), 514–523. doi:10.1016/j.media.2008.02.004 PMID:18381247

Manjón, J. V., Coupe, P., Martí-Bonmatí, L., Collins, D. L., & Robles, M. (2010). Adaptive non-local means denoising of MR images with spatially varying noise levels. *Magnetic Resonance Imaging*, *31*(1), 192–203. doi:10.1002/jmri.22003 PMID:20027588

Mao, W., & Chu, W. (2007). The phrase-based vector space model for automatic retrieval of free-text medical documents. *Data & Knowledge Engineering*, *61*, 76–92.

Marciani, M. G., Stefanini, F., Stefani, N., Maschio, M. C. E., Gigli, G. L., Roncacci, S., & Bernardi, G. et al. (1992). Lateralization of the epileptogenic focus by çomputerized EEG study and neuropsychological evaluation. *The International Journal of Neuroscience*, *66*(1–2), 53–60. doi:10.3109/00207459208999789 PMID:1304570

Mariappan, P. M., Raghavan, D. R., Aleem, S. H. A., & Zobaa, A. F. (2016). Effects of electromagnetic interference on the functional usage of medical equipment by 2G/3G/4G cellular phones: A review. *Journal of Advanced Research*, 7(5), 727-738.

Markiewicz, T., Osowski, S., Marianska, B., & Moszczynski, L. (2005). Automatic recognition of the blood cells of myelogenous leukemia using SVM. *IEEE International Joint Conference on Neural Networks*, 4, 2496-2501. doi:10.1109/IJCNN.2005.1556295

Martínez-Fernández, J., Serrano, A., Villena, J., Sáenz, V., Tortosa, S., Castagnone, M., & Alonso, J. (2004, September). MIRACLE at ImageCLEF 2004. *Working Notes for the CLEF 2004 Workshop*, 545-553.

Martis, R. J., Acharya, U. R., Tan, J. H., Petznick, A., Yanti, R., Chua, C. K., Ng, E. Y. K., and Tong, L. (2012). Application of empirical mode decomposition (EMD) for automated detection of epilepsy using EEG signals. *International Journal of Neural Systems*, 22(6), 1–16.

Ma, W., Deng, Y., & Manjunath, B. (1997, June). Tools for texture-and color-based search of images. *Human Vision and Electronic Imaging II, SPIE*, *3016*, 496–507.

McGibney, G., & Smith, M. (1993). Unbiased signal-to-noise ratio measure for magnetic resonance images. *Medical Physics*, *20*(4), 1077–1078. doi:10.1118/1.597004 PMID:8413015

McPherson, C. (n.d.). *Video lecture on "Image guided Surgery"*. Mayfield Clinic and UC Brain Tumor Center. Retrieved from www.youtube.com

McVeigh, E. R., Henkelman, R. M., & Bronskill, M. J. (1985). Noise and filtration in magnetic resonance imaging. *Medical Physics*, *12*(5), 586–591. doi:10.1118/1.595679 PMID:4046992

Medi, B. M., & Singh, J. (2003). Electronically facilitated transdermal delivery of human parathyroid hormone (1–34). *International Journal of Pharmaceutics*, *263*(1), 25–33. doi:10.1016/S0378-5173(03)00337-5 PMID:12954177

Mejia-Guevara, I., Morales, A., & Kuri, F. (2007). MP-Polynomial Kernel for Training Support Vector Machines. In *CIARP of Lecture Notes in Computer Science* (Vol. 4756, pp. 584–593). Springer.

Melgani, F., & Bazi, Y. (2008). Classification of electrocardiogram signals with support vector machines and particle swarm optimization. *IEEE Transactions on Information Technology in Biomedicine*, *12*(5), 667–677. doi:10.1109/TITB.2008.923147 PMID:18779082

Mercier, L., Fonov, V., Haegelen, C., Maestro, R.F.D., Petrecca, K., & Collins, D. L. (2012). Comparing two approaches to rigid registration of three-dimensional ultrasound and magnetic resonance images for neurosurgery. *Int J Comput Assist Radiol Surg.*, *7*(1), 125-36.

Mercier, L., Maestro, R. F. Del, Petrecca, K., Kochanowska, A., Drouin, S., Yan, C. X. B., … Collins, L. (2011). New prototype neuronavigation system based on preoperative imaging and intraoperative freehand ultrasound: system description and validation. *Int J CARS, 6*, 507–522.

Mercier, L., Araujo, D., Haegelen, C., Maestro, R. F. D., Petrecca, K., & Collins, D. L. (2013, January). Registering pre- and postresection 3-dimensional ultrasound for improved visualization of residual brain tumor. *Ultrasound in Medicine & Biology*, *39*(1), 16–29. doi:10.1016/j.ultrasmedbio.2012.08.004 PMID:23200177

Mercier, L., DelMaestro, R. F., Petrecca, K., Araujo, D., Haegelen, C., & Collins, D. L. (2012, June). Online database of clinical MR and ultrasound images of brain tumors. *Medical Physics*, *6*(39), 3253–3261. doi:10.1118/1.4709600 PMID:22755708

Meyer, R. E. (1996). Neuropsychopharmacology: Are we ready for a paradigm shift? *Neuropsychopharmacology*, *14*(3), 169–179. doi:10.1016/0893-133X(95)00074-N PMID:8866700

Michailovich, O. V., & Tannenbaum, A. (2006). De-speckling of medical ultrasound images. *IEEE Transactions on Ultrasonics, Ferroelectrics, and Frequency Control, 53*(1).

Michailovich, O., & Adam, D. (2003). Robust Estimation of Ultrasound Pulses Using Outlier-Resistant De-Noising. *IEEE Transactions on Medical Imaging, 22*(3).

Millar, E., Shen, D., Liu, J., & Nicholas, C. (2006). Performance and scalability of a large-scale n-gram based information retrieval system. *Journal of Digital Information*, *1*(5), 1–25.

Mina, T., Behzad, A., & Rassoul, A. (2009). Assessment of depth of anes-thesia using principal component analysis. *J Biomedical Science and Engineering*, *96*(2), 9–15.

MIPAV. (2005). Labeling and Measuring Brain Components in Talairach Space. National Institutes of Health Center for Information Technology.

Miranda, J. G. V., Montero, E., Alves, M. C., González, A. P., & Vázquez, E. V. (2006). Multifractal characterization of saprolite particle-size distributions after topsoil removal. *Geoderma*, *134*(3), 373–385. doi:10.1016/j.geoderma.2006.03.014

Mitchell, P., Parsons, S., & Leonard, A. (2007). Using virtual environments for teaching social understanding to 6 adolescents with autistic spectrum disorders. *Journal of Autism and Developmental Disorders*, *37*(3), 589–600. doi:10.1007/s10803-006-0189-8 PMID:16900403

Mitra, M., Bera, J. N., & Gupta, R. (2012). Electrocardiogram compression technique for global system of mobile-based offline telecardiology application for rural clinics in India. *IET Science. Measurement Techniques*, *6*(6), 412–419.

Mittelstadt, B. D., & Floridi, L. (2016). *The ethics of biomedical big data*. Springer. doi:10.1007/978-3-319-33525-4

Mladenic, D. (2006). Feature Selection for Dimensionality Reduction. In *Subspace, Latent Structure and Feature Selection* (Vol. 3940, pp. 84–102). Berlin: Springer. doi:10.1007/11752790_5

Modarresi, M., & Oveisi, I. S. (2014, June). A Contourlet Transform Based for Features Fusion in Retina and Iris Multimodal Biometric System. In *International Workshop on Biometric Authentication* (pp. 75-90). Springer International Publishing. doi:10.1007/978-3-319-13386-7_7

Moffat, S. D. (2009). Aging and spatial navigation: What do we know and where do we go? *Neuropsychology Review*, *19*(4), 478–489. doi:10.1007/s11065-009-9120-3 PMID:19936933

Mohamed, M., Far, B., & Guaily, A. (2012). An efficient technique for white blood cells nuclei automatic segmentation. *IEEE International Conference on Systems, Man, and Cybernetics*, 220-225. doi:10.1109/ICSMC.2012.6377703

Mohapatra, S., Patra, D., & Satpathy, S. (2010). Image analysis of blood microscopic images for acute leukemia detection. *International Conference on Industrial Electronics, Control Robotics*, 215-219. doi:10.1109/IECR.2010.5720171

Mohapatra, S., Patra, D., & Satpathy, S. (2013). An ensemble classifier system for early diagnosis of acute lymphoblastic leukemia in blood microscopic images. *Neural Computing & Applications*, 1–18.

Moiyadi, A., Shetty, V., & Shetty, P. (2016). Direct navigated 3d ultrasound for resection of brain tumors: A useful tool for intraoperative image guidance. *Neurosurgical Focus*, *40*(3), E5. doi:10.3171/2015.12.FOCUS15529 PMID:26926063

Montani, S., & Bellazzi, R. (2002). Supporting decisions in medical applications: The knowledge management perspective. *International Journal of Medical Informatics*, *68*(1), 79–90. doi:10.1016/S1386-5056(02)00067-9 PMID:12467793

Moody, G. B., & Mark, R. G. (2001). The impact of the MIT-BIH arrhythmia database. *IEEE Engineering in Medicine and Biology Magazine*, *20*(3), 45–50. doi:10.1109/51.932724 PMID:11446209

Mookiah, M. R. K., Acharya, U. R., Chua, C. K., Lim, C. M., Ng, E. Y. K., & Laude, A. (2013). Computer-aided diagnosis of diabetic retinopathy: A review. *Computers in Biology and Medicine*, *43*(12), 2136–2155. doi:10.1016/j.compbiomed.2013.10.007 PMID:24290931

Moore, K., & Kim, L. (2009). Primary Brain Tumors: Characteristics, Practical Diagnostic and Treatment Approaches. *Glioblastoma*, 43-75.

Moore, D., Cheng, Y., McGrath, P., & Powell, N. J. (2005). Collaborative virtual environment technology for people with autism. *Focus on Autism and Other Developmental Disabilities*, *20*(4), 231–243. doi:10.1177/10883576050200040501

Morales-Carbajal, C., Bravo-Zanoguera, M. E., Vera-Perez, M., Arriola, H., Lopez-Avitia, R., & Reyna-Carranza, M. A. (2010). *Identification of tuberculosis bacillus in direct smears with low image quality. Pan American Health Care Exchange*. PAHCE.

Morel, J.-M., & Yu, G. (2009). ASIFT: A new framework for fully affine invariant image comparison. *SIAM Journal on Imaging Sciences*, *2*(2), 438–469. doi:10.1137/080732730

Mori, Y., Takahashi, H., & Oka, R. (1999, October). Image-to-word transformation based on dividing and vector quantizing images with words. *First International Workshop on Multimedia Intelligent Storage and Retrieval Management*.

Morrow, D., McCarron, P., Woolfson, A., & Donnelly, R. (2007). Innovative strategies for enhancing topical and transdermal drug delivery. *The Open Drug Delivery Journal, 1*, 36-59.

Mott, J., Bucolo, S., Cuttle, L., Mill, J., Hilder, M., Miller, K., & Kimble, R. M. (2008). The efficacy of an augmented virtual reality system to alleviate pain in children undergoing burns dressing changes: A randomised controlled trial. *Burns*, *34*(6), 803–808. doi:10.1016/j.burns.2007.10.010 PMID:18325675

Moulin, C., Barat, C., Géry, M., Ducottet, C., & Largeron, C. (2009). UJM at ImageCLEFwiki 2008. In *Evaluating Systems for Multilingual and Multimodal Information Access* (pp. 779–786). Berlin: Springer. doi:10.1007/978-3-642-04447-2_101

Mukhopadhyay, S., Gupta, A., & Bansal, R. (2014). Needs/Requirements and Design of Retinal Imaging and Image Processing Methods for Diabetic Retinopathy in the Indian Context. In *Ophthalmological Imaging and Applications* (pp. 127–134). CRC Press. doi:10.1201/b17026-8

Müller, H. (2013). Medical (visual) information retrieval. In *Information Retrieval Meets Information Visualization* (pp. 155–166). Berlin: Springer. doi:10.1007/978-3-642-36415-0_10

Müller, H., Clough, P., Deselaers, T., & Caputo, B. (Eds.). (2010). *ImageCLEF: Experimental Evaluation in Visual Information Retrieval.* Springer. doi:10.1007/978-3-642-15181-1

Müller, H., Michoux, N., Bandon, D., & Geissbuhler, A. (2004). A review of content-based image retrieval systems in medical applications—clinical benefits and future directions. *International Journal of Medical Informatics*, *73*(1), 1–23. doi:10.1016/j.ijmedinf.2003.11.024 PMID:15036075

Müller, H., Rosset, A., Vallée, J., & Geissbuhler, A. (2002). Integrating content-based visual access methods into a medical case database. *Studies in Health Technology and Informatics*, *95*, 480–485. PMID:14664033

Muñoz-Diosdado, A., & Del Río-Correa, J. L. (2006, August). Further study of the asymmetry for multifractal spectra of heartbeat time series. *Engineering in Medicine and Biology Society, 2006. EMBS'06. 28th Annual International Conference of the IEEE*, 1450-1453. doi:10.1109/IEMBS.2006.260166

Muramatsu, C., Schmidt, R., Shiraishi, J., Li, Q., & Doi, K. (2010). Presentation of similar images as a reference for distinction between benign and malignant masses on mammograms: Analysis of initial observer study. *Journal of Digital Imaging*, *23*(5), 592–602. doi:10.1007/s10278-009-9263-z PMID:20054606

Muramatsu, C., Suzuki, K., Schmidt, R., Shiraishi, J., Newstead, G., & Doi, K. (2005). Investigation of psychophysical measure for evaluation of similar images for mammographic masses: Preliminary results. *Medical Physics*, *32*(7), 2295–2304. doi:10.1118/1.1944913 PMID:16121585

Nadkarni, P., Ohno-Machado, L., & Chapman, W. (2011). Natural language processing: An introduction. *Journal of the American Medical Informatics Association*, *18*(5), 544–551. doi:10.1136/amiajnl-2011-000464 PMID:21846786

Naik, A., Kalia, Y. N., & Guy, R. H. (2000). Transdermal drug delivery: Overcoming the skins barrier function. *Pharmaceutical Science & Technology Today*, *3*(9), 318–326. doi:10.1016/S1461-5347(00)00295-9 PMID:10996573

Nair, V., Pillai, O., Poduri, R., & Panchagnula, R. (1999). Transdermal iontophoresis. Part I: Basic principles and considerations. *Methods and Findings in Experimental and Clinical Pharmacology*, *21*(2), 139–151. doi:10.1358/mf.1999.21.2.529241 PMID:10327395

Nakayama, R., Abe, H., Shiraishi, J., & Doi, K. (2009). Potential usefulness of similar images in the differential diagnosis of clustered Microcalcifications on Mammograms. *Radiology, 253*(3), 625–631. doi:10.1148/radiol.2533090373 PMID:19789245

Napel, S., Beaulieu, C., Rodriguez, C., Cui, J., Xu, J., Gupta, A., & Rubin, D. (2010). Automated retrieval of CT images of liver lesions on the basis of image similarity: Method and preliminary results. *Radiology, 256*(1), 243–252. doi:10.1148/radiol.10091694 PMID:20505065

Nassif, H., Woods, R., Burnside, E., Ayvaci, M., Shavlik, J., & Page, D. (2009, December). Information extraction for clinical data mining: A mammography case study. *IEEE International Conference on Data Mining Workshops*, 37-42. doi:10.1109/ICDMW.2009.63

National Library of Medicine NLM. (2014). Retrieved from http://www.nlm.nih.gov/

Nayak, R., Shenoy, V. P., & Galigekere, R. R. (2010). A new algorithm for automatic assessment of the degree of TB-infection using images of ZN-stained sputum smear. *Proceedings of International Conference on Systems in Medicine and Biology (ICSMB)*, 294–299. doi:10.1109/ICSMB.2010.5735390

NCD Risk Factor Collaboration. (2016). Worldwide trends in diabetes since 1980: A pooled analysis of 751 population-based studies with 4· 4 million participants. *Lancet, 387*(10027), 1513–1530. doi:10.1016/S0140-6736(16)00618-8 PMID:27061677

Niblack, C., Barber, R., Equitz, W., Flickner, M., Glasman, E., Petkovic, D., & Taubin, G. (1993, April). QBIC project: Querying images by content, using color, texture, and shape. *IS&T/SPIE's Symposium on Electronic Imaging: Science and Technology*, 173-187.

Niemeijer, M., Van Ginneken, B., Cree, M. J., Mizutani, A., Quellec, G., Sánchez, C. I., & Wu, X. (2010). Retinopathy online challenge: Automatic detection of microaneurysms in digital color fundus photographs. *IEEE Transactions on Medical Imaging, 29*(1), 185–195. doi:10.1109/TMI.2009.2033909 PMID:19822469

Niemeijer, M., van Ginneken, B., Russell, S. R., Suttorp-Schulten, M. S., & Abramoff, M. D. (2007). Automated detection and differentiation of drusen, exudates, and cotton-wool spots in digital color fundus photographs for diabetic retinopathy diagnosis. *Investigative Ophthalmology & Visual Science, 48*(5), 2260–2267. doi:10.1167/iovs.06-0996 PMID:17460289

Nigris, D. D., Collins, D. L., & Arbel, T. (2012). Multi-Modal Image Registration Based on Gradient Orientations of Minimal Uncertainty. *IEEE Transactions on Medical Imaging, 31*(12), 2343-2354.

Nigris, D. D., Mercier, L., Maestro, R. D., Collins, D. L., & Arbel, T. (2010). Hierarchical Multimodal Image Registration Based on Adaptive Local Mutual Information. *LNCS, 6362*, 643–651.

Nilsson, E. (2007). *Multifractal-based image analysis with applications in medical imaging*. Umea, Sweden: Umea Univ.

Nilsson, S., Finnström, B., Kokinsky, E., & Enskär, K. (2009). The use of Virtual Reality for needle-related procedural pain and distress in children and adolescents in a paediatric oncology unit. *European Journal of Oncology Nursing, 13*(2), 102–109. doi:10.1016/j.ejon.2009.01.003 PMID:19230769

Nister, D., & Stewenius, H. (2006). Scalable recognition with a vocabulary tree. *IEEE Computer Society Conference on Computer Vision and Pattern Recognition, 2*, 2161-2168.

Novianto, S., Guimaraes, L., Suzuki, Y., Maeda, J., & Anh, V. V. (1999). Multiwindowed approach to the optimum estimation of the local fractal dimension for natural image segmentation. *International Conference on Image Processing*, 3, 222-226. doi:10.1109/ICIP.1999.817105

Nowak, R. D. (1999). Wavelet-based Rician noise removal for magnetic resonance imaging. *IEEE Transactions on Image Processing*, *8*(10), 1408–1419. doi:10.1109/83.791966 PMID:18267412

Ojala, T., Pietikinen, M., & Harwood, D. (1994). Performance evaluation of texture measures with classification based on Kullback discrimination of distributions. *Proceedings of the 12th IAPR International Conference on Pattern Recognition*, 582-585. doi:10.1109/ICPR.1994.576366

Okabe, K., Yamaguchi, H., & Kawai, Y. (1986). New iontophoretic transdermal administration of the beta-blocker metoprolol. *Journal of Controlled Release*, *4*(2), 79–85. doi:10.1016/0168-3659(86)90043-X

Olmos, S., Millan, M., Garcia, J., & Laguna, P. (1996, September). ECG data compression with the Karhunen-Loeve transform. In Computers in Cardiology, 1996 (pp. 253-256). IEEE.

Optale, G., Urgesi, C., Busato, V., Marin, S., Piron, L., Priftis, K., & Bordin, A. et al. (2010). Controlling memory impairment in elderly adults using virtual reality memory training: A randomized controlled pilot study. *Neurorehabilitation and Neural Repair*, *24*(4), 348–357. doi:10.1177/1545968309353328 PMID:19934445

Osman, M. K., Mashor, M. Y., & Jaafar, H. (2010). Detection of mycobacterium tuberculosis in Ziehl Neelsen stained tissue images using Zernike moments and hybrid multilayered perceptron network. *Proceedings of IEEE International Conference on Systems Man and Cybernetics*, 4049-4055. doi:10.1109/ICSMC.2010.5642191

Osman, M. K., Mashor, M. Y., & Jaafar, H. (2012). Performance comparison of extreme learning machine algorithms for mycobacterium tuberculosis detection in tissue sections. *Journal of Medical Imaging and Health Informatics*, *2*(3), 307–312. doi:10.1166/jmihi.2012.1100

Osowski, S., Hoai, L. T., & Markiewicz, T. (2004). Support vector machine-based expert system for reliable heartbeat recognition. *IEEE Transactions on Bio-Medical Engineering*, *51*(4), 582–589. doi:10.1109/TBME.2004.824138 PMID:15072212

Oudejans, R. R., & Nieuwenhuys, A. (2009). Perceiving and moving in sports and other high-pressure contexts. *Progress in Brain Research*, *174*, 35–48. doi:10.1016/S0079-6123(09)01304-1 PMID:19477328

Oweis, R. J., & Abdulhay, E. W. (2011). Seizure classification in EEG signals utilizing Hilbert-Huang transform. *Biomedical Engineering Online*, *10*(38), 1–15. PMID:21609459

Oza & Joshi. (2017). Performance Analysis of Denoising Filters for MR Images. Advances in Computing Applications, 87-96.

Pachori, R. B. (2008). Discrimination between ictal and seizure-free EEG signals using empirical mode decomposition. *Research Letters in Signal Processing*, *293056*, 1–5. doi:10.1155/2008/293056

Pachori, R. B., & Patidar, S. (2014). Epileptic seizure classification in EEG signals using second-order difference plot of intrinsic mode functions. *Computer Methods and Programs in Biomedicine*, *113*(2), 494–502. doi:10.1016/j.cmpb.2013.11.014 PMID:24377902

Pagoulatos, N., Edwards, W. S., Haynor, D. R., & Kim, Y. (1999). Interactive 3-D Registration of Ultrasound and Magnetic Resonance Images Based on a Magnetic Position Sensor. IEEE Transactions on Information Technology in Biomedicine, 3(4).

Palomino, J. C., Leao, S. C., & Ritacco, V. (2007). *Tuberculosis 2007. From basic science to patient care*. Institute of Tropical Medicine.

Panet-Raymond, D., & Gotman, J. (1990). Asymmetry in delta activity in patients with focal epilepsy. *Electroencephalography and Clinical Neurophysiology*, *75*(6), 474–481. doi:10.1016/0013-4694(90)90134-6 PMID:1693892

Panicker, R. O., Soman, B., Saini, G., & Rajan, G. (2016). A Review of Automatic Methods Based on Image Processing Techniques for Tuberculosis Detection from Microscopic Sputum Smear Images. *Journal of Medical Systems, 40*(17), 1-13.

Pan, J., & Tompkins, W. J. (1985). A real-time QRS detection algorithm. *IEEE Transactions on Bio-Medical Engineering, BME-32*(3), 230–236. doi:10.1109/TBME.1985.325532 PMID:3997178

Pantic, I., Dacic, S., Brkic, P., Lavrnja, I., Pantic, S., Jovanovic, T., & Pekovic, S. (2014). Application of fractal and grey level co-occurrence matrix analysis in evaluation of brain corpus callosum and cingulum architecture. *Microscopy and Microanalysis, 20*(05), 1373–1381. doi:10.1017/S1431927614012811 PMID:24967845

Parekar, J., Porwal, P., & Kokare, M. (2016, October). Automatic retinal image registration using fully connected vascular tree. In *Signal and Information Processing (IConSIP), International Conference on* (pp. 1-5). IEEE. doi:10.1109/ICONSIP.2016.7857498

Paris, S., Kornprobst, P., Tumblin, J. T., & Durand, F. (2008). Bilateral Filtering: Theory and Applications. *Computer Graphics and Vision, 4*(1), 1–73. doi:10.1561/0600000020

Park, C., Looney, D., Kidmose, P., Ungstrup, M., & Mandic, D. P. (2011). Time-frequency analysis of EEG asymmetry using bivariate empirical mode decomposition. *IEEE Transactions on Neural Systems and Rehabilitation Engineering, 19*(4), 366–373. doi:10.1109/TNSRE.2011.2116805 PMID:21342855

Parsons, T. D. (2011a). Neuropsychological assessment using virtual environments: enhanced assessment technology for improved ecological validity. In Advanced Computational Intelligence Paradigms in Healthcare 6. Virtual Reality in Psychotherapy, Rehabilitation, and Assessment (pp. 271-289). Springer Berlin Heidelberg. doi:10.1007/978-3-642-17824-5_13

Parsons, T. D. (2015). Ecological validity in virtual reality-based neuropsychological assessment. *Information Science and Technology,*, 214-223.

Parsons, T. D., Courtney, C. G., Dawson, M. E., Rizzo, A. A., & Arizmendi, B. J. (2013, July). Visuospatial processing and learning effects in virtual reality based mental rotation and navigational tasks. In *International Conference on Engineering Psychology and Cognitive Ergonomics* (pp. 75-83). Springer Berlin Heidelberg. doi:10.1007/978-3-642-39360-0_9

Parsons, T. D., McPherson, S., & Interrante, V. (2013, March). Enhancing neurocognitive assessment using immersive virtual reality. In *Virtual and Augmented Assistive Technology (VAAT), 2013 1st Workshop on* (pp. 27-34). IEEE. doi:10.1109/VAAT.2013.6786190

Parsons, T. D., Bowerly, T., Buckwalter, J. G., & Rizzo, A. A. (2007). A controlled clinical comparison of attention performance in children with ADHD in a virtual reality classroom compared to standard neuropsychological methods. *Child Neuropsychology, 13*(4), 363–381. doi:10.1080/13825580600943473 PMID:17564852

Parsons, T. D., Courtney, C. G., Arizmendi, B. J., & Dawson, M. E. (2011, February). *Virtual Reality Stroop Task for neurocognitive assessment*. MMVR.

Parsons, T. D., Iyer, A., Cosand, L., Courtney, C., & Rizzo, A. A. (2009). Neurocognitive and psychophysiological analysis of human performance within virtual reality environments. *Studies in Health Technology and Informatics, 142*, 247–252. PMID:19377160

Parsons, T. D., & Reinebold, J. L. (2012). Adaptive virtual environments for neuropsychological assessment in serious games. *IEEE Transactions on Consumer Electronics, 58*(2), 197–204. doi:10.1109/TCE.2012.6227413

Parsons, T. D., & Rizzo, A. A. (2008). Affective outcomes of virtual reality exposure therapy for anxiety and specific phobias: A meta-analysis. *Journal of Behavior Therapy and Experimental Psychiatry*, *39*(3), 250–261. doi:10.1016/j.jbtep.2007.07.007 PMID:17720136

Parsons, T. D., & Rizzo, A. A. (2008). Initial validation of a virtual environment for assessment of memory functioning: Virtual reality cognitive performance assessment test. *Cyberpsychology & Behavior*, *11*(1), 17–25. doi:10.1089/cpb.2007.9934 PMID:18275308

Patidar, S., & Pachori, R. B. (2014). Classification of cardiac sound signals using constrained tunable-Q wavelet transform. *Expert Systems with Applications*, *41*(16), 7161–7170. doi:10.1016/j.eswa.2014.05.052

Patidar, S., Pachori, R. B., & Garg, N. (2015). Automatic diagnosis of septal defects based on tunable-Q wavelet transform of cardiac sound signals. *Expert Systems with Applications*, *42*(7), 3315–3326. doi:10.1016/j.eswa.2014.11.046

Patil, S. A., & Udupi, V. R. (2011). Geometrical and texture features estimation of lung cancer and TB images using chest X-ray database. *International Journal of Biomedical Engineering and Technology*, *6*(1), 58–75. doi:10.1504/IJBET.2011.040453

Pati, S., & Alexopoulos, A. V. (2010). Pharmacoresistant epilepsy: From pathogenesis to current and emerging therapies. *Cleveland Clinic Journal of Medicine*, *77*(7), 457–467. doi:10.3949/ccjm.77a.09061 PMID:20601619

Paul, V., & William, M. W. (1997). Alignment by Maximization of Mutual Information. *International Journal of Computer Vision*, *24*(2), 137–154. doi:10.1023/A:1007958904918

Pearson, K. (1901). On Lines and Planes of Closest Fit to Systems of Points in Space. *Philosophical Magazine*, *11*(1), 559–572. doi:10.1080/14786440109462720

Pedrosa, G., & Traina, A. (2013, August). From Bag-of-Visual-Words to Bag-of-Visual-Phrases Using n-Grams. *SIBGRAPI-Conference on Graphics, Patterns and Images,* 304-311. doi:10.1109/SIBGRAPI.2013.49

Pennec, X., Roche, A., Cathier, P., & Ayache, N. (2005). Non-Rigid MR/US Registration for Tracking Brain Deformations. In Multi-Sensor Image Fusion and Its Applications. CRC Press - Taylor and Francis.

Penney, G.P, Blackall, J.M., Hamady, M.S., Sabharwal, T., Adam, A., & Hawkes, D.J. (2004). Registration of freehand 3D ultrasound and magnetic resonance liver images. *Medical Image Analysis, 8*, 81–91.

Penney, G. P., Blackall, J. M., Hamady, M. S., Sabharwal, T., Adam, A., & Hawkes, D. J. (2004). Registration of freehand 3D ultrasound and magnetic resonance liver images. *Medical Image Analysis*, *8*(1), 81–91. doi:10.1016/j.media.2003.07.003 PMID:14644148

Pentland, A., Picard, R., & Sclaroff, S. (1996). Photobook: Content-based manipulation of image databases. *International Journal of Computer Vision, 18*(3), 233–254.

Perona, P., & Malik, J. (1990). Scale-space and edge detection using anisotropic diffusion. *IEEE Transactions on Pattern Analysis and Machine Intelligence*, *12*(7), 629–639. doi:10.1109/34.56205

Petridis, A. K., Anokhin, M., Vavruska, J., Mahvash, M., & Scholz, M. (2015). The value of intraoperative sonography in low grade glioma surgery. *Clinical Neurology and Neurosurgery*, *131*, 64–68. doi:10.1016/j.clineuro.2015.02.004 PMID:25704192

Pham, D., Xu, C., & Prince, J. (2000). Current methods in medical image segmentation 1. *Annual Review of Biomedical Engineering Arequipa, Peru, 2*(1), 315-337.

Philbin, J., Chum, O., Isard, M., Sivic, J., & Zisserman, A. (2007, June). Object retrieval with large vocabularies and fast spatial matching. *Proceedings of IEEE Conference on Computer Vision and Pattern Recognition*, 1-8. doi:10.1109/CVPR.2007.383172

Phipps, J., Padmanabhan, R., & Lattin, G. (1989). Iontophoretic delivery model inorganic and drug ions. *Journal of Pharmaceutical Sciences*, *78*(5), 365–369. doi:10.1002/jps.2600780505 PMID:2746475

Pikal, M. J. (1990). Transport mechanisms in iontophoresis. I. A theoretical model for the effect of electroosmotic flow on flux enhancement in transdermal iontophoresis. *Pharmaceutical Research*, *7*(2), 118–126. doi:10.1023/A:1015816532532 PMID:2308891

Pikal, M. J., & Shah, S. (1990a). Transport mechanisms in iontophoresis. II. Electroosmotic flow and transference number measurements for hairless mouse skin. *Pharmaceutical Research*, *7*(3), 213–221. doi:10.1023/A:1015857608850 PMID:2339092

Pikal, M. J., & Shah, S. (1990b). Transport mechanisms in iontophoresis. III. An experimental study of the contributions of electroosmotic flow and permeability change in transport of low and high molecular weight solutes. *Pharmaceutical Research*, *7*(3), 222–229. doi:10.1023/A:1015809725688 PMID:2339093

Pillai, O., Nair, V., Poduri, R., & Panchagnula, R. (1999). Transdermal iontophoresis. Part II: Peptide and protein delivery. *Methods and Findings in Experimental and Clinical Pharmacology*, *21*(3), 229–240. doi:10.1358/mf.1999.21.3.534833 PMID:10389126

Piraino, D. (2013). *Evaluation of Free text search of radiology reports for clinical decision support during radiology reporting using open source software.* Society for Imaging Informatics In Medicine Annual Meeting, Grapevine, TX.

Pires, R., Jelinek, H., Wainer, J., Goldenstein, S., Valle, E., & Rocha, A. (2013). Assessing the Need for Referral in Automatic Diabetic Retinopathy Detection. *IEEE Transactions on Bio-Medical Engineering*, *60*(12), 3391–3398. doi:10.1109/TBME.2013.2278845 PMID:23963192

Pittarello, F., & De Faveri, A. (2006, May). Improving access of elderly people to real environments: a semantic based approach. In *Proceedings of the working conference on Advanced visual interfaces* (pp. 364-368). ACM. doi:10.1145/1133265.1133341

Piuri, V., & Scotti, F. (2004). Morphological classification of blood leucocytes by microscope images. *IEEE International Conference on Computational Intelligence for Measurement Systems and Applications*, 103-108. doi:10.1109/CIMSA.2004.1397242

Pluim, J. P. W., Maintz, J. B. A., & Viergever, M. A. (2003). Mutual information based registration of medical images: A survey. *IEEE Transactions on Medical Imaging*.

Pollak, Y., Shomaly, H. B., Weiss, P. L., Rizzo, A. A., & Gross-Tsur, V. (2010). Methylphenidate effect in children with ADHD can be measured by an ecologically valid continuous performance test embedded in virtual reality. *CNS Spectrums*, *15*(02), 125–130. doi:10.1017/S109285290002736X PMID:20414157

Porter, M. (1980). An algorithm for suffix stripping. *Program: Electronic Library and Information Systems, 14*(3), 130-137.

Porwal, P., & Kokare, M. (2016, October). A novel method to remove bright artifacts for enhancing lesion detection in retinal images. In *Signal and Information Processing (IConSIP), International Conference on* (pp. 1-5). IEEE. doi:10.1109/ICONSIP.2016.7857474

Potts, R. O., & Francoeur, M. L. (1991). The influence of stratum corneum morphology on water permeability. *The Journal of Investigative Dermatology*, *96*(4), 495–499. doi:10.1111/1523-1747.ep12470197 PMID:2007788

Priya, E., Srinivasan, S., & Ramakrishnan, S. (2014). Retrospective Non-Uniform Illumination Correction Techniques in Images of Tuberculosis. *Microscopy and Microanalysis*, *20*(05), 1382–1391. doi:10.1017/S1431927614012896 PMID:25115957

Purwanti, E., & Widiyanti, P. (2012). Using learning vector quantization method for automated identification of mycobacterium tuberculosis. *Indonesian Journal of Tropical and Infectious Disease*, 3(1), 26-29.

Quellec, G., Lamard, M., Cazuguel, G., Cochener, B., & Roux, C. (2010). Wavelet optimization for content-based image retrieval in medical databases. *Medical Image Analysis*, *14*(2), 227–241. doi:10.1016/j.media.2009.11.004 PMID:20007020

Rabin, L. A., Burton, L. A., & Barr, W. B. (2007). Utilization rates of ecologically oriented instruments among clinical neuropsychologists. *The Clinical Neuropsychologist*, *21*(5), 727–743. doi:10.1080/13854040600888776 PMID:17676540

Racoceanu, D., Lacoste, C., Teodorescu, R., & Vuillemenot, N. (2006). A semantic fusion approach between medical images and reports using UMLS. In *Information Retrieval Technology* (pp. 460–475). Berlin: Springer. doi:10.1007/11880592_35

Radha, M. L. (2004). *The Essential Guide to Brain Tumors*. San Francisco, CA: National Brain Tumor Foundation.

Rahman, M., Antani, S., & Thoma, G. (2011, June). Biomedical CBIR using "bag of keypoints" in a modified inverted index. *IEEE 24th International Symposium on Computer-Based Medical Systems (CBMS)*, 1-6.

Raiman, J., Koljonen, M., Huikko, K., Kostiainen, R., & Hirvonen, J. (2004). Delivery and stability of LHRH and Nafarelin in human skin: The effect of constant/pulsed iontophoresis. *European Journal of Pharmaceutical Sciences*, *21*(2), 371–377. doi:10.1016/j.ejps.2003.11.003 PMID:14757511

Rajan, J., Jeurissen, B., Verhoye, M., Audekerke, J. V., & Sijbers, J. (2011). Maximum like-lihood estimation-based denoising of magnetic resonance images using restriced local neighborhoods. *Physics in Medicine and Biology*, *56*(16), 5221–5234. doi:10.1088/0031-9155/56/16/009 PMID:21791732

Rajan, J., Poot, D., Juntu, J., & Sijbers, J. (2010). Noise measurement from magnitude MRI using local estimates of variance and skewness. *Physics in Medicine and Biology*, *55*(16), 441–449. doi:10.1088/0031-9155/55/16/N02 PMID:20679694

Rajan, J., Veraat, J., Audekerke, J. V., Verhoye, M., & Sijbers, J. (2012). Nonlocal maximum likelihood estimation method for denoising multiple-coil magnetic resonance images. *Magnetic Resonance Imaging*, *30*(10), 1512–1518. doi:10.1016/j.mri.2012.04.021 PMID:22819583

Rajoub, B. A. (2002). An efficient coding algorithm for the compression of ECG signals using the wavelet transform. *IEEE Transactions on Bio-Medical Engineering*, *49*(4), 355–362. doi:10.1109/10.991163 PMID:11942727

Raman, R., Gella, L., Srinivasan, S., & Sharma, T. (2016). Diabetic retinopathy: An epidemic at home and around the world. *Indian Journal of Ophthalmology*, *64*(1), 69. doi:10.4103/0301-4738.178150 PMID:26953027

Ramaswamy, M., Patterson, D., Yin, L., & Goodacre, B. W. (1996). MoSearch: A radiologist-friendly tool for finding-based diagnostic report and image retrieval. *Radiographics*, *16*(4), 923–933. doi:10.1148/radiographics.16.4.8835980 PMID:8835980

Raof, R. A. A., Mashor, M. Y., Ahmad, R. B., & Noor, S. S. M. (2011). *Image Segmentation of Ziehl-Neelsen Sputum Slide Images for Tubercle Bacilli Detection*. INTECH Open Access Publisher.

Rasiwasia, N., Costa Pereira, J., Coviello, E., Doyle, G., Lanckriet, G., Levy, R., & Vasconcelos, N. (2010, October). A new approach to cross-modal multimedia retrieval. *Proceedings of the international conference on Multimedia*, 251-260. doi:10.1145/1873951.1873987

Rasmussen, I. A. Jr, Lindseth, F., Rygh, O. M., Berntsen, E. M., Selbekk, T., Xu, J., & Unsgaard, G. et al. (2007). Functional neuronavigation combined with intra-operative 3D ultrasound: Initial experiences during surgical resections close to eloquent brain areas and future directions in automatic brain shift compensation of preoperative data. *Acta Neurochirurgica*, *149*(4), 365–378. doi:10.1007/s00701-006-1110-0 PMID:17308976

Rawat, J., Singh, A., Bhadauria, H. S., & Kumar, I. (2014). Comparative analysis of segmentation algorithms for leukocyte extraction in the acute Lymphoblastic Leukemia images. *International Conference on Parallel, Distributed and Grid Computing*, 245-250. doi:10.1109/PDGC.2014.7030750

Reddy, B. S., & Murthy, I. S. N. (1986). ECG data compression using Fourier descriptors. *IEEE Transactions on Bio-Medical Engineering*, *BME-33*(4), 428–434. doi:10.1109/TBME.1986.325799 PMID:3957398

Reid, D. (2004). The influence of virtual reality on playfulness in children with cerebral palsy: A pilot study. *Occupational Therapy International*, *11*(3), 131–144. doi:10.1002/oti.202 PMID:15297894

Reid, D. T. (2002). Benefits of a virtual play rehabilitation environment for children with cerebral palsy on perceptions of self-efficacy: A pilot study. *Pediatric Rehabilitation*, *5*(3), 141–148. doi:10.1080/1363849021000039344 PMID:12581476

Ren, J. (2012). ANN vs. SVM: Which one performs better in classification of MCCs in mammogram imaging. *Knowledge-Based Systems*, *26*, 144–153. doi:10.1016/j.knosys.2011.07.016

Renovanz, M., Hickmann, A. K., Henkel, C., Nadji-Ohl, M., & Hopf, N. J. (2014). Navigated versus non-navigated intraoperative ultrasound: is there any impact on the extent of resection of high-grade gliomas? a retrospective clinical analysis. Journal of Neurological Surgery. Part A, Central European Neurosurgery, 75(3), 224–230.

Rezatofighi, S., Soltanian-Zadeh, H., Sharifian, R., & Zoroofi, R. (2009). A New Approach to White Blood Cell Nucleus Segmentation Based on Gram-Schmidt Orthogonalization. *International Conference on Digital Image Processing*, 107-111. doi:10.1109/ICDIP.2009.19

Ries, L. A. G., Melbert, D., Krapcho, M., Mariotto, A., Miller, B. A., Feuer, E. J., . . . Edwards, B. K. (Eds.). (1975-2004). *SEER Cancer Statistics Review*. National Cancer Institute. Retrieved from http://seer.cancer.gov/csr/1975-2004/

Riji, R., Rajan, J., Sijbers, J., & Nair, M. S. (2015). Iterative Bilateral Filter for Rician Noise Reduction in MR Images, *Signal. Image and Video Processing*, *9*(7), 1543–1548. doi:10.1007/s11760-013-0611-6

Rilling, G., Flandrin, P., Gonçalves, P., & Lilly, J. M. (2007). Bivariate empirical mode decomposition. *IEEE Signal Processing Letters*, *14*(12), 936–939. doi:10.1109/LSP.2007.904710

Rivaz, H., Chen, S.J.S., & Collins, D. L. (2015). Automatic Deformable MR-Ultrasound Registration for Image-Guided Neurosurgery. *IEEE Transactions on Medical Imaging, 34*(2), 366-380.

Rivaz, H., & Collins, D. L. (2014). Near real-time robust nonrigid registration of volumetric ultrasound images for neurosurgery. *Ultrasound in Medicine & Biology*, *2014*. doi:10.1016/j.ultrasmedbio.2014.08.013 PMID:25542482

Rivaz, H., & Collins, D. L. (2015, July). Deformable registration of preoperative MR, pre-resection ultrasound, and post-resection ultrasound images of neurosurgery. *International Journal of Computer Assisted Radiology and Surgery*, *10*(7), 1017–1028. doi:10.1007/s11548-014-1099-4 PMID:25373447

Rizzo, A. A., Buckwalter, J. G., Bowerly, T., Van Der Zaag, C., Humphrey, L., Neumann, U., & Sisemore, D. et al. (2000). The virtual classroom: A virtual reality environment for the assessment and rehabilitation of attention deficits. *Cyberpsychology & Behavior*, *3*(3), 483–499. doi:10.1089/10949310050078940

Rizzo, A. A., Schultheis, M., Kerns, K. A., & Mateer, C. (2004). Analysis of assets for virtual reality applications in neuropsychology. *Neuropsychological Rehabilitation*, *14*(1-2), 207–239. doi:10.1080/09602010343000183

Robertson, S. E., & Jones, K. S. (1997). *Simple, proven approaches to text retrieval.* UK Computer Laboratory, University of Cambridge.

Roche, A., Malandain, G., & Ayache, N. (1999). *Unifying maximum likelihood approaches in medical image registration.* RR-3741 1999. Retrieved from https://hal.inria.fr/inria-00072923

Roche, A., Pennec, X., Malandain, G., & Ayache, N. (2001, October). Rigid Registration of 3D Ultrasound with MR Images: A New Approach Combining Intensity and Gradient Information. *IEEE Transactions on Medical Imaging, 20*(10), 1038–1049. doi:10.1109/42.959301 PMID:11686439

Rogers, E., & Arkin, R. C. (1991, October). Visual interaction: A link between perception and problem solving. *Proceedings of IEEE International Conference on Systems, Man, and Cybernetics, Decision Aiding for Complex Systems,* 1265-1270. doi:10.1109/ICSMC.1991.169861

Romero, I., & Serrano, L. (2001). ECG frequency domain features extraction: a new characteristic for arrhythmias classification. In *Engineering in Medicine and Biology Society, 2001. Proceedings of the 23rd Annual International Conference of the IEEE* (*Vol. 2*, pp. 2006-2008). IEEE. doi:10.1109/IEMBS.2001.1020624

Rosenbaum, P., Paneth, N., Leviton, A., Goldstein, M., Bax, M., Damiano, D., & Jacobsson, B. et al. (2007). A report: The definition and classification of cerebral palsy April 2006. *Developmental Medicine and Child Neurology. Supplement, 109*(suppl 109), 8–14. PMID:17370477

Rosenow, F. (2001). Rosenow, F. and Lüders, H. (2001). Presurgical evaluation of epilepsy. *Brain, 124*(9), 1683–1700. doi:10.1093/brain/124.9.1683 PMID:11522572

Rosse, C., & Mejino, J. Jr. (2003). A reference ontology for biomedical informatics: The Foundational Model of Anatomy. *Journal of Biomedical Informatics, 36*(6), 478–500. doi:10.1016/j.jbi.2003.11.007 PMID:14759820

Royer, A. S., Doud, A. J., Rose, M. L., & He, B. (2010). EEG control of a virtual helicopter in 3-dimensional space using intelligent control strategies. *IEEE Transactions on Neural Systems and Rehabilitation Engineering, 18*(6), 581–589. doi:10.1109/TNSRE.2010.2077654 PMID:20876032

Rubin, G. (2000). Data explosion: The challenge of multidetector-row CT. *European Journal of Radiology, 36*(2), 74–80. doi:10.1016/S0720-048X(00)00270-9 PMID:11116170

Ruiz-Manzano, J., Blanquer, R., Calpe, J. L., Caminero, J. A., Caylà, J., Domínguez, J. A., & Vidal, R. et al. (2008). Diagnosis and treatment of tuberculosis. *Archivos de Bronconeumologia, 44*(10), 551–566. PMID:19006636

Rulaningtyas, R., Suksmono, A. B., Mengko, T. L. R., & Saptawati, P. (2015). Identification of mycobacterium tuberculosis in sputum smear slide using automatic scanning microscope. *AIP Conference Proceedings, 1656,* 060011. doi:10.1063/1.4917142

Sabesan, S., Good, L. B., Tsakalis, K. S., Spanias, A., Treiman, D. M., & Iasemidis, L. D. (2009). Information flow and application to epileptogenic focus localization from intracranial EEG. *IEEE Transactions on Neural Systems and Rehabilitation Engineering, 17*(3), 244–253. doi:10.1109/TNSRE.2009.2023291 PMID:19497831

Sai Sateesh, S., Prasanjit, P., Kunal, P., & Sirsendu Sekhar, R. (2015). *Drug Delivery: Iontophoretic. In Encyclopedia of Biomedical Polymers and Polymeric Biomaterials* (pp. 2726–2740). CRC Press.

Sakamoto, T., Miyazaki, E., Aramaki, Y., Arima, H., Takahashi, M., Kato, Y., & Tsuchiya, S. et al. (2004). Improvement of dermatitis by iontophoretically delivered antisense oligonucleotides for interleukin-10 in NC/Nga mice. *Gene Therapy, 11*(3), 317–324. doi:10.1038/sj.gt.3302171 PMID:14737092

Salton, G. (1971). *The SMART retrieval system—experiments in automatic document processing.* Academic Press.

Samanta, B., & Nataraj, C. (2009). Application of particle swarm optimization and proximal support vector machines for fault detection. *Swarm Intelligence*, *3*(4), 303–325. doi:10.1007/s11721-009-0028-6

Samson, E., & Marchand, J. (1999). Numerical solution of the extended Nernst–Planck model. *Journal of Colloid and Interface Science*, *215*(1), 1–8. doi:10.1006/jcis.1999.6145 PMID:10362465

Samsonov, A., & Johnson, C. (2004). Noise-adaptive nonlinear diffusion filtering of MR images with spatially varying noise levels. *Magnetic Resonance in Medicine*, *52*(4), 798–806. doi:10.1002/mrm.20207 PMID:15389962

Santiago-Mozos, R., Fernandez-Lorenzana, R., Perez-Cruz, F., & Artes-Rodriguez, A. (2008). On the uncertainty in sequential hypothesis testing. *Proceedings of IEEE International Symposium on Biomedical Imaging: From Nano to Macro*, 1223-1226. doi:10.1109/ISBI.2008.4541223

Saravia, L. A. (2014). mfSBA: Multifractal analysis of spatial patterns in ecological communities. *F1000 Research*, *3*, 14. doi:10.12688/f1000research.3-14.v2 PMID:25324962

Sawyers, C. L., Denny, C. T., & Witte, O. N. (1991). Leukemia and the disruption of normal hematopoiesis. *Cell*, *64*(2), 337–350. doi:10.1016/0092-8674(91)90643-D PMID:1988151

Scanlon, P. H., Wilkinson, C. P., Aldington, S. J., & Matthews, D. R. (2009). *A practical manual of diabetic retinopathy management*. Academic Press.

Schevon, C. A., Cappell, J., Emerson, R., Isler, J., Grieve, P., Goodman, R., & Gilliam, F. et al. (2007). Cortical abnormalities in epilepsy revealed by local EEG synchrony. *NeuroImage*, *35*(1), 140–148. doi:10.1016/j.neuroimage.2006.11.009 PMID:17224281

Scholkopf, B., Sung, K. K., Burges, C. J., Girosi, F., Niyogi, P., Poggio, T., & Vapnik, V. (1997). Comparing support vector machines with Gaussian kernels to radial basis function classifiers. *IEEE Transactions on Signal Processing*, *45*(11), 2758–2765. doi:10.1109/78.650102

Schreiber, M. (1999). Potential of an interactive computer-based training in the rehabilitation of dementia: An initial study. *Neuropsychological Rehabilitation*, *9*(2), 155–167. doi:10.1080/713755596

Schwarz, L. A. (2007). *Non-rigid Registration Using Free-form Deformations* (Thesis). Siemens Corporate Research, Inc.

Scotti, F. (2010). *ALL-IDB, Acute Lymphoblastic Leukemia Image Database for Image Processing*. Retrieved from http://www.dti.unimi.it/fscotti/all/results.php

Scotti, F. (2005). Automatic morphological analysis for acute leukemia identification in peripheral blood microscope images. *IEEE International Conference on Computational Intelligence for Measurement Systems and Applications*, 96-101. doi:10.1109/CIMSA.2005.1522835

Selesnick, I. W., Baraniuk, R. G., & Kingsbury, N. C. (2005). The dual-tree complex wavelet transforms. *IEEE Signal Processing Magazine, 22*(6), 123-151.

Sharan, D., Ajeesh, P. S., Rameshkumar, R., Mathankumar, M., Paulina, R. J., & Manjula, M. (2012). Virtual reality based therapy for post operative rehabilitation of children with cerebral palsy. *Work (Reading, Mass.)*, *41*(Supplement 1), 3612–3615. PMID:22317271

Sharma, R., Pachori, R. B., & Acharya, U. R. (2015). An integrated index for the identification of focal electroencephalogram signals using discrete wavelet transform and entropy measures. *Entropy, 17*(8), 5218-5240.

Sharma, M., Dhere, A., Pachori, R. B., & Acharya, U. R. (2017). An automatic detection of focal EEG signals using new class of time-frequency localized orthogonal wavelet filter banks. *Knowledge-Based Systems*, *118*, 217–227. doi:10.1016/j.knosys.2016.11.024

Sharma, R., & Pachori, R. B. (2015). Classification of epileptic seizures in EEG signals based on phase space representation of intrinsic mode functions. *Expert Systems with Applications*, *42*(3), 1106–1117. doi:10.1016/j.eswa.2014.08.030

Sharma, R., Pachori, R. B., & Acharya, U. R. (2015a). Application of entropy measures on intrinsic mode functions for the automated identification of focal electroencephalogram signals. *Entropy*, *17*(2), 669–691. doi:10.3390/e17020669

Sharma, R., Pachori, R. B., & Acharya, U. R. (2015b). An integrated index for the identification of focal electroencephalogram signals using discrete wavelet transform and entropy measures. *Entropy*, *17*(8), 5218–5240. doi:10.3390/e17085218

Sharma, R., Pachori, R. B., & Gautam, S. (2014). Empirical mode decomposition based classification of focal and non-focal EEG signals. In *International Conference on Medical Biometrics*, (pp. 135–140). Shenzhen, China. IEEE. doi:10.1109/ICMB.2014.31

Shaw, J., & Fox, E. (1995). Combination of multiple searches. *NIST Special Publication SP*, 105-105.

Shyu, C., Brodley, C., Kak, A., Kosaka, A., Aisen, A., & Broderick, L. (1999). ASSERT, A physician-in-the-loop content-based image retrieval system for HRCT image databases. *Computer Vision and Image Understanding*, *75*(1), 111–132. doi:10.1006/cviu.1999.0768

Sickles, E., Miglioretti, D., Ballard-Barbash, R., Geller, B., Leung, J., Rosenberg, R., & Yankaskas, B. et al. (2005). Performance benchmarks for diagnostic mammography. *Radiology*, *235*(3), 775–790. doi:10.1148/radiol.2353040738 PMID:15914475

Siegle, R., Baram, E., Reuter, S., Clarke, E., Lancaster, J., & McMahan, C. (1998). Rates of disagreement in imaging interpretation in a group of community hospitals. *Academic Radiology*, *5*(3), 148–154. doi:10.1016/S1076-6332(98)80277-8 PMID:9522880

Sijbers, J., & den Dekker, A. J. (2004). Maximum likelihood estimation of signal amplitude and noise variance form MR data. *Magnetic Resonance Imaging*, *51*, 586–594. PMID:15004801

Sijbers, J., den Dekker, A. J., Scheunders, P., & Van Dyck, D. (1998). Maximum likelihood destimation of Rician distribution parameters. *IEEE Transactions on Medical Imaging*, *17*(3), 357–361. doi:10.1109/42.712125 PMID:9735899

Sijbers, J., den Dekker, A. J., Van Audekerke, J., Verhoye, M., & Van Dyck, D. (1998). Estimation of the noise in magnitude MR images. *Magnetic Resonance Imaging*, *16*(1), 87–90. doi:10.1016/S0730-725X(97)00199-9 PMID:9436952

Simpson, M., Rahman, M., Demner-Fushman, D., Antani, S., & Thoma, G. (2009, September). Text-and content-based approaches to image retrieval for the ImageCLEF 2009 medical retrieval track. *CLEF2009 Working Notes. CLEF 2009 Workshop,* (30).

Singhal, V., & Singh, P. (2014). Local Binary Pattern for Automatic Detection of Acute Lymphoblastic Leukemia. *Twentieth National Conference on Communications*, 1-5. doi:10.1109/NCC.2014.6811261

Singh, P., & Maibach, H. I. (1993). Iontophoresis in drug delivery: Basic principles and applications. *Critical Reviews in Therapeutic Drug Carrier Systems*, *11*(2-3), 161–213. PMID:7600587

Siuly, L., Li, Y., & Wen, P. P. (2011). Clustering technique-based least square support vector machine for EEG signal classification. *Computer Methods and Programs in Biomedicine*, *104*(3), 358–372. doi:10.1016/j.cmpb.2010.11.014 PMID:21168234

Sivic, J., & Zisserman, A. (2003, October). Video Google: A text retrieval approach to object matching in videos. *Proceedings of Ninth IEEE International Conference on Computer Vision*, 1470-1477. doi:10.1109/ICCV.2003.1238663

Sklansky, J., Tao, E., Bazargan, M., Ornes, C., Murchison, R., & Teklehaimanot, S. (2000). Computer-aided, case-based diagnosis of mammographic regions of interest containing microcalcifications. *Academic Radiology*, *7*(6), 395–405. doi:10.1016/S1076-6332(00)80379-7 PMID:10845398

Sloan, J. B., & Soltani, K. (1986). Iontophoresis in dermatology: A review. *Journal of the American Academy of Dermatology*, *15*(4), 671–684. doi:10.1016/S0190-9622(86)70223-5 PMID:3534013

Smeulders, A., Worring, M., Santini, S., Gupta, A., & Jain, R. (2000). Content-based image retrieval at the end of the early years. *IEEE Transactions on Pattern Analysis and Machine Intelligence*, *22*(12), 1349–1380. doi:10.1109/34.895972

Smith, J. D., & Steel, M. J. (2001). *The use of virtual simulation for dismounted infantry training.* Cranfield University/ RMCS Shrivenham. (Unpublished)

Snider, L., Majnemer, A., & Darsaklis, V. (2010). Virtual reality as a therapeutic modality for children with cerebral palsy. *Developmental Neurorehabilitation*, *13*(2), 120–128. doi:10.3109/17518420903357753 PMID:20222773

Snoek, C., Worring, M., & Smeulders, A. (2005, November). Early versus late fusion in semantic video analysis. *Proceedings of the 13th annual ACM international conference on Multimedia*, 399-402. doi:10.1145/1101149.1101236

Soares, F., Freire, M. M., Pereira, M., Janela, F., & Seabra, J. (2009, August). Towards the detection of microcalcifications on mammograms through multifractal detrended fluctuation analysis. *2009 IEEE Pacific Rim Conference on Communications, Computers and Signal Processing*, 677-681. doi:10.1109/PACRIM.2009.5291288

Soffa, D., Lewis, R., Sunshine, J., & Bhargavan, M. (2004). Disagreement in interpretation: A method for the development of benchmarks for quality assurance in imaging. *Journal of the American College of Radiology*, *1*(3), 212–217. doi:10.1016/j.jacr.2003.12.017 PMID:17411562

Sokalski, T., Lingenfelter, P., & Lewenstam, A. (2003). Numerical solution of the coupled Nernst-Planck and Poisson equations for liquid junction and ion selective membrane potentials. *The Journal of Physical Chemistry B*, *107*(11), 2443–2452. doi:10.1021/jp026406a

Sopharak, A., Uyyanonvara, B., Barman, S., & Williamson, T. H. (2008). Automatic detection of diabetic retinopathy exudates from non-dilated retinal images using mathematical morphology methods. *Computerized Medical Imaging and Graphics*, *32*(8), 720–727. doi:10.1016/j.compmedimag.2008.08.009 PMID:18930631

Sotaquira, M., Rueda, L., & Narvaez, R. (2009). Detection and quantification of bacilli and clusters present in sputum smear samples: a novel algorithm for pulmonary tuberculosis diagnosis. *Proceedings of International Conference on Digital Image Processing*, 117-121. doi:10.1109/ICDIP.2009.59

Sotiras, A., Christos, D., & Paragios, N. (2013). Deformable Medical Image Registration: A Survey. *IEEE Transactions on Medical Imaging*, *32*(7), 1153–1190. doi:10.1109/TMI.2013.2265603 PMID:23739795

Srinivasan, S., Rindflesch, T., Hole, W., Aronson, A., & Mork, J. (2002). Finding UMLS Metathesaurus concepts in MEDLINE. *Proceedings of AMIA Symposium*, 727–31.

Srinivasan, V., & Higuchi, W. (1990). A model for iontophoresis incroporating the effect of convective solvent flow. *International Journal of Pharmaceutics*, *60*(2), 133–138. doi:10.1016/0378-5173(90)90298-I

Stearns, M., Price, C., Spackman, K., & Wang, A. (2001). SNOMED clinical terms: Overview of the development process and project status. *Proceedings of the* American Medical Informatics Association *(AMIA) Symposium*, 662.

Steingart, K. R., Henry, M., Ng, V., Hopewell, P. C., Ramsay, A., Cunningham, J., & Pai, M. et al. (2006). Fluorescence versus conventional sputum smear microscopy for tuberculosis: A systematic review. *The Lancet Infectious Diseases*, *6*(9), 570–581. doi:10.1016/S1473-3099(06)70578-3 PMID:16931408

Sternberg, R. J. (1997). Intelligence and lifelong learning: Whats new and how can we use it? *The American Psychologist*, *52*(10), 1134–1139. doi:10.1037/0003-066X.52.10.1134 PMID:9329294

Stewart, C. V., Tsai, C. L., & Roysam, B. (2003). The dual-bootstrap iterative closest point algorithm with application to retinal image registration. *IEEE Transactions on Medical Imaging*, *22*(11), 1379–1394. doi:10.1109/TMI.2003.819276 PMID:14606672

Stinson, C. A. (2013). *Virtual Reality for Sport Training* (Doctoral dissertation). Virginia Tech.

Stojić, T., Reljin, I., & Reljin, B. (2006). Adaptation of multifractal analysis to segmentation of microcalcifications in digital mammograms. *Physica A: Statistical Mechanics and its Applications, 367*, 494-508.

Stosic, T., & Stosic, B. D. (2006). Multifractal analysis of human retinal vessels. *IEEE Transactions on Medical Imaging*, *25*(8), 1101–1107. doi:10.1109/TMI.2006.879316 PMID:16895002

Suckling, J., Parker, J., Dance, D., Astley, S., Hutt, I., Boggis, C., & Savage, J. (1994). The mammographic image analysis society digital mammogram database. In *Proceedings of Second International Workshop on Digital Mammography*. Excerta Medica.

Sung-Hyuk, C. (2007). Comprehensive Survey on Distance/Similarity Measures between Probability Density Function. *International Journal of Mathematical Models and Methods in Applied Sciences*, *1*(4), 2007.

Suykens, J. A. K., & Vandewalle, J. (1999). Least squares support vector machine classifiers. *Neural Processing Letters*, *9*(3), 293–300. doi:10.1023/A:1018628609742

Swami, P., Gandhi, T.K., Panigrahi, B.K., Tripathi, M., & Anand, S. (2016). A novel robust diagnostic model to detect seizures in electroencephalography. *Expert Systems With Applications, 56*, 116–130.

Swett, H., Fisher, P., Cohn, A., Miller, P., & Mutalik, P. (1989). Expert system-controlled image display. *Radiology*, *172*(2), 487–493. doi:10.1148/radiology.172.2.2664871 PMID:2664871

Tadrous, P. J. (2010). Computer-Assisted Screening of Ziehl-Neelsen–Stained Tissue for Mycobacteria. *American Journal of Clinical Pathology*, *133*(6), 849–858. doi:10.1309/AJCPMR3BLVBH8THV PMID:20472842

Tai, S. C., Sun, C., & Yan, W. C. (2005). A 2-D ECG compression method based on wavelet transform and modified SPIHT. *IEEE Transactions on Bio-Medical Engineering*, *52*(6), 999–1008. doi:10.1109/TBME.2005.846727 PMID:15977730

Takahashi, T., Murata, T., Narita, K., Hamada, T., Kosaka, H., Omori, M., & Wada, Y. et al. (2006). Multifractal analysis of deep white matter microstructural changes on MRI in relation to early-stage atherosclerosis. *NeuroImage*, *32*(3), 1158–1166. doi:10.1016/j.neuroimage.2006.04.218 PMID:16815037

Takane, Y., Kawasumi, Y., Horie, T., & Ishibashi, T. (2013, March). Does image reduction affect the diagnostic accuracy of digital mammograms? In *SPIE Medical Imaging* (p. 867319–867319). International Society for Optics and Photonics. doi:10.1117/12.2008169

Ţălu, Ş. (2012). Mathematical methods used in monofractal and multifractal analysis for the processing of biological and medical data and images. *ABAH Bioflux*, *4*(1), 1–4.

Tang, J., Sun, Q., Liu, J., & Cao, Y. (2007). An adaptive anisotropic diffusion filter for noise reduction in MR images. *Proceedings of IEEE International Conference on Mechatronics and Automation*, 1299–1304. doi:10.1109/ICMA.2007.4303737

Tarnanas, I., Tsolaki, M., Nef, T., Müri, R. M., & Mosimann, U. P. (2014). Can a novel computerized cognitive screening test provide additional information for early detection of Alzheimers disease? *Alzheimers & Dementia*, *10*(6), 790–798. doi:10.1016/j.jalz.2014.01.002 PMID:24656838

Tasoulis, S. K., Doukas, C. N., Maglogiannis, I., & Plagianakos, V. P. (2010, August). Classification of apoptosis using advanced clustering techniques on digital microscopic images. *2010 Annual International Conference of the IEEE Engineering in Medicine and Biology*, 5565-5568. doi:10.1109/IEMBS.2010.5626777

Tavakoli, Nazar, & Mehdizadeh. (2017). Effect of two different preprocessing steps in detection of optic nerve head in fundus images. *Proc. SPIE 10134, Medical Imaging 2017: Computer-Aided Diagnosis*. doi:10.1117/12.2254841

Tedesco, M., Hamelers, H., & Biesheuvel, P. (2016). Nernst-Planck transport theory for (reverse) electrodialysis: I. Effect of co-ion transport through the membranes. *Journal of Membrane Science*, *510*, 370–381. doi:10.1016/j.memsci.2016.03.012

Teng, S., & Lu, G. (2007). Image indexing and retrieval based on vector quantization. *Pattern Recognition*, *40*(11), 3299–3316. doi:10.1016/j.patcog.2007.01.029

Tirilly, P., Claveau, V., & Gros, P. (2008, July). Language modeling for bag-of-visual words image categorization. In *Proceedings of the 2008 international conference on Content-based image and video retrieval* (pp. 249-258). ACM doi:10.1145/1386352.1386388

Tomasi, C., & Manduchi, R. (1998). Bilateral Filtering for Gray and Color Images. *Proc. Int. Conf. Computer Vision*, 839-846. doi:10.1109/ICCV.1998.710815

Tommasi, T., Orabona, F., & Caputo, B. (2008). CLEF2008 image annotation task: An SVM confidence-based approach. Working Notes of the 2008 CLEF Workshop.

Traina, A., Castanon, C., & Traina, C. Jr. (2003, June). Multiwavemed: A system for medical image retrieval through wavelets transformations. *Proceedings of 16th IEEE Symposium on Computer-Based Medical Systems*, 150-155. doi:10.1109/CBMS.2003.1212781

Trobaugh, J. W., Richard, W. D., Smith, K. R., & Bucholz, R. D. (1994). Frameless stereotactic ultrasonography: Method and applications. *Computerized Medical Imaging and Graphics, 18*(4), 235-246.

Tsuru, T., Urairi, M., Nakao, S.-i., & Kimura, S. (1991). Reverse osmosis of single and mixed electrolytes with charged membranes: Experiment and analysis. *Journal of Chemical Engineering of Japan*, *24*(4), 518–524. doi:10.1252/jcej.24.518

Tuberculosis Facts. (2007). Stop TB Partnership, World Health Organization.

Unified Medical Language System. (2014). Retrieved from http://www.nlm.nih.gov/research/umls/

Unsgaard, G., Gronningsaeter, A., Ommedal, S., & Hernes. T. A. N. (2002). Brain operations guided by real-time two-dimensional ultrasound: New possibilities as a result of improved image quality. *Neurosurgery, 51*(2), 402–412.

Unsgaard, G., Ommedal, S., Muller, T., Gronningsaeter, A., & Hernes, N.TA. (2002). Neuronavigation by intraoperative three-dimensional ultrasound: Initial experience during brain tumor resection. *Neurosurgery, 50*, 804–812.

Unsgaard, G., Selbekk, T., Brostrup, M. T., Ommedal, S., Torp, S. H., Myhr, G., & Hernes, N. T. A. et al. (2005). Ability of navigated 3D ultrasound to delineate gliomas and metastases–comparison of image interpretations with histopathology. *Acta Neurochirurgica*, *147*(12), 1259–1269, discussion 1269. doi:10.1007/s00701-005-0624-1 PMID:16172831

Ustun, B., Melssen, W., & Buydens, L. (2006). Facilitating the application of Support Vector Regression by using a universal Pearson VII function based kernel. *Chemometrics and Intelligent Laboratory Systems*, *81*(1), 29–40. doi:10.1016/j.chemolab.2005.09.003

Uwimana, E., & Ruiz, M. E. (2008). Integrating an automatic classification method into the medical image retrieval process. *AMIA ... Annual Symposium Proceedings / AMIA Symposium. AMIA Symposium*, *2008*, 747. PMID:18999165

Valente, F., Costa, C., & Silva, A. (2013). Dicoogle, a PACS featuring profiled content based image retrieval. *PLoS ONE*, *8*(5), e61888. doi:10.1371/journal.pone.0061888 PMID:23671578

Van Erp, M., & Schomaker, L. (2000). Variants of the borda count method for combining ranked classifier hypotheses. *Seventh International Workshop on Frontiers in Handwriting Recognition.*

van Mierlo, P., Carrette, E., Hallez, H., Raedt, R., Meurs, A., Vandenberghe, S., & Vonck, K. et al. (2013). Ictal-onset localization through connectivity analysis of intracranial EEG signals in patients with refractory epilepsy. *Epilepsia*, *54*(8), 1409–1418. doi:10.1111/epi.12206 PMID:23647147

van Mierlo, P., Papadopoulou, M., Carrette, E., Boon, P., Vandenberghe, S., Vonck, K., & Marinazzo, D. (2014). Functional brain connectivity from EEG in epilepsy: Seizure prediction and epileptogenic focus localization. *Progress in Neurobiology*, *121*, 19–35. doi:10.1016/j.pneurobio.2014.06.004 PMID:25014528

van Zaanen, & de Croon. (2005). Multi-modal information retrieval using FINT. In *Multilingual Information Access for Text, Speech and Images* (pp. 728-739). Berlin: Springer.

Vapnik, V. (1995). *The nature of statistical learning theory*. New York: Springer. doi:10.1007/978-1-4757-2440-0

Veropoulos, K., Campbell, C., Learmonth, G., Knight, B., & Simpson, J. (1998). The automated identification of tubercle bacilli using image processing and neural computing techniques. In ICANN 98 (pp. 797-802). Springer London. doi:10.1007/978-1-4471-1599-1_123

Villena Román, J., González Cristóbal, J., Goñi Menoyo, J., Martínez Fernández, J., & Fernández, J. (2005). MIRACLE's combination of visual and textual queries for medical images retrieval. *Working Notes for the CLEF 2005 Workshop.*

Villena-Román, J., Lana-Serrano, S., & González-Cristóbal, J. (2008). MIRACLE at ImageCLEFmed 2007: Merging textual and visual strategies to improve medical image retrieval. In *Advances in Multilingual and Multimodal Information Retrieval* (pp. 593–596). Berlin: Springer. doi:10.1007/978-3-540-85760-0_74

Vinokourov, A., Hardoon, D., & Shawe-Taylor, J. (2003). Learning the semantics of multimedia content with application to web image retrieval and classification. *Fourth International Symposium on Independent Component Analysis and Blind Source Separation.*

Wählby, C., Lindblad, J., Vondrus, M., Bengtsson, E., & Björkesten, L. (2002). Algorithms for cytoplasm segmentation of fluorescence labelled cells. *Analytical Cellular Pathology*, *24*(2-3), 101-111.

Walker, S. A., Miller, D., & Tanabe, J. (2006). Bilateral spatial filtering: Refining methods for localizing brain activation in the presence of parenchymal abnormalities. *NeuroImage*, *33*(2), 564–569. doi:10.1016/j.neuroimage.2006.06.051 PMID:16942890

Walter, T., Klein, J. C., Massin, P., & Erginay, A. (2002). A contribution of image processing to the diagnosis of diabetic retinopathy-detection of exudates in color fundus images of the human retina. *IEEE Transactions on Medical Imaging*, *21*(10), 1236–1243. doi:10.1109/TMI.2002.806290 PMID:12585705

Wang, J., Chen, Q., & Chen, Y. (2003). RBF Kernel Based Support Vector Machine with Universal Approximation and its Applications. In F. Yin, J. Wang, & C. Guo (Eds.), Lecture Notes in Computer Science: Vol. 3173. Advances in Neural Networks (pp. 512–517). Springer.

Wang, J., Li, Y., Zhang, Y., Xie, H., & Wang, C. (2011, August). Bag-of-features based classification of breast parenchymal tissue in the mammogram via jointly selecting and weighting visual words. *Sixth IEEE International Conference on Image and Graphics (ICIG)*, 622-627. doi:10.1109/ICIG.2011.192

Wang, X., & Meng, J. (2008). A 2-D ECG compression algorithm based on wavelet transform and vector quantization. *Digital Signal Processing*, *18*(2), 179–188. doi:10.1016/j.dsp.2007.03.003

Wang, Y., Thakur, R., Fan, Q., & Michniak, B. (2005). Transdermal iontophoresis: Combination strategies to improve transdermal iontophoretic drug delivery. *European Journal of Pharmaceutics and Biopharmaceutics*, *60*(2), 179–191. doi:10.1016/j.ejpb.2004.12.008 PMID:15939232

Wang, Z. (2002). A Universal Image Quality Index. *IEEE Signal Processing Letters*, *20*.

Wang, Z., Bovik, A. C., Sheikh, H. R., & Simoncelli, E. P. (2004). Image Quality Assessment: From Error Visibility to Structural Similarity. *IEEE Transactions on Image Processing*, *13*(4), 600–612. doi:10.1109/TIP.2003.819861 PMID:15376593

Warren, C. P., Hu, S., Stead, M., Brinkmann, B. H., Bower, M. R., & Worrell, G. A. (2010). Synchrony in normal and focal epileptic brain: The seizure onset zone is functionally disconnected. *Journal of Neurophysiology*, *104*(6), 3530–3539. doi:10.1152/jn.00368.2010 PMID:20926610

Wee, C., & Paramesran, R. (2007). On the computational aspects of Zernike moments. *Image and Vision Computing*, *25*(6), 967–980. doi:10.1016/j.imavis.2006.07.010

Wei, C., Chen, S., & Liu, X. (2012). Mammogram retrieval on similar mass lesions. *Computer Methods and Programs in Biomedicine*, *106*(3), 234–248. doi:10.1016/j.cmpb.2010.09.002 PMID:20933295

Wei, C., Li, C., & Wilson, R. (2005, April). A general framework for content-based medical image retrieval with its application to mammograms. In *Medical Imaging* (pp. 134–143). International Society for Optics and Photonics. doi:10.1117/12.594929

Wei, C., Li, Y., & Huang, P. (2011). Mammogram retrieval through machine learning within BI-RADS standards. *Journal of Biomedical Informatics*, *44*(4), 607–614. doi:10.1016/j.jbi.2011.01.012 PMID:21277387

Welter, P., Deserno, T. M., Fischer, B., Günther, R. W., & Spreckelsen, C. (2011). Towards case-based medical learning in radiological decision making using content-based image retrieval. *BMC Medical Informatics and Decision Making*, *11*(1), 68. doi:10.1186/1472-6947-11-68 PMID:22032775

Westbrook, C. (2008). Handbook of MRI Technique. John Wiley & Sons, Ltd.

Weyand, T., & Deselaers, T. (2005, October). *Combining Content-based Image Retrieval with Textual Information Retrieval*. RWTH Aachen.

Widman, G., Lehnertz, K., Urbach, H., & Elger, C. E. (2000). Spatial distribution of neuronal complexity loss in neocortical lesional epilepsies. *Epilepsia*, *41*(7), 811–817. doi:10.1111/j.1528-1157.2000.tb00247.x PMID:10897151

Wiest-Daesslé, N., Prima, S., Coupé, P., Morrissey, S. P., & Barillot, C. (2007). *Nonlocal means variants for denoising of diffusion-weighted and diffusion tensor MRI*. Med. Image Comput. Comput. Assist. Interv.

Wilhelm, T., Kürsten, J., Eibl, M., & der Nationen, S. (2007). *Experiments for the ImageCLEF 2007 photographic retrieval task. Working Notes for the CLEF.*

Wilkinson, C. P., Ferris, F. L., Klein, R. E., Lee, P. P., Agardh, C. D., Davis, M., & Group, G. D. R. P. (2003). Proposed international clinical diabetic retinopathy and diabetic macular edema disease severity scales. *Ophthalmology, 110*(9), 1677–1682. doi:10.1016/S0161-6420(03)00475-5 PMID:13129861

Wong, T. Y., Klein, R., Islam, F. A., Cotch, M. F., Folsom, A. R., Klein, B. E., & Shea, S. et al. (2006). Diabetic retinopathy in a multi-ethnic cohort in the United States. *American Journal of Ophthalmology, 141*(3), 446–455. doi:10.1016/j.ajo.2005.08.063 PMID:16490489

Wong, W. C. K., & Chung, A. C. S. (2004). A nonlinear and non-iterative noise reduction technique for medical images: Concept and methods comparison. *Elsevier International Congress Series, 1268*, 171–176. doi:10.1016/j.ics.2004.03.143

Wong, W. C. K., Chung, A. C. S., & Yu, S. C. H. (2004). Trilateral filter for biomedical images. *Proceedings of ISBI*, 820–823.

Wood, J. C., & Johnson, K. M. (1999). Wavelet packet denoising of magnetic resonance images: Importance of Rician noise at low SNR. *Magnetic Resonance in Medicine, 41*(3), 631–635. doi:10.1002/(SICI)1522-2594(199903)41:3<631::AID-MRM29>3.0.CO;2-Q PMID:10204890

World Health Organization (WHO). (2010). *Tuberculosis Fact Sheet No. 104*. WHO.

Worrell, G. A., Parish, L., Cranstoun, S. D., Jonas, R., Baltuch, G., & Litt, B. (2004). High frequency oscillations and seizure generation in neocortical epilepsy. *Brain, 127*(7), 1496–1506. doi:10.1093/brain/awh149 PMID:15155522

Worsley, D., & Simmons, D. (2010). Diabetic retinopathy and public health. *Automated Image Detection of Retinal Pathology*, 27-66.

Wu, H., Sun, T., Wang, J., Li, X., Wang, W., Huo, D., & Guo, X. (2013). Combination of radiological and gray level co-occurrence matrix textural features used to distinguish solitary pulmonary nodules by computed tomography. *Journal of Digital Imaging, 26*(4), 797–802. doi:10.1007/s10278-012-9547-6 PMID:23325122

Wu, Q., Merchant, F., & Castleman, K. (2010). *Microscope image processing*. Academic Press.

Xie, H. B., He, W. X., & Liu, H. (2008). Measuring time series regularity using nonlinear similarity-based sample entropy. *Physics Letters A, 372*(48), 7140-7146.

Xie, J., Heng, P. A., & Shah, M. (2008). Image diffusion using saliency bilateral filter. *IEEE Transactions on Information Technology in Biomedicine, 12*(6), 768–771. doi:10.1109/TITB.2008.926462 PMID:19000957

Xie, Z., & Farin, G. E. (2004, January/February). Image Registration Using Hierarchical B-Splines. *IEEE Transactions on Visualization and Computer Graphics, 10*(1). PMID:15382700

Xu, Y., Huang, S., Ji, H., & Fermuller, C. (2009). Combining powerful local and global statistics for texture description. In *IEEE Conference on* In *Computer Vision and Pattern Recognition*, 573-580.

Xue, Z., Antani, S., Long, L., & Thoma, G. (2009, August). A system for searching uterine cervix images by visual attributes. *22nd IEEE International Symposium on Computer-Based Medical Systems (CBMS 2009)*, 1-5. doi:10.1109/CBMS.2009.5255319

Xu, Y., Ji, H., & Fermuller, C. (2006). A projective invariant for textures. *IEEE Computer Society Conference on Computer Vision and Pattern Recognition, 2*, 1932-1939.

Xu, Y., Ji, H., & Fermüller, C. (2009). Viewpoint invariant texture description using fractal analysis. *International Journal of Computer Vision*, *83*(1), 85–100. doi:10.1007/s11263-009-0220-6

Yampri, P., Pintavirooj, C., Daochai, S., & Teartulakarn, S. (2006). White Blood Cell Classification based on the Combination of Eigen Cell and Parametric Feature Detection. *IEEE Conference on Industrial Electronics and Applications*, 1-4. doi:10.1109/ICIEA.2006.257341

Yan, A., Wang, Z., & Cai, Z. (2008). Prediction of human intestinal absorption by GA feature selection and support vector machine regression. *International Journal of Molecular Sciences*, *9*(10), 1961–1976. doi:10.3390/ijms9101961 PMID:19325729

Yanasak et al. (2015). *Parallel Imaging in MRI: Technology, Applications, and Quality Control.* American Association of Physicists in Medicine.

Yoshika, H. (n.d.). *Magnetic resonance imaging.* Retrieved from www.intl.elsevierhealth.com/media/us/samplechapters

Young, B. L., Mlamla, Z., Gqamana, P. P., Smit, S., Roberts, T., Peter, J., & Blackburn, J. et al. (2014). The identification of tuberculosis biomarkers in human urine samples. *The European Respiratory Journal*, *43*(6), 1719–1729. doi:10.1183/09031936.00175113 PMID:24743962

You, S. H., Jang, S. H., Kim, Y. H., Kwon, Y. H., Barrow, I., & Hallett, M. (2005). Cortical reorganization induced by virtual reality therapy in a child with hemiparetic cerebral palsy. *Developmental Medicine and Child Neurology*, *47*(09), 628–635. doi:10.1111/j.1469-8749.2005.tb01216.x PMID:16138671

Yuan, Q., Cai, C., Xiao, H., Liu, X., & Wen, Y. (2007). Diagnosis of breast tumours and evaluation of prognostic risk by using machine learning approaches. In D.-S. Huang, L. Heutte, & M. Loog (Eds.), *Advanced Intelligent Computing Theories and Applications. With Aspects of Contemporary Intelligent Computing Techniques* (pp. 1250–1260). Springer. doi:10.1007/978-3-540-74282-1_141

Zavar, M., Rahati, S., Akbarzadeh-T, M.-R., & Ghasemifard, H. (2011). Evolutionary model selection in a wavelet-based support vector machine for automated seizure detection. *Expert Systems with Applications*, *38*(9), 10751–10758. doi:10.1016/j.eswa.2011.01.087

Zeybek, E. H., Fournier, R., & Na, A. (2012). Multimodal compression applied to biomedical data. *Journal of Biomedical Science and Engineering*, *5*(12), 755–761. doi:10.4236/jbise.2012.512094

Zhai, Y., Liu, Y., Zhou, D., & Liu, S. (2010). Automatic identification of mycobacterium tuberculosis from ZN-stained sputum smear: algorithm and system design. *Proceedings of IEEE International Conference on Robotics and Biomimetrics*, 41-46. doi:10.1109/ROBIO.2010.5723300

Zhang, X., Thibault, G., Decencière, E., Marcotegui, B., Laÿ, B., Danno, R., & Chabouis, A. (2014). Exudate detection in color retinal images for mass screening of diabetic retinopathy. *Medical Image Analysis*, *18*(7), 1026–1043. doi:10.1016/j.media.2014.05.004 PMID:24972380

Zha, Z., Wang, M., Shen, J., & Chua, T. (2012). Text Mining in Multimedia. In *Mining Text Data* (pp. 361–384). Springer. doi:10.1007/978-1-4614-3223-4_11

Zheng, Q., Wang, W., & Gao, W. (2006, October). Effective and efficient object-based image retrieval using visual phrases. *Proceedings of the 14th annual ACM international conference on Multimedia*, 77-80. doi:10.1145/1180639.1180664

Zhou, H., & Rivaz, H. (2016). Registration of Pre- and Postresection Ultrasound Volumes With Noncorresponding Regions in Neurosurgery. *IEEE Journal of Biomedical and Health Informatics, 20*(5).

Zhou, X., Gobeill, J., & Müller, H. (2008). *MedGIFT at ImageCLEF 2008. Working Notes of CLEF.*

Zhou, X., Stern, R., & Müller, H. (2012). Case-based fracture image retrieval. *International Journal of Computer Assisted Radiology and Surgery*, *7*(3), 401–411. doi:10.1007/s11548-011-0643-8 PMID:21800188

Zhu, G., Li, Y., Wen, P. P., Wang, S., & Xi, M. (2013). Epileptogenic focus detection in intracranial EEG based on delay permutation entropy. *Proceedings of AIP Conference*, 1559, 31–36. doi:10.1063/1.4824993

Zitova, B., & Flusser, J. (2003). Image registration methods: A survey. *Image and Vision Computing, Vol*, *21*(11), 977–1000. doi:10.1016/S0262-8856(03)00137-9

About the Contributors

Maheshkumar H. Kolekar was born in Satara, India. He received the Ph.D. degree in Electronics and Electrical Communication Engineering from the Indian Institute of Technology Kharagpur in 2007. From 2008 to 2009, he was a Post-Doctoral Research Fellow with the Department of Computer Science, University of Missouri, Columbia, USA. Since 2010, he has been working as faculty member in the Department of Electrical Engineering with the Indian Institute of Technology Patna (IIT Patna), where he is presently Associate Professor. He has served as a Coordinator (Head) of the department of Electrical Engineering, in 2013 and Head of the Center for Advanced Systems Engineering from 2014 to 2016. He was a recipient of the Best Paper Award from the Computer Society of India for his research paper. In 2012, he was an Organizing Chair of the IEEE sponsored International Conference on Signal, Image and Video Processing at the IIT Patna, a Guest Editor of the Journal of Medical Imaging and Health Informatics (American Scientific) for Special Issue on Biomedical Signal and Image Processing, a Tutorial Chair of the 4th IEEE International Conference on Intelligent Human Computer Interaction, a Keynote Speaker of the International conference on Biomedical Systems, Signals and Images at the IIT Madras, an Editorial Board Member of the American Journal of Signal Processing (Scientific and Academic). In 2014, he successfully organized Special Session on Intelligent Video Surveillance Systems at the International Conference on Systems Engineering, Las Vegas, NV, USA. In 2016, he organized special session on video surveillance successfully during TENCON 2016 which was held at Singapore. He is program chair of Fourth International Symposium on Computer Vision and the Internet (VisionNet'17), going to be held at Manipal University, Karnataka, India during September 13-16, 2017. He is a life fellow of IETE, CSI, and ISTE, and senior member of IEEE USA. His research interests are in digital image and video processing, video surveillance, bio-medical signal and image processing, and machine learning.

Vinod Kumar was Deputy Director and Professor of Electrical Engineering at IIT Roorkee. He received his B.Tech degree from Punjab Engineering College, Chandigarh and M.Tech. and Ph.D. from IIT Roorkee (erstwhile University of Roorkee). He has many academic awards, distinctions and scholarships to his credit including the Khosla Research Awards of University of Roorkee, Ist IETE-R S Khandpur Medical Instrumentation Gold Medal in recognition of life time achievements and outstanding contribution in the field of Biomedical Instrumentation 2006, Railways Board Award for the best paper by IE(I) 2006, KS Krishna Memorial Award of IETE, The Brij Mohanlal Award of IE (I), The Corps of Engineers Prize of IR(I), best paper certificates of Awards of IE (I). He is the best teacher awardee of IIT Roorkee. Prof. Vinod Kumar has about 180 research papers to his credit in the area of Medical Instrumentation and Signal Processing. He has guided 28 PhD.s, more than 150 M. Tech dissertations and more than 150 B.

Tech. Projects in the area of medical instrumentation and digital signal and image processing. He held many positions in IIT Roorkee administration such as Dean Faculty Affairs, Heads of Electrical Engineering Department, Continuing Education Centre, Quality Improvement Program Centre, Information Super Highway Centre and Audio Visual Centre. He was also Associate Dean Academic, Chairperson of many Committees and member of several academic committees of other educational institutions of higher learning and councils. He was National Coordinator QIP. He has widely travelled in India and abroad namely USA, UK, Germany, France, Canada, Singapore, Dubai, Thailand, Finland, Switzerland for invited key notes, research collaborations and discussions. He has taken more that 90 assignments as consultant in diverse fields which includes development of instruments, signal processing packages, residual life assessment of power plants and e-governance. He has 41 years of rich experience of teaching & research and technical education management. He is a life fellow of IETE and IE (I), member IEI UK and senior member of IEEE USA. His areas of interest are Medical Instrumentation, Digital Signal Processing, Telemedicine and e-Governance.

* * *

Haradhan Chel has completed his M.Tech in 2009 from the National Institute of Technology Durgapur, India. He has served few years for Indian Railway, BSNL and NCSM, reputed organizations in India. Presently he is working with Central Institute of Technology Kokrajhar as an assistant professor since 2012. He is currently pursuing his PHD in the department of EEE, IIT Guwahati. His research interest is Medical image processing, Pattern recognition and machine learning.

Deba Prasad Dash was born in Bhubaneswar, Odisha, India in 4th February, 1989. He has completed his M.tech in Bio-medical Engineering from MIT, Manipal. Presently he is pursuing PhD from Indian Institute of Technology, Patna in Electrical Engineering Department. His research area includes neuro-signal processing and video processing.

Girish Deshmukh has done M.B.B.S in 1991 and M.S.(Ophthalmology) in 1995 from Government Medical College, Aurangabad. He was the Vitro-Retinal fellow at Aravind Eye Hospital and PG institute of Ophthalmology, Madurai between 1995 - 1997. Since then, he is working as Vitero-Retinal Surgeon at Nanded.

Vijay R. Ghorpade received his M.E. and PhD in Computer Engineering. Currently, he is working as a Principal and Professor at D. Y. Patil College of Engineering and Technology, Kolhapur. His research interests are mobile adhoc networks and network security. He has published papers in various reputed journals. He is a PhD guide in Computer Science and Engineering. Being an experienced academician and administrator for years, he is bestowed with the responsibility to work as a chairman/co-ordinator for the Board of Studies in Computer Science and Engineering at Shivaji University, Kolhapur.

Chandan Kumar Jha is currently pursuing Ph.D. from Indian Institute of Technology Patna in the Department of Electrical Engineering. He worked as Assistant Professor of Electronics and Communication Engineering at Institute of Information Technology and Management, Gwalior during March 2013 to Dec. 2014. He received Master degree with distinction in Electronics and Communication Engineering from Birla Institute of Technology Mesra in 2012. He received Bachelor degree in Electronics and Communication Engineering from West Bengal University of Technology Kolkata in 2010. His research interests include biomedical signal processing, ECG signal analysis and telemedicine.

Kamlesh Jha is working presently as an assistant professor in the department of Physiology of AIIMS Patna. Besides his 8 years of experience of teaching human physiology to medical nursing students, he also has good experience in the research and clinical services. The area of interest of Dr. Jha is the field of Neurophysiology and cardio-vascular physiology. He is having more than 8 national/international paper publication in his name in various national and international journals. Presently he is working in the field of EEG.

Kalyani Joshi is Principal, Professor & Head of Electronics and Telecommunication Department at PES"s MCOE, Pune affiliated to Savitribai Phule Pune University (SPPU). She has more than 26 years of teaching experience and 12 years of research experience. She is a recognized Ph.D. Guide under SPPU. Her research interests are Signal Processing, Medical Imaging, and Image quality analysis. She has worked as Principal Investigator for Board of College and University Development (BCUD) funded projects under SPPU for the projects viz "Implementation of Spectrum Sensing Algorithm for Cognitive Radio", "Independent Component Analysis and Support Vector Machines in MRI", "Analysis of De Noising MR Images", "FPGA Based HWA for Transform Techniques" and "Qualitative and Quantitative Analysis of medical Images for Better diagnostic Purpose". Her current research work includes implementing denoising filters for MRI using hardware accelerators like FPGA and parallel computing architectures like CUDA. The research work emphasizes on analyzing the filter performance using various image quality assessment metrics. Other research work being executed under her guidance is in the field of cognitive radio and Identification of Ragas and Singer in Indian Classical Music. More than 40 national and international research paper publications are to her credit. Dr. Joshi has co-authored a book titled "Image and Video Compression: Fundamentals, Techniques and Applications" Published by CRC Press. Dr Joshi was "IEEE Senior Member", IEEE in the year 2015 and was Chair, Signal Processing Chapter, IEEE Pune section for three consecutive years from 2013 to 2016.

Manesh B. Kokare earned his Ph.D. from the Department of Electronics and Electrical Communication Engineering, Indian Institute of Technology, Kharagpur, India, in 2005 and completed Post Doctoral research work in 2011-12 from University of California Santa Barbara USA. Presently he is holding position of Associate Professor and Dean Research and Development, Coordinator of Center of Excellence in Signal and Image Processing at SGGSIE&T, Nanded. He has published about 80 papers in international and national journals and conferences. He received the prestigious Career Award for Young Teachers (CAYT) for the year 2005 from All India Council for Technical Education (AICTE), New Delhi, India. Recently Dr. Kokare has been awarded "BOYSCAST: Better Opportunity for Young Scientist in Chosen Area of Science and Technology" Fellowship for year 2010-2011 by Department of Science and Technology, Government of India to Carryout Post Doctoral Research Work at University of California USA. Under his supervision nine research scholars completed PhD in Electronics and Computer Engineering and presently eight research scholars are working towards their PhD. He is a life member of System Society of India, Indian Society for Technical Education (ISTE), and The Institution of Electronics and Telecommunication Engineers (IETE) and Member of IEEE, Member of IEEE Signal Processing Society, Member of IEEE Computer Society. Dr. Kokare was Program Chair of IEEE International Conference on Signal and Information Processing (IConSIP-2016) held at Nanded, India during 6th to 8th October 2016.

Pradnya Kulkarni is currently a PhD student at Centre for Informatics and Applied Optimization, Federation University, Australia. She has completed postgraduate diploma in information technology from University of Ballarat, Australia and Bachelors of Electronics Engineering from India. She possesses ten years of international experience in teaching, research and software development. She has published ten research papers in international conferences and reputed journals. She won Most Outstanding Paper Award at UB Research conference 2013 and Best Presentation Award at IEEE International Conference on Signal and Image Processing 2016 held at Beijing, China. She has also served as reviewer for several international conferences and a journal. Her research interests are Medical Image Retrieval, Health Informatics, and Artificial Intelligence.

Siddhivinayak Kulkarni (Sid) has completed his Masters and PhD in Information Technology from Griffith University, Australia. He has worked as an Assistant Professor at Nipissing University, Canada for four years and later at Federation University, Australia for ten years. Dr. Kulkarni is an Honorary Research Fellow (HRF) from School of Engineering and Information Technology, Federation University Australia. Currently he is working as an Associate Professor at the Department of Computer Engineering, Maharashtra Academy of Engineering Education and Research (MAEER), Pune. He is also a Coordinator for Centre of Excellence for Machine Intelligence and High Performance Computing at MIT-College of Engineering. Dr. Kulkarni has organized couple of workshops on Machine Learning and Algorithms in conjunction with Intelligent Sensors, Sensor Networks and Information Processing (ISSNIP) Australia, and attracted many research papers from various countries. He has served as an organizer and program committee member for more than sixty International conferences organized in various countries and editorial board member and reviewer for many reputed journals. He has published two books at an International level, along with fifty five research papers in reputable peer reviewed journals and presented many papers at International conferences. He obtained research grants from Canadian and Australian Universities for projects related to image processing, biometrics and Health Informatics. He has experience of supervising Masters and PhD students. His research interests include computational intelligence, pattern recognition, sensor networks (IOT) and its application in image/video retrieval, and health informatics.

Prabin Kumar Bora received his M.E. and PhD degrees from Indian Institute of Science, Bangalore, both in Electrical Engineering. Since 1997, he has been associated with the Department of Electrical and Electronics Engineering, Indian Institute of Technology Guwahati where he is a professor now. His area of interest includes image processing and computer vision and the application of signal processing techniques to process physiological and communication signals. He has guided 10 PhD students and over 60 M.Tech. students. He has published more than 120 journal and international conference publications.

Suraj Kumar Nayak received his B. Tech in Electrical Engineering from Government College of Engineering Keonjhar, Odisha, India (formerly known as OSME Keonjhar) and M. Tech in Biomedical Engineering from National Institute of Technology Rourkela, Odisha, India. Currently, he is pursuing his PhD degree in Biomedical Engineering from National Institute of Technology Rourkela, Odisha, India. His research interests include Biomedical Instrumentation, Biomedical Signal & Image Processing, Artificial Neural Network and Controlled Drug Delivery.

Shraddha Oza is working as an assistant professor in the department of E&Tc at Army Institute of Technology, Pune, India. She has 26 years of teaching experience and 3 years of industrial experience. Her areas of specialization are Advanced Computer Architecture, Embedded Systems, and Instrumentation. She has completed her BE from Bharati Vidyapeeth's College of Engineering, Pune and done her Masters from VJTI, Mumbai. Presently she is pursuing her PhD in the domain of medical imaging and parallel computing at College of Engineering Pune, under Savitribai Phule Pune University.

Samiksha Pachade received the B.E. degree in Electronics and Telecommunication Engineering from Sant Gadge Baba Amravati University, India, in 2014. Presently, she is pursuing the M.Tech degree from Shri Guru Gobind Singhji Institute of Engineering and Technology, Nanded, India. Her major field of interest is Biomedical Image Processing.

Ram Bilas Pachori received the BE degree with honors in Electronics and Communication Engineering from Rajiv Gandhi Technological University, Bhopal, India in 2001, the M. Tech and PhD degrees in Electrical Engineering from Indian Institute of Technology Kanpur, Kanpur, India in 2003 and 2008, respectively. He worked as a Postdoctoral Fellow at Charles Delaunay Institute, University of Technology of Troyes, Troyes, France during 2007-2008. He served as an Assistant Professor at Communication Research Center, International Institute of Information Technology, Hyderabad, India during 2008-2009. He served as an Assistant Professor at Discipline of Electrical Engineering, Indian Institute of Technology Indore, Indore, India during 2009- 2013, where presently he has been working as an Associate Professor since 2013. He worked as a Visiting Scholar at Intelligent Systems Research Center, Ulster University, Northern Ireland, UK during December 2014. His research interests are in the areas of biomedical signal processing, non-stationary signal processing, speech signal processing, signal processing for communications, computer aided medical diagnosis, and signal processing applications.

Kunal Pal pursued his graduation in Pharmacy from University of Delhi, New Delhi, India in the year 2002 followed by post-graduation in Biomedical Engineering from Jadavpur University, Kolkata, India in the year 2004. Later, he did his Ph.D. in Materials Science from Indian Institute of Technology, Kharagpur, India in the year 2006. Subsequently, he joined Ryerson University, Toronto, Canada as a post-doctoral fellow in the year 2007. During his tenure at Ryerson University, he served as Vice-Chair (Elect), HQPA, AFMNet Network of Excellence, Canada. He joined National Institute of Technology, Rourkela, India in the year 2009 as an Assistant Professor in Biomedical Engineering. He is currently the Professor-in-Charge of Medical Electronics and Instrumentation Laboratory in the Department of Biotechnology and Medical Engineering, National Institute of technology, Rourkela, India. His major research interests revolve around Biomedical Signal Processing and Biomedical Equipment Design. He is also working in the fields of soft materials and controlled drug delivery. He has more than 140 publications in SCI cited journals of high repute, Book Chapters and peer-reviewed conferences. He is a very well cited researcher having more than 2000 citations.

Preeti Madhuri Pandey received her M.Tech. in Biomedical Engineering from National Institute of Technology Rourkela, Odisha, India. Her research interests include biomedical instrumentation and fabrication of wireless devices for medical applications.

Prasanna Porwal received B.E. degree in Electronics and Telecommunication Engineering from MSS's College of Engineering and Technology, Jalna, India, in 2011 and M.Tech. in Electronics engineering from SGGS Institute of Engineering and Technology, Nanded, India, in 2014. He is currently a Doctoral candidate in the Department of Electronics and Telecommunication Engineering, SGGS Institute of Engineering and Technology, Nanded. His research interests include image processing, signal processing, pattern recognition, machine learning, and artificial intelligence.

Ebenezer Priya received her B.E degree in Electronics and Communication Engineering from University of Madras in 1994 and M.E degree in 2008 from Madras Institute of Technology, Anna University. She completed her Ph.D in November 2013 under the faculty of Information and Communication from Anna University in the field of Biomedical Engineering. She has 14 years of teaching experience and 3 years of industrial experience. She is a recipient of DST-PURSE fellow, which is awarded for meritorious candidates pursuing research in the areas of Science, Engineering and Technology. She has presented her research paper at the 49th Annual Rocky Mountain Bio-Engineering Symposium, Virginia Tech, Blacksburg, USA in 2012. She is a project participant of India-South African collaborative project titled "Development of computing tools for decision support in health assessment in rural areas" during the period 16.07.2009 to 30.03.2012. She has published papers in International Journals and Conferences in the area of medical imaging and infectious diseases. Her areas of interest include bio-medical imaging, image processing, signal processing, application of artificial intelligence and machine learning techniques.

Vivek Sahasrabuddhe, M.B.B.S, M.S. (Ophthalmology), is Professor & Head, Department of Ophthalmology in Dr. S. C. Government Medical College, Vishnupuri. Nanded. He has teaching experience of 30 years. He is recognized PG teacher of Maharashtra University of Health Sciences, Nashik and recognized UG & PG examiner and inspector of Medical Council of India. He has published 8 papers in last 3 years and delivered several keynote speeches at various conferences. He has received many awards like Rotary club award, 2015, Best Paper Award, MOSCON, 2004. He is also a trained & qualified yoga teacher.

Amit Savyanavar is currently working as Associate Professor at MAEER's MIT College of Engineering, Kothrud, Pune in Computer department. He has a teaching experience of almost 15 years, during which he taught subjects like Operating systems, Distributed Computing and Software Engineering at the undergraduate and postgraduate level. He has a Masters degree in Computer Science and Engineering, and currently pursuing PhD in Computer Science and Engineering at Shivaji University, Kolhapur, India. His research interests include Mobile Computing, Health Informatics and Image Processing. He is a life member of Computer Society of India. To his credit, he has published his research work in renowned journals.

Greeshma Sharma has joined Defence R&D Organisation of Indian Ministry of Defence in 2012 after completing her masters in cognitive science from University of Rajasthan. She has worked on the project in cognitive assessment and enhancement using virtual reality. Currently, she is about to submit her PhD thesis on "Performance evaluation in navigation through psychophysiological assessment". Her research interest includes the development of cognitive test battery using virtual reality. She is also keen for looking out neural correlates of individual differences in the navigation performance.

Rajeev Sharma received Ph.D. degree in the Electrical Engineering from Indian Institute of Technology Indore, Indore, India in 2017. He has completed B.E. degree in Electronics and Communication Engineering from Rajiv Gandhi Proudyogiki Vishwavidyalaya, Bhopal, India in 2009, and M.Tech. degree in Electronic Instrumentation from National Institute of Technology, Warangal, India in 2011. His research interest is Signal Processing and its application in bio-medical signals like EEG and ECG, pattern recognition, and machine learning etc.

Preety Singh did her Bachelors in Electrical Engineering from MNREC, Allahabad followed by her Masters in Integrated Circuits and Electronics from IIT Delhi. She completed her PhD from MNIT Jaipur in the area of image processing.

Vanika Singhal completed her Masters in Computer Science from LNMIIT, Jaipur and is currently pursuing her Ph.D. from IIIT Delhi.

Subramanian Srinivasan is currently working as Associate Professor in the Department of Instrumentation Engineering, Madras Institute of Technology, Anna University, Chennai. He received his B.E. from Annamalai University in 1991, M.E. from University of Roorkee (Presently IIT Roorkee) in 1997 and PhD from Anna University in the area of fault diagnosis in December 2008. His area of interest is fault diagnosis, Application of Neural network and fuzzy logic systems in the area of Biomedical. He has been instrumental in organizing various national level conferences, workshops and faculty development programs. He is one of the principal investigator of India-South African collaborative project titled "Development of computing tools for decision support in health assessment in rural areas" during the period 16.07.2009 to 30.03.2012. He has published papers in renowned International Journals and Conferences in the area of medical imaging and infectious diseases, fault tolerance and control.

Andrew Stranieri is the leader of the Health Informatics Laboratory within the Centre for Informatics and Applied Optimisation at Federation University, Australia. His research in combining argumentation theory with machine learning led to a new approach for modelling discretionary reasoning and numerous commercial decision support systems. This formed the basis of approaches to support group reasoning. Currently, he performs research in health informatics in data mining, decision support, complementary medicine informatics and telemedicine. He is the author of over 150 peer reviewed articles and has authored two books.

D. N. Tibarewala is presently a Professor of Biomedical Engineering at Jadavpur University, Kolkata, India since August 1996, Dr. D. N. Tibarewala has earlier served as Director in the School of Bioscience & Engineering of the same University during the period May 2004-November 2011. He did his BSc (Honours) in 1971 and B. Tech (Applied Physics) in 1974 from the Calcutta University, India. He was admitted to the Ph.D. (Tech) degree of the Calcutta University in 1980. Having professional, academic and research experience of about 40 years, Dr. Tibarewala has contributed more than 250 research publications in the areas of Rehabilitation Technology, Biomedical Instrumentation & Signal Processing, Human Computer Interfaces and, related branches of Biomedical Engineering.

Index

K

L

M

N

O

P

Q

R

S

T

V

W

Z

www.ingramcontent.com/pod-product-compliance
Lightning Source LLC
LaVergne TN
LVHW060304011026
849161LV00011B/2772